45–

D1537668

CONTEMPORARY
Chiropractic

CONTEMPORARY
Chiropractic

Edited by

DANIEL REDWOOD, D.C.
Private Practice
Virginia Beach, Virginia

Editorial Adviser

Marc S. Micozzi, M.D., Ph.D.
Executive Director
The College of Physicians of Philadelphia
Philadelphia, Pennsylvania

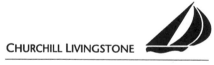

CHURCHILL LIVINGSTONE

New York, Edinburgh, London, Madrid, Melbourne, San Francisco, Tokyo

Library of Congress Cataloging-in-Publication Data

Contemporary chiropractic/edited by Daniel Redwood; editorial adviser, Marc S. Micozzi.

     p.   cm.
   Includes bibliographical references and index.
   ISBN 0-443-07809-2 (alk. paper)
   1. Chiropractic   I. Redwood, Daniel, Date.
   [DNLM: 1. Chiropractic. WB 905 C761 1997]
RZ232.2.C66   1997
615.5′34—dc21
DNLM/DLC
for Library of Congress   97-18583
                                                CIP

© Churchill Livingstone Inc. 1997

All rights reserved. No part of this publication may be reproduced, stored in a retrieval system, or transmitted in any form or by any means, electronic, mechanical, photocopying, recording, or otherwise, without prior permission of the publisher (Churchill Livingstone, 650 Avenue of the Americas, New York, NY 10011).

Distributed in the United Kingdom by Churchill Livingstone, Robert Stevenson House, 1–3 Baxter's Place, Leith Walk, Edinburgh EH1 3AF, and by associated companies, branches, and representatives throughout the world.

Medical knowledge is constantly changing. As new information becomes available, changes in treatment, procedures, equipment and the use of drugs become necessary. The editors/authors/contributors and the publishers have, as far as it is possible, taken care to ensure that the information given in this text is accurate and up to date. However, readers are strongly advised to confirm that the information, especially with regard to drug usage, complies with the latest legislation and standards of practice.

The Publishers have made every effort to trace the copyright holders for borrowed material. If they have inadvertently overlooked any, they will be pleased to make the necessary arrangements at the first opportunity.

Acquisitions Editor: *Carol Bader*
Production Editor: *Elizabeth A. Lipp*
Production Supervisor: *Sharon Tuder*
Cover Design: *Jeannette Jacobs*
Desktop Coordinator: *Alice Terry*

Printed in the United States of America

First published in 1997   7 6 5 4 3 2 1

For Daniel David Palmer, who lives on

Contributors

Geoffrey Bove, D.C., Ph.D.
Visiting Professor, Department of Biomechanics, Odense University, Odense, Denmark

Jon Buriak, D.C.
Chairman, ACA Hospital Relations Committee; Private Practice, Brentwood, Missouri

Carl S. Cleveland III, D.C.
President, Cleveland Chiropractic College, Kansas City, Missouri and Los Angeles, California

Alan Dumoff, J.D., M.S.W.
Adjunct Professor, Department of Justice, Law & Society, American University, Washington D.C.; Attorney at Law, Executive Director, LifeTree Medical Center, Rockville, Maryland

Joan Fallon, D.C., F.I.C.C.P.
Assistant Professor, Natural Sciences and Mathematics, Yeshiva University; Fellow, International Council of Chiropractic Pediatrics; Private practice, New Rochelle, New York

Ed Feinberg, D.C., C.C.S.P.
Professor, Departments of Diagnosis and Chiropractic Technique, Palmer College of Chiropractic-West, San Jose, California; Private Practice, St. Claire Chiropractic, Santa Clara, California

Robert S. Francis, D.C.
Associate Professor, Post Graduate Education, University of Bridgeport College of Chiropractic, Wilmington, Delaware; Former Dean, Clinical Sciences, Texas Chiropractic College, Pasadena, Texas; Director, Physical Medicine, Medical Industrial Center, Houston, Texas; Chairman, Chiropractic Medicine, Amedisys Surgery Centers, Houston, Texas

Russell W. Gibbons, Litt.D.(h.c.)
Editor Emeritus, *Chiropractic History*, Pittsburgh, Pennsylvania

David P. Gilkey, D.C., C.C.S.P., D.A.B.C.O., D.A.C.B.O.H., F.I.C.C.
Past President, ACA Council on Occupational Health, Westminster, Colorado

Warren Hammer, D.C., M.S., D.A.B.C.O.
Lecturer, Postgraduate Department, Cleveland Chiropractic College, Kansas City, Missouri

Christopher Kent, D.C., F.C.C.I.
Postgraduate Faculty, Life Chiropractic College, Marietta, Georgia and San Lorenzo, California; Chair, ICA Council on Imaging

C. Jacob Ladenheim
Attorney at Law, Fincastle, Virginia

William J. Lauretti, D.C.
Private Practice, Bethesda, Maryland

Charles Masarsky, D.C.
Co-editor, *Neurological Fitness*, Vienna, Virginia, Postgraduate Lecturer, Postgraduate Education Department, Life Chiropractic College, Marietta, Georgia; Continuing Education Lecturer, Continuing Education Department, Palmer College of Davenport, Iowa; Co-Director, Vienna Chiropractic Associates, Vienna, Virginia

J.F. McAndrews, D.C.
Board member, National Chiropractic Mutual Insurance Company; Past President, Palmer College of Chiropractic, Davenport, Iowa; Past Vice President, Professional Affairs, American Chiropractic Association

Daniel Redwood, D.C.
Private Practice, Virginia Beach, Virginia

Anthony L. Rosner, Ph.D.
Director of Research and Education, Foundation for Chiropractic Education and Research, Arlington, Virginia

John Scaringe, D.C., D.A.C.B.S.P.
Professor, Department of Diagnosis, Los Angeles College of Chiropractic, Whittier, California; Center for Research and Spine Care, Los Angeles College of Chiropractic, Anaheim, California

Henry W. Shull, D.C.
Associate Professor, Department of Diagnosis, Palmer College of Chiropractic, Davenport, Iowa

David Sikorski, D.C.
Assistant Professor, Department of Chiropractic Procedures, Los Angeles College of Chiropractic, Whittier, California; Private Practice, La Crescenta, California

Jerrold Simon, D.C., D.A.C.B.N., C.C.N.
Postgraduate Instructor, Department of Clinical Nutrition, National College of Chiropractic, Lombard, Illinois; President, ACA Council on Nutrition; Director, Lancaster Chiropractic Clinic, Lancaster, Ohio

Juanee Surprise, R.N., D.C., D.A.A.P.M., D.A.C.B.N., C.C.N.
Director, Diplomate and Special Certification Programs, Center for Postgraduate and Continuing Education, Parker College of Chiropractic, Dallas, Texas; President, Chiropractic Board on Nutrition; Director of Education, Council on Nutrition; Private Practice, Denton, Texas

Herbert Vear, D.C., L.L.D.
Dean Emeritus, Canadian Memorial Chiropractic College, Toronto, Canada; President Emeritus, Western States Chiropractic College, Portland, Oregon

Marion Weber, D.C.
Co-editor, *Neurological Fitness*; Co-director, Vienna Chiropractic Associates, Vienna, Virginia

Holly A. Williams, D.C., C.C.S.P., D.A.B.C.O.
Past President, ACA Council on Chiropractic Orthopedics, Westminster, Colorado

Foreword

*C*ontemporary Chiropractic is a textbook of high quality that I strongly recommend to chiropractors, chiropractic educators, and members of other health professions who are seeking to better understand chiropractic. I have the greatest respect for this text—its conception, its chapter authors, and its editor. Dr. Redwood is a skilled organizer, author, and editor with outstanding dedication to his chosen profession. The birth of a book on chiropractic is not an easy labor. The literary tasks, the persuading, the cajoling, and the deadlines are such that any book must be a labor of total love, something that Daniel Redwood has in great abundance.

Aside from providing a well balanced and wide ranging introduction to current chiropractic concepts and methodologies, *Contemporary Chiropractic* is unique among chiropractic textbooks in its in-depth coverage of social and economic issues. Numerous chapters are marked by analytical thinking that encourages readers to reflect more deeply about questions crucial to the profession and the society of which it is a part. History provides a framework to explain the present and predict the future, and the insightful opening chapters describe the colorful and turbulent socioeconomic and political history of the profession. This is followed by cogent presentations on the development of chiropractic concepts of health and disease, and the evolution of the practice arts of chiropractic. I was also particularly pleased to see the section on the small but growing body of scientific research that may eventually allow chiropractic to integrate as a full and equal partner in the health care system.

The section on controversies is highly instructive as it frankly addresses issues the profession must grapple with in order to progress. Whether or not one agrees with all the authors' conclusions (and I personally disagree with some), this section will certainly provide grist for countless interesting and ultimately useful discussions on the past, present, and future of chiropractic.

The closing section, Chiropractic in Special Situations, offers a gratifying demonstration of chiropractors' professional involvement in important arenas such as sports medicine, pediatrics, and occupational medicine in ways that integrate the best of all perspectives for the benefit of patients. Finally, Dr. Redwood's forward-looking closing chapter lays out clear directions for future chiropractors.

Chiropractic has never been easily defined. Providing an accurate picture of the profession at this time in history, when the clinical, economic, and social fabric of our health care system is undergoing rapid change, is a major intellectual challenge. This text ably meets that challenge.

William C. Meeker, DC, MPH
Director of Research
Palmer College of Chiropractic
Davenport, Iowa
Palmer College of Chiropractic-West
San Jose, California

*C*hiropractic, having started a century ago as an alternative to the medical mainstream based on the relations of the spine and nervous system to the overall function of the body, is in the process of becoming mainstream in the late twentieth century, just as the social movement behind popular medicine sees medical alternatives in a renewed, positive light. Many of the chapters in this volume illustrate the clinical and basic science that has been developed to support chiropractic within the biomedical model. This research has been a primary driving force behind the enhanced cooperation between chiropractors and medical physicians in recent years.

A new medical paradigm is on the horizon that leaves room for the core concepts of chiropractic—the link between structure and function, the effectiveness of manual adjustment and manipulation, and the crucial mediating role of the nervous system—as well as other non-allopathic approaches. This new perspective may allow consideration of various alternative methods as part of a more inclusive and expansive model that accommodates rather than subsumes these alternatives, and that is coming to see allopathic "medicine" as one alternative among many. Chiropractic is on the very cusp of this potentially significant transition as we approach the new millennium.

Marc S. Micozzi, M.D., Ph.D.
Executive Director
The College of Physicians of Philadelphia
Philadelphia, Pennsylvania

Preface

Chiropractic has undergone profound changes in the past generation, and is now in the position of having in many ways scaled the walls of the health care establishment (with licensure, an increasingly strong scientific research base, widespread insurance coverage, and approximately 22 million patients per year in the United States). At the same time, it has maintained strong roots in the "alternative" or holistic health community (with a philosophy that emphasizes healing without drugs). Chiropractors may thus be able to play a bridging role in this time of transition.

Contemporary Chiropractic seeks to provide solid grounding in the essential principles and practices of chiropractic and natural healing, to furnish current data that informs and inspires, and perhaps most importantly, to stimulate both critical and creative thinking.

Contemporary developments can only be fully understood against the backdrop of history. Particularly in times of significant change, it is essential to know our roots in order to properly evaluate and appreciate newly emerging shoots and blossoms. This book's opening section—Chiropractic: Past and Present—has two chapters that trace the development of chiropractic from its beginnings to the present. In "Chiropractic and the Natural Health Movement," Russell Gibbons, founding editor of the journal *Chiropractic History*, examines chiropractic in the context of the broader natural health movement that began with the Popular Health Movement of the 1830s and lives on today in the alternative health movement of the 1990s. Herbert Vear, formerly dean at Canadian Memorial Chiropractic College and president of Western States Chiropractic College, demonstrates in "Chiropractic Education and Accreditation: A Century of Progress" that immense changes have swept through chiropractic education in the past century. An increasingly strong and reputable system of higher education has been built from what began as an informal tutorial system and

for many years consisted of trade schools with poorly defined standards.

The History and Development of Chiropractic Concepts section contains two chapters by Carl Cleveland III, a fourth generation chiropractor and third generation chiropractic college president. "Vertebral Subluxation," follows the progress of this quintessential chiropractic concept through its many passages, up to and including contemporary models of the vertebral subluxation complex. "Neurobiologic Relationships," offers a wide-ranging presentation of the chiropractic theories and research that at the dawn of the twenty-first century are opening new vistas of understanding and possibilities for interdisciplinary study.

The Principles and Practice section opens with Henry Shull's unique "Physical Examination and Diagnosis" chapter. Shull, who has chaired the diagnosis department and curriculum committee at Palmer College of Chiropractic, largely bypasses the usual long list of proper-named orthopedic tests (readers should consult other texts for these), focusing instead on how chiropractors can develop the physical and mental clarity and acuity that are the foundation of diagnostic skills. The keys, according to Shull, are an engaged patient interview and keen observation, along with classical methods such as inspection, palpation, percussion, auscultation, and motion.

Christopher Kent, chair of the ICA Council on Imaging, offers in his "Diagnostic Imaging" chapter a well-constructed introduction to this crucial diagnostic area, covering basic concepts and practical applications of radiography, videofluoroscopy, computed tomography, magnetic resonance imaging, and sonographic imaging. In 'The Art of Manual Palpation and Adjustment,' John Scaringe and David Sikorski of Los Angeles College of Chiropractic provide an informative entree to a topic at the core of chiropractic concerns, discussing the identification of the adjustive lesion and various methods for its correction. In "Soft Tissue Therapies," Warren Hammer, the premier chiropractic instructor in this field, provides both the rationale for soft tissue work and a well-guided tour through many of the most widely used contemporary methods.

Long before nutrition attained mainstream respectability, chiropractors insisted on its central role as a health determinant. In their chapter, "Clinical Nutrition," Jerrold Simon and Juanee Surprise of the ACA Council on Nutrition, present a compelling case for including nutritional counseling in chiropractic practice, both as a method to help patients achieve and maintain wellness and to treat ailments amenable to nutritional intervention.

Research is a linchpin of professional growth and development. This text's Research section offers up-to-date summaries of the relevant literature, along with interpretations of its significance. In his "Musculoskeletal Disorders Research" chapter, Anthony Rosner, Director of Research and Education for the Foundation for Chiropractic Education and Research, demonstrates clearly how and why chiropractic has made such dramatic strides in the past generation. Chiropractic research on visceral disorders is currently at a much earlier stage than musculoskeletal research, but as Charles Masarsky and Marion Weber, editors of the newsletter *Neurological Fitness*, show in their chapter, "Research on Visceral Disorders," there exists a promising basis for what may be a most fertile area for chiropractic research in the twenty-first century. Geoffrey Bove wrote his chapter, "Nociceptors, Pain and Chiropractic," while a research fellow in neurosurgery and anesthesiology at Harvard Medical School and Beth Israel Hospital, and is now teaching in the new chiropractic department at the University of Odense in Denmark. Bove offers a state of the art presentation on the neurophysiology of pain, culminating in a final section that offers a scientific rationale for chiropractic treatment.

The Controversies section is intended to provoke thought and discussion. J.F. McAndrews, a past president of Palmer College who has also held leadership positions at ICA and ACA, has been a leading political figure in chiropractic in the second half of the twentieth century. In "Appropriate Care, Ethics and Practice Guidelines," McAndrews contends that while the profession has made great strides toward maturity, substantial improvement is still required in two pivotal areas: respect for reasonable, objectively based practice guidelines, and development of a profession-wide ethic of financial fairness. William Lauretti's "The Comparative Safety of Chiropractic," is a solidly documented summary of critical safety issues, with special emphasis on cerebrovascular accidents. Lauretti's key original contribution is his logically drawn, statistically cogent comparison between chiropractic neck adjustments and the most common medical treatment for neck pain, nonsteroidal anti-inflammatory drugs. Lauretti powerfully demonstrates the relative safety of chiropractic, while offering cautionary instruction on how to minimize the likelihood of negative reactions to chiropractic care. Attorney Alan Dumoff's "Chiropractic and the Law" covers the essentials of legal matters including licensure, scope of practice, insurance reimbursement, and malpractice, as well as the landmark *Wilk v. AMA* case.

The Chiropractic in Special Situations section is designed to showcase a variety of possibilities open to chiropractors at the start of the profession's second century. Ed Feinberg, a chiropractic sports physician and professor at Palmer College-West, discusses in his "Sports Chiropractic" chapter the unique and important role of chiropractors in helping athletes to perform safely and recover from injuries. Joan Fallon, vice chair of the ICA Council on Pediatrics, in her chapter, "Chiropractic Pediatrics," illustrates the value of chiropractic care at this special stage of the life cycle. David Gilkey and Holly Williams, who have chaired the ACA councils on occupational health and orthopedics, respectively, offer a wide-ranging discussion of occupational health in "Chiropractic in the Workplace." They demonstrate that traditional chiropractic emphasis on after-the-fact treatment of work-related injuries has been enlarged to include prevention, ergonomic analysis, and interdisciplinary case management. "Hospitals and Integrated Settings," by Robert Francis and John Buriak, of the ACA Hospital Relations Committee, and attorney C. Jacob Ladenheim, illustrates the opportunities and the potential pitfalls of multidisciplinary collaboration. The authors address a variety of issues chiropractors should consider before entering a multidisciplinary practice or seeking hospital privileges. Their chapter offers guidance that should spare numerous chiropractors from repeating the mistakes of others.

My closing chapter, "Pathways for an Evolving Profession," begins with this question: "How can chiropractors and chiropractic students help the profession evolve so that it more fully reflects our noblest aspirations?" I offer ten touchstones to guide the process, including distinguishing clearly among the proven, the probable, and the speculative; promoting a healing partnership with patients; recognizing that the doctor must strive to model the healthy lifestyle choices he or she recommends; cultivating an attitude of tolerance and openmindedness; minimizing patient dependency; and serving those who cannot afford our services.

At the end of each chapter is a series of review questions and 'concept' questions, along with a list of key terms which are defined in an extensive, user-friendly glossary. The review questions are factual, while the concept questions do not necessarily have a correct answer and call for in-depth thought about what in many cases are provocative questions.

I am aware that readers outside the United States will have to contend with parts of a few chapters (particularly those relating to legal matters) where the focus is on issues specific to the United States. Since most of the world's chiropractors are in the United States, I think this emphasis is justified. The vast majority of the text should be directly relevant to students and practitioners from all nations.

Daniel Redwood, DC

Acknowledgments

I would like to acknowledge the help of the following people: my wife Beth, for her encouragement, support, and creative ideas; all the chapter authors, for the time and energy they devoted to this project; Marc Micozzi, for his skillful yet nonintrusive editing, and his pioneering role in bridging the gap between alternative and mainstream health care; Alan Gaby and Sandra McLanahan, for help with specialized references; Ron Hendrickson, J.F. McAndrews, and Carl Cleveland III, for sage advice and extending the hand of friendship; Margaret Sendak and Meryl Ann Butler, for their artful line drawings; Carol Bader and Elizabeth Lipp of Churchill Livingstone, for faithfully answering my phone calls, faxes, and e-mails; Jeannette Jacobs for her cover design; Mark Rhodes, for his cover photographs; and Daniel David Palmer, for starting the wheels turning.

Contents

About the Author

*D*aniel Redwood, D.C., lectures on chiropractic in complementary medicine courses at the Medical College of Virginia and the National Institutes of Health. He is also a member of the editorial board of a complementary medicine journal.

A graduate of Palmer College of Chiropractic where he was student council president, Dr. Redwood is a former vice president and legislative committee chairman for the chiropractic state association in the District of Columbia. He has a private practice in Virginia Beach, Virginia.

1

The Natural Health Movement

Russell W. Gibbons

*C*hiropractic, which has always identified itself as an alternative to conventional allopathic medicine, is part of a broader natural health movement with roots reaching deep into the bedrock of American and European healing traditions. The history of chiropractic is best understood not in isolation but with full appreciation of pioneers who preceded it, healing arts that developed alongside it, and conventional medicine that staunchly opposed it.

Social historians who have traced the evolution of contemporary medical practice in America from the early nineteenth century to the present have noted the relationships of political, economic, and religious dissent with reform in the healing arts. The French Revolution, the Napoleonic era and its codes, the midcentury revolts in central Europe—all would compare with the American Revolution, the period of Jacksonian democracy, and the successive waves of European and Asian immigrants who brought medical alternatives to American shores.

Paul Starr,[1] who won a Pulitzer Prize for his seminal work in this field, *The Social Transformation of American Medicine*, captured the convergence of these forces when he wrote of the role of medicine in a democratic culture:

> By the nineteenth century in America, popular belief reflected an extreme form of rationalism that demanded science be democratic ... it had become an article of faith in America that every sphere of social life—law, government, religion, science, industry—obeyed principles of natural reason that were intelligible to ordinary men and women of common sense.

This democratic, populist climate survived the Civil War and proved a fertile seedbed for dissenting ideas about therapeutics in treating disease. The American experience in medical unorthodoxy is distinct from its European counterparts. Its advocates could channel that dissent within the framework of a pluralistic state that tolerated challenges to authority.

Medicine in the United States experienced its own civil war and reconstruction, according to Starr, in parallel with the larger trauma that tore at the fabric of the young republic and gradually mended itself through the end of the Victorian period and the start of the industrial age at the dawn of the new century.[1] For much of the nineteenth century, various medical and health reformers competed with mainstream practitioners for the loyalty of the citizen-patients.

THE POPULAR HEALTH MOVEMENT: VARIETIES OF NATURAL HEALING

What Ehrenreich and English[2] call the "Popular Health Movement" began in the 1830s, a period noteworthy for dissenting religious revival and the

1

early feminist movement. When feminists gathered at their historic Seneca Falls, New York, convention, they traded medical horror stories about abuse suffered at the hands of physicians. Women's study groups challenged the mainstream "heroic" medicine that used bloodletting and purges and deemed most women's "complaints" unworthy of serious attention. The subsequent Ladies Physiological Societies of the 1850s also found common ground with early advocates of alternative healing.

ALTERNATIVES TO "HEROIC" MEDICINE

Hydropathy, introduced from Europe during the 1840s, stressed the curative power of water and offered a counterpoint to the excessive drugging of the regular school of physicians in that period.[1] Russell Trall, a pioneer of hydropathy, opened a water cure sanitarium and published a journal advocating the practice. The comprehensive water cure was touted as a veritable panacea for all ills, and according to Robert Fuller,[3] for its practitioners, "water had an almost sacramental power to remove impurities." The movement was ideologically opposed to the regular school, which was condemned for its use of excessive drugs, emetics, and bleedings.

Fuller describes hydropathy as one of four "countervailing" healing systems of the first part of the nineteenth century, the theoretical basis of which survived in the early twentieth century alternative schools, especially naturopathy. The other three were Grahamism, founded by an ordained Presbyterian minister, Sylvester Graham; Thomsonianism, the brainchild of a lay itinerant healer, Samuel Thomson; and homeopathy, a European import founded by German physician Samuel Hahnemann that mounted a serious challenge to the mainline "allopaths" (physicians who utilize substances or procedures to suppress or counteract symptoms) in this period of sectarian warfare.

Medical historian John Duffy[4] stated that, during this era, the public favored the alternative schools because of the acceptance of dissent in the new republic, and that "as much as anything, it was the public's decision to turn to the herbalists, homeopaths, hydropaths and other medical sects eschew-

ing heroic practices which literally forced orthodox physicians to reconsider their position."

EARLY REFORM EFFORTS: SUCCESSES AND FAILURES

Like political reform movements in general, the alternative therapy movement influenced the established school to reform itself. Just as third parties, antislavery movements, suffragettes, and trade unions moved the traditional political parties to adopt their platforms, so too the sectarians exerted influence far beyond their numbers and patient constituencies.

Rise of the American Medical Association

One lesson that was not learned by all the alternative sects was the necessity of organizing societies on a state and national level to influence legislative action and protect their socioeconomic position. This was the pattern followed by the allopaths, who were able to standardize medical practice according to their philosophy and ideology and to eventually overwhelm the assault by the dissenters. It was actually the homeopaths who organized the first national medical society, in 1844—the American Institute of Homeopathy—three years before the American Medical Association (AMA) was founded.[5]

The AMA's physician code and mission statement[5] was a unique combination of humanistic concerns coupled with the desire to achieve cultural status. It called on physicians to "study also in their deportment, so to unite tenderness with firmness, and condescension with authority, as to inspire in the minds of the patients with gratitude, respect and confidence … [and to] inspire obedience to the prescriptions of his physician to be prompt and implicit."

Partnership Model and the Democratic Instinct

Rather than seeking control of their patient constituency, alternative practitioners saw themselves as partners with those who needed health care. The Thomsonians organized around the concepts of botanic medicine, gaining repute as "root and herb doctors." Not formally trained, they had broad appeal, Fuller[3] writes, for they "gave succinct popular expression to the fierce democratizing spirit of Jacksonian America." The Thomsonians published journals and claimed millions of adherents in the Northeast and Midwest in the pre-Civil War decades. The movement was dedicated to "make every man his physician" and, as one writer concluded, "played well in an era in which the common person yearned for common remedies to common ailments."[1]

Not coincidentally, in the third decade of the nineteenth century, the American religious revival movement began, with the emergence of the Seventh Day Adventists, Millennium sects, and Mormonism. Later, during the 1880s, New Thought and Christian Science emerged as the concept of spiritual healing spread like a brushfire across the American heartland. Each of these groups advocated principles of natural healing. In time, the holistic awareness and mind–body–spirit concept they embodied would intertwine the surviving alternative sects.

Harvey Kellogg and Grahamism

Grahamism had the broadest constituency of the nineteenth century health philosophies, and perhaps the most prominent convert, physician John Harvey Kellogg, who took over a former Adventist Health Reform Institute in Battle Creek, Michigan, and turned it into a nationwide mecca of natural healing.

Its growth and popularity were attested to by famous patrons, a veritable "Who's Who" of American mercantile and financial luminaries at the turn of the century, including J.C. Penney, Montgomery Ward, Alfred DuPont, and John D. Rockefeller. President Taft was also a frequent guest. Battle Creek, Kellogg, and Graham's cracker soon became part of American consumer culture. Later Kellogg and C.W. Post developed the dry, prepackaged breakfast cereals that became synonomous with Americana itself.[5]

Rise and Decline of the Sectarians

Grahamism and its other three counterparts followed the curve line of alternative medicine throughout most of the nineteenth century, gaining public favor but eventually descending into the obscurity that appeared to be the fate of all schools challenging the orthodox medical mainstream. The sectarians' popularity was due in part to the fact that their services were less costly than those of the "-regulars." Yet common sense also was a factor; the sectarian irregulars did not assault the body with questionable, and sometimes poisonous, drugs and refrained as well from using the leeches which were important allopathic remedies. The "every man his own physician" concept also played well in a society that remained largely rural until the twentieth century. But the gulf between rural America and the rising urban class with its industrial and professional status was growing, and it gradually became clear that the urban centers would dominate medicine and other aspects of the changing society.[1]

Spiritualizing of Alternative Medicine

During the period following the Civil War, Mesmerism, evolving from the teachings of Viennese physician Anton Mesmer, and Swedenborgianism, named for the prolific Swedish nobleman who wrote 30 volumes about his metaphysical concepts, had a small but significant American intellectual following that joined the streams of religious and medical dissent, in what Fuller calls "the spiritualizing of alternative medicine." Its lasting importance is reflected in two dissenting schools that weathered the storm—osteopathy and chiropractic.[1] The metaphysical healing vision was also an integral part of another European import, naturopathy, which arrived literally at the turn of the century and soon joined forces with the more modern sectarian challenges.

Organized Medicine's Response
The Flexner Report
Organized medicine, having consolidated its authority and unquestioned professional dominance through the AMA, adopted a challenging posture toward the alternative schools. The elimination of medical "cults" became a policy goal of the association, which used the 1910 Flexner Report—the Report of the Carnegie Foundation for the Advancement of Teaching on Medical Education—as an instrument to ameliorate the problem of substandard schools and to eliminate remaining homeo-

pathic and botanic (now termed eclectic medicine) teaching institutions.[6]

The watershed survey and report by educator Abraham Flexner was an opportunity for organized medicine to perform a sweeping self-examination. The medical profession was growing at a faster rate than the nation as a whole and was experiencing significant growing pains. The burgeoning numbers of new physicians were seen by concerned officials of the old school as "coarse and common elements." Writing about the state of medical education, Harvard President Charles Eliot minced no words: "The ignorance and general incompetency of the average graduate of American medical schools, at a time when he receives the degree which turns him loose upon the community, is something very horrible to contemplate."[1]

Eliot's concerns were reflected in the prolification of medical schools, of which there were more than 160 by the year 1900, with 35 sectarian institutions. This was a period in which young men without a high school diploma could register for classes in fully half of these institutions, dropping out to apprentice with their own doctors and obtain MD degrees in about two calendar years. This pattern was also followed by the first osteopathic and chiropractic schools, where requirements for actual classroom attendance of lectures were minimal at best.

The reformation period of medical education coincided with the formative years of the osteopathic and chiropractic professions, whose survival through this century provided a significant ongoing alternative to medical orthodoxy. That survival— and its impact on the health care system at a time when health has become a primary social and political issue (Fig. 1-1)—justifies a review of the careers of osteopathy's founder Andrew Taylor Still and of Daniel David Palmer, the founder of chiropractic.

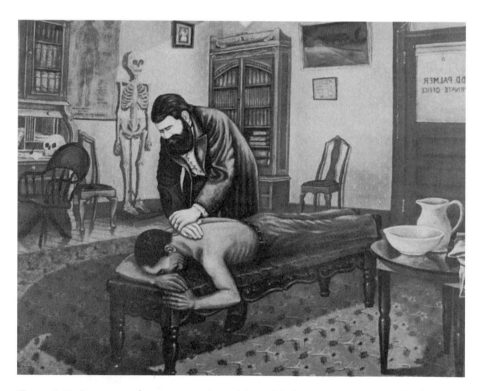

Figure 1-1. Present at the creation: Daniel David Palmer gives Harvey Lillard the first chiropractic adjustment in the Ryan Building, Davenport, Iowa, on September 18, 1895. (Courtesy of C. Paciorek, the artist.)

OSTEOPATHY AND CHIROPRACTIC: THE EARLY YEARS

Still and Palmer: Parallel Paths of the Founders

Brantingham[7] and others have shown the similarities between Still and Palmer, "bone doctors" in the post-frontier Midwest who through difficult but methodical clinical trials in thriving small town practices evolved separate concepts as to the cause of disease and formulated philosophies that provided a framework for their followers. They came—first few in number and curious, but later a small tide of what Gaucher-Peslherbe[8] has called "a particular kind, who had almost spent their lives searching."

The "coarse and common elements" that had offended the guardians of old-school orthodoxy in assessing the homeopaths and eclectic/botanical physicians appeared again in the classrooms and laboratories at Kirksville, Missouri, and Davenport, Iowa, the respective therapeutic meccas of Still and Palmer. Yet among those searching for alternatives to allopathic medicine were a surprising number of well-trained physicians of the regular school, as well as other professionals from the sciences, education, and the liberal arts. In fact, the first two decades of the twentieth century would show more "MD, DO" and "MD, DC" listings within the new professions than in later years.[9] Inevitably, the two manipulative therapy schools came into conflict with each other, while the regulars pointed disdainfully at the "new sectarians" who had rejected, they declared, the fundamentals of science and the biological truths that now fueled a medicine flush with power, influence, and increasing public favor.

Still, the "Old Doctor" of osteopathy, and Palmer, who was "Old Dad Chiro" to his followers, did in fact share a metaphysical footing in their new schools of healing, though by the time of their deaths (1917 and 1913, respectively), this was placed on the back burner by their followers. Still and Palmer met on a few documented occasions, not at a "bonesetter's summit" but at spiritualist camp meetings on the banks of the Mississippi. A mini-debate continues to this day as to whether Palmer actually visited Still at Kirksville (Still's family said he did, Palmer's son denied it).[10] Their similarities were on record: both

were born in log cabins (Still in Virginia, Palmer in Ontario). Both practiced what they called magnetic healing (Still in Missouri, Palmer in Iowa). Both wrote of the spiritual and metaphysical nature of healing (Still called the body a machine run by unseen forces; Palmer said that "innate intelligence" governed healing). Some of these concepts are similar to those of Asian medical systems.

Changing Course: William Smith and B.J. Palmer

The initial philosophies of chiropractic and osteopathy were altered by two men who made crucial decisions in the formative years of their professions as the influence of the founders was waning. These decisions would chart the course of both professions and greatly affect their relations with other alternative movements and what would evolve as complementary medicine.

The contrasts were marked. Few osteopathic physicians today know of a Scottish-trained physician named William Smith. Yet Smith, traveling through upstate Missouri during the early 1890s, became the Jefferson of Still's medical revolution. Convinced that osteopathy had merit, he became one of the first professors at the American School of Osteopathy and soon was hiring competent faculty, developing the curriculum, and seeking a medical presence in osteopathic theory. Surgery, obstetrics, and materia medica soon became standard at the Kirksville mother school and at others that had mushroomed across the country. The Old Doctor protested about the "medicalization" of his osteopathy but, by the time he died, few osteopaths would claim to be "drugless" physicians using manipulation only.[11]

Palmer's story was more dramatic. The person who would most alter the course of his profession was his only son, Bartlett Joshua. Like his father, without formal training and controversial and colorful, he was in constant conflict with the founder of chiropractic for the last 7 years of D.D.'s life. Their separation in April 1906 was both personal and professional—B.J. having bought out his father's interest in the first school after the senior Palmer's conviction and imprisonment in the county jail at Davenport for having "practiced medicine without a license." Bitter, feeling betrayed, and convinced that he was losing control of the profession he had founded, Gaucher-Peslherbe writes that Palmer

realized that the profession was escaping him: it was developing not only without him, but also at times in opposition to him, and many of his former pupils had parted company with him … in some cases, they went so far as to suggest that he did not understand what he was doing, in the hope of claiming for themselves the honor of being recognized as the founders, if not the discoverers, of the new science.[8]

B.J. Palmer and the Palmer School: Dynamism and Controversy

The younger Palmer had attributes not known or understood by the father. Whether B.J. ever approached his father's level of intellectual thought and formulation, he was an undenied advocate of everything chiropractic, flamboyant and contemptuous of orthodoxy in any form. Although uneducated in the classic sense, he attracted well-educated associates, faculty, students, and patients. Typesetters at the Palmer School printing press had difficulty keeping up with the rolled-paper pronouncements churned out from B.J.'s Underwood. He edited the publication that echoed the words of the self-styled "Developer of Chiropractic," or "B.J. Himself," *The Fountainhead News*. The younger Palmer also edited the monthly journal founded by his father, *The Chiropractor* (later *The Chiropractor and Clinical Journal*), until his death in 1961, for well over half a century.[11] While the founder authored two large volumes and one book published posthumously, B.J. claimed more than 30 books on clinical thought, marketing, philosophy, travel, social commentary, and technique. Most titles meshed all of these together, becoming known to devoted students, alumni, and collectors as "The Green Books," from their original Palmer School printery binding.

Dissent Among the Pioneers

B.J. Palmer became the dominant force in early chiropractic, but the rebellious nature of the profession soon introduced further dissent among its pioneers. Some carried with them an association with "Old

Dad Chiro," among them John F. Allen Howard, who launched a new school in the watershed year of 1906, when D.D. emerged from jail, sold his school interests, and set out for Oklahoma. Other early Palmer students—Solon Massey Langworthy, Andrew P. Davis (Fig. 1-2) and Charles Ray Parker—also opened rival teaching institutions, as did graduates of the rival schools such as Willard Carver, D.D.'s attorney[12] (for further details, see Ch. 2).

Although this intraprofessional dissent was rooted in both philosophical and technical considerations, in many instances there was a strong personal element. Feuds arose not unlike those that

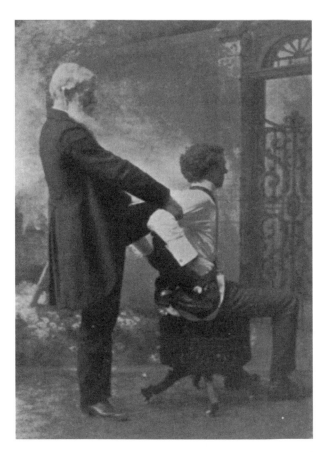

Figure 1-2. Andrew P. Davis, the first physician-osteopath graduate under Daniel D. Palmer, founded at least eight schools, authored a large volume on "Neuropathy," and carried on a dialogue with the founder about adjustive thrusts and modalities. Davis termed this his "knee-chest expansion" thrust

had plagued the medical profession in the previous century. Their model was the ongoing series of diatribes and acrimonious exchanges between the Palmers themselves, father and son. The schools founded by their rivals had little impact on the fortunes of the Palmer School. Many recreated the conditions prevalent in American medical education a generation earlier[1]:

> Touted laboratories were nowhere to be found, or consisted of a few vagrant test tubes squirreled away in a cigar box; corpses reeked because of the failure to use disinfectant in the dissecting room. Libraries had no books; alleged faculty members were busily occupied in private practice. Requirements for admission were waived for anyone who would pay.

The ideological and even missionary fervor that characterized early graduates partially overshadowed their academic shortcomings. The Palmer School of Chiropractic sent thousands into "the field" convinced that theirs was a mission as much as a healing art. During this period, the relations between chiropractic and its medical and osteopathic adversaries—and its smaller allies in the alternative field who had survived the Flexner era assault on the sectarians—were established.

Legacy of Civil Disobedience

Chiropractic survived—and actually thrived in much of its second and third decades—in virtually total isolation from the mainstream health care community, and for part of that time in violation of the medical practice laws. Following D.D. Palmer's conviction and jailing, literally thousands of chiropractors made similar sacrifices for their chosen calling. Their legacy occupies a small yet significant place in the history of American reform[13]:

> Like the abolitionists, they were victims of a systematic persecution and were literally driven from one town to another. Like the feminists and suffragettes, they were ridiculed and ostracized in the community. Like the union organizers, they were arrested on trumped-up charges and jailed. And like the civil rights workers, they were intimidated and

subverted by *agent provocateurs*. And in the finest tradition of reform movements, they were imprisoned for their beliefs.

Straights and Mixers

Armed with a sense of purpose, these chiropractors gathered strength in their isolation. In time, a growing part of the chiropractic profession reached out to the larger "drugless" community, which embraced those who stood in opposition to the regulars. The evolutionary process in chiropractic was complicated by the interminable "straight-mixer" controversy, which had its inception almost with the first of the pioneer graduates of the senior Palmer. Those adhering to the "straight" philosophy of the Palmers generally avoided any interchange with naturopaths, osteopaths, naprapaths, and other healers. The implication was that such association would introduce straights to the "mixing" modalities of heat, light, water, electricity, and the supplements of nonprescription drugs that characterized the drugless physicians.

In truth, "mixing" in chiropractic may have had its roots in the nineteenth century, with ancillary procedures used by some of the original "fifteen disciples," so termed to designate the lonely students who sat under Old Dad Chiro at Davenport through the graduation of B.J. in 1902. Some were already practitioners—four physicians and osteopaths, one who would become an osteopath, one who was a medical student, another a "manual therapist," and one a midwife. Better than half of D.D.'s first pupils had previous exposure to medical or sectarian instruction and clinical experiences.[14]

Formation of New Chiropractic Schools

It is not surprising, then, that of this original group, one-third either founded or became involved in rival schools during the lifetime of the founder. Physician-osteopath Andrew P. Davis, then 9 years D.D.'s senior and his second graduate in 1898, had already had a varied career as an allopath, homeopath, osteopath, and ophthalmologist and in a few years would coin the term *neuropathy* as a catch-all for these combined practices. He was later joined by a 1901 graduate, onetime minister Alan Raymond, in school ventures in Michigan and California. Davis was a classic itinerant alternative doctor and "school-man," having established schools of neuropathy, chiropractic, osteopathy, or all of those disciplines together in half a dozen states through 1911 (Oregon, Michigan, Texas, Missouri, Pennsylvania, and California). While Davis stressed manipulation—and engaged in ongoing correspondence with the founder about the merits of various thrusts—he was anything but a "straight" chiropractor.[15]

Three graduates of the successive years 1899, 1900, and 1901—Oakley Smith, Minora Paxson, and Solon Massey Langworthy—comprise the researchers and practitioners who kept counsel with D.D. during that first decade and then in 1903 formed the first known rival institution—the American School of

=THE=
AMERICAN SCHOOL
OF CHIROPRACTIC

(INCORPORATED)

603-605 First Ave., Cedar Rapids, Iowa.

The American School of Chiropractic has recently been reorganized and will re-open Sept. 6th. It is prepared to better fit students to successfully combat disease than any other system, drugless or otherwise.

The course of study extends over a period of two years divided into four terms of five months each.

Course of Study.

FIRST YEAR—FRESHMAN TERM. Anatomy, Histology and Microscopy, Physiology, Inorganic and Organic Chemistry.

SOPHMORE TERM. Anatomy, Physiology, Principles of Chiropractic. Physiological Chemistry, Urinalysis, Histology, Tracing and Record Work.

SECOND YEAR—JUNIOR TERM. Anatomy with Dissection, Principles of Chiropractic, Technique of Adjusting with actual practice, Symptomatology and Pathology.

SENIOR TERM. Anatomy, Pathology, Fractures and Dislocations, Bandaging, Hygiene and Dietetics, Gynecology, Chemical Diagnosis and Adjusting, Obstetrics and Medical Jurisprudence.

For School Announcement or other information, write

DR. S. M. LANGWORTHY, Pres.
Cedar Rapids, Iowa, U. S. A.

Figure 1-3. The American School of Chiropractic, founded in 1903, was the first "mixer" institution to challenge the Palmers. This curriculum met the requirements of the first Minnesota Practice Act of 1905, which was vetoed at the behest of D.D. Palmer.

Chiropractic and Nature Cure in Cedar Rapids, Iowa (Fig. 1-3). Smith, who had studied at the University of Iowa medical school and Paxson, a former school teacher and practicing midwife, followed D.D. Palmer to California in 1903, where he organized schools in Pasadena and Santa Barbara.[13]

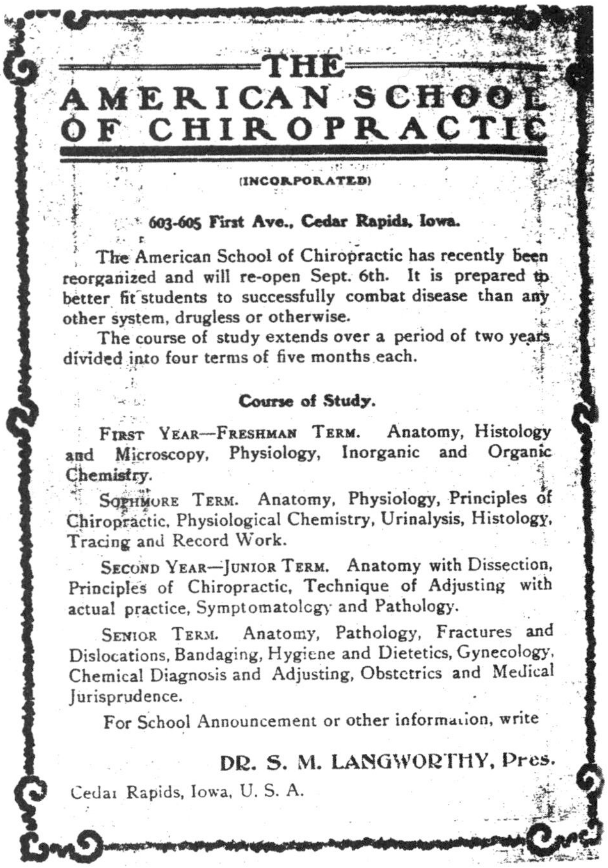

Both were present when D.D. announced on July 1, 1903 that the thermoregulation of the body was a neural, rather than a circulatory, phenomenon, having demonstrated this process on a patient attending a clinic "with eight witnesses" in the Aiken building in Santa Barbara. Keating[16] provides an extensive review of this little known event in chiropractic, which he calls "the first major reduction in chiropractic theory," suggesting that "in the fullness of time, chiropractors would re-discover the 'bloodless surgery' concepts of Palmer's first stage of chiropractic theory (Fig. 1-4)." Shown in a group photo of "the witnesses," Smith and Paxson soon returned to Iowa, where with Langworthy they launched their own school, with the first "mixer" curriculum.

The American School saga, although brief, has been widely discussed in the literature of chiropractic history. What is significant is that "nature cure," a term also used by the pioneer naturopaths, was a catch-all for the "mixing" that the Palmers decried. The American school advertised in *The Naturopath* and other sectarian journals, while Langworthy promoted "traction tables" and accepted advertisements for botanical medicines and other adjuncts in his own journal, *The Backbone*.[17]

In the years preceding the senior Palmer's death in 1913, other dissenters from Davenport, and Palmer alumni who in turn began schools, dotted the chiropractic landscape. While all were based on fundamental chiropractic theory, many were sympathetic to alternative therapies. Howard's National School, founded in Davenport and soon relocated in Chicago, in time became the flagship of what he and his associates termed "rational, progressive chiropractic," while B.J. Palmer denounced the school as a hotbed of "mixing." A strong basic science and medical faculty, an informal visitation arrangement with Cook County Hospital (enjoyed by all sectarian schools in Chicago in that period), and pronounced use of "physiological therapeutics" made the National School a serious counterpoint to Palmer academic leadership (Fig. 1-5). A new group of field

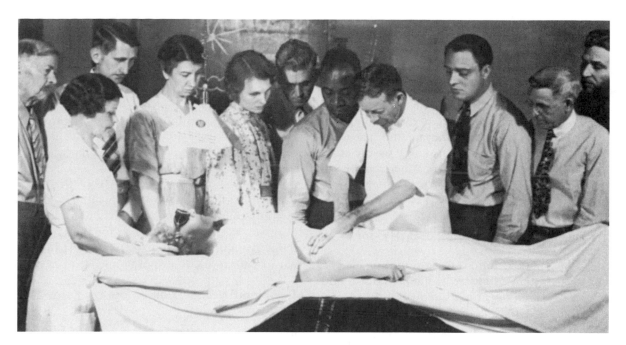

Figure 1-4. Chiropractic "bloodless surgery," circa 1938. Soft tissue manipulation was considered "mixing" by purist chiropractors, yet had legitimate origins in the early days of the profession. (Courtesy R.W. Gibbons Collection.)

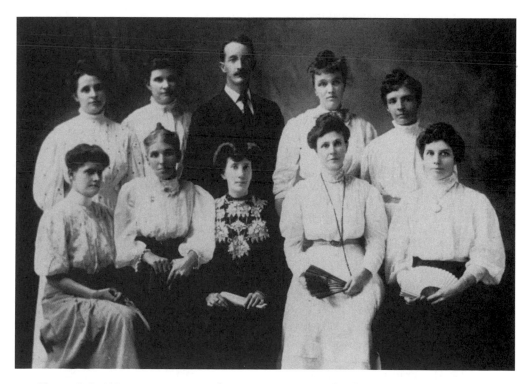

Figure 1-5. Women were a significant presence in early chiropractic, teaching and authoring textbooks. Above, the second graduating class of the National School of Chiropractic in Davenport, with founding president John F. Howard. (Courtesy National College of Chiropractic)

doctors, although decidedly a minority (Palmer graduates numerically dominated practice until the mid-1930s) engaged in nonstraight practices while still maintaining the adjustment as the central therapy. Modalities began to dominate the pages of many state association journals as well as the non-Palmer national groups, the first American Chiropractic Association (1922–1930) and the National Chiropractic Association (1930–1963).

CHIROPRACTIC AND NATUROPATHY

Some of the major training institutions outside the Palmer solar system of allied "straight" schools and associations offered naturopathic degrees for nearly half a century. These included the National College, the Los Angeles College (LACC), and Western States College in Portland, Oregon (the direct descendant of a school founded by D.D. Palmer in 1908).[5] Other institutions that graduated significant numbers of chiropractors also offered Doctor of Naturopathy (ND) postgraduate degrees for a few additional months of residence and clinical training. The University of Natural Healing Arts in Colorado, several California institutions that later merged into LACC, the Nashville College in Tennessee, and a few others offered DC and ND courses.

Parting of the Ways

By the mid-1950s, aware that the United States Office of Education looked with disfavor on such dual programs, the National Chiropractic Association Council on Education and its director, John J. Nugent (see Ch. 2), urged abolition of ND programs at accredited and provisionally accredited chiropractic institutions.

This development may have turned out to be a blessing for naturopathic medicine, which had been virtually eliminated in many jurisdictions (in some—such as Tennessee and Florida—by adverse legislative action) and reduced to a presence in the Pacific northwest and a half-dozen other states. The discontinued naturopathic program at Western States in Portland became the National College of Naturopathic Medicine (NCNM), graduates of which later founded the John Bastyr College (now Bastyr University) in Seattle, Washington. NCNM and Bastyr are now naturopathy's flagship institutions, having gained accreditation as the naturopathic profession

has undergone a late-twentieth century renaissance in practice and acceptance.[6]

In 1995, Bastyr University received a grant of nearly $1 million from the new National Institutes of Health Office of Alternative Medicine to create a center for the study of natural therapeutics for human immunodeficiency virus/acquired immunodeficiency syndrome (HIV/AIDS). In 1996, King County, Washington (in the Seattle metropolitan area) became the first jurisdiction in the United States to allocate public funds for the creation of a natural medicine clinic, and the first to appoint a naturopath to the Board of Public Health.

Traditional Values, Contemporary Forms

The chiropractic-naturopathic association and dialogue from the 1960s onward has offered new perspectives to alternative healing. The political and social discontent for which the 1960s are remembered was accompanied by a rebirth of nineteenth century "popular health" concepts, with renewed interest in nutrition, vegetarianism, natural birth, holistic health principles, Asian medicine and acupuncture, mind–body awareness, and self-help. Chiropractors have been instrumental in bringing public attention to these concepts, exploring these areas and in some cases incorporating them into chiropractic practice and education. This in turn has provided an expanded audience for chiropractic and a newly revitalized naturopathic medicine.

Orthodoxy has also relaxed some of its prohibitions, permitting physician members of the AMA (who now constitute less than one-half of practicing physicians in the United States) to enter into relations with non-allopathic practitioners.[18] Aided by the landmark 1991 Wilk decision, organized medicine has allowed the once unthinkable—professional cooperation with chiropractors, some of whom have become part of hospital staffs (see Ch. 19) and have been invited to join faculties of medical schools and publish in specialty journals.

"DRUGLESS ALLIANCES": PAST AND PRESENT

The contemporary alternative health movement hearkens back to the "drugless alliances" between alternative practitioners in the period between World Wars I and II. These alliances were more than

ALMA ARNOLD: HEALING ARTS PIONEER

Alma Arnold (Fig. 1-6) provides a classic early-twentieth century study of what Wardwell[12] has called the kaleidoscope of therapeutic offerings. Like some of the other early pioneers, little has survived about her personal life, yet she claimed several accomplishments following her graduation from Langworthy's American School in 1903. Going to New York City, she became the first known chiropractor in that state. She corresponded with D.D. Palmer, who cites her more than a dozen times in his 1910 book, especially criticizing the Arnold "painless" system of adjusting.

Remarkably, this German-born woman from the rural Midwest established dual practices in Manhattan and Washington, DC, and headed an institution in New York City that taught chiropractic, becoming the first known woman president of a chiropractic college (1908). Ten years later, Alfred A. Knopf, the old and respected New York publishing house, published her book, *The Triangle of Health*, which reflected the marriage between chiropractic and alternative therapies. Well written, it expounded on mind–body–spirit concepts of holistic thought.[19]

If Arnold's name survives, it was because of her most famous patient, Clara Barton, founder of the American Red Cross and perhaps the most admired woman in the United States before World War I. Arnold said, "I was privileged to be [Miss Barton's] physician for the last four years of her life, and I prize the friendship and confidences of this great woman highly." Arnold writes in her book, "I had studied medicine and osteopathy (in Chicago)" but provides no other information as to her career before she met Langworthy, to whom she credits the restoration of her own chronic ill-health, as well as that of her daughter.[19]

(Continues)

Langworthy, Arnold[20] wrote, "taught that spinal freedom should be supplemented by right living in hygiene and diet." She praised "the broadness of the curriculum in his school," which influenced her practice as much as the spinal adustment concept of Palmer. After Arnold had established her New York and Washington practices in 1908, she published a small booklet titled "Cosmotherapy," which embraced chiropractic, hydrotherapy, hygiene, and dietetics. She was listed as president of the Columbia College of Cosmotherapy. That designation did not survive for long, but Arnold as a cosmopolitan chiropractor did. A chiropractic directory lists her as still practicing in Manhattan in 1938.

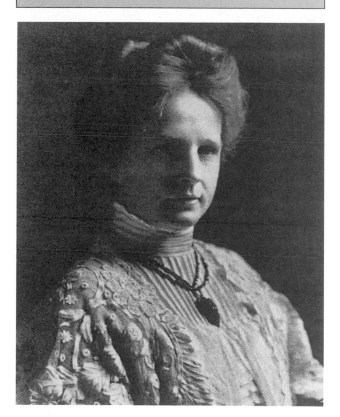

Figure 1-6. Alma Cusian Arnold, circa 1909. Within a decade of her graduation from the American School of Chiropractic, she had a dual practice in Manhattan and Washington, D.C., conducted a school, and authored a book issued by a prominent publisher. She was the personal physician for Clara Barton, founder of the American Red Cross.

a wagon-circling reaction to the consolidation of medical power and more than a fleeting aberration. The intellectual dialogue engaged in by D.D. Palmer before the publication of his massive 1910 tome, *The Chiropractor's Adjustor*, was with former students and graduates of schools started by onetime students, most of whom would be considered "mixers" in the pre-1950 chiropractic lexicon. They included Howard and Langworthy and Willard Carver.[21] Carver, who saw himself as "The Constructor" of chiropractic (as counterpoint to B.J. Palmer as "The Developer") was an attorney who conducted a school in Oklahoma (and in three other states and the District of Columbia) and wrote papers and books with a strong concentration on biopsychology and "suggestion therapy," a metaphysical concept that D.D. Palmer had rejected. While Carver aligned himself politically with the "straights," his schools offered obstetrics and minor surgery, and ultimately physical therapy adjuncts.[22,23]

The Palmers—and especially B.J. Palmer for his years as the dominant figure in the profession— were fearful of the "medicalization" of chiropractic, just as Still in his final years had warned that this process was subverting osteopathy. However one views these events, the evidence is that early chiropractors—straight and mixer alike—developed split personality characteristics in their search for professionalization, sometimes moving in two different directions at the same time.

For example, while B.J. Palmer was actively seeking legislative recognition for chiropractors as professional health care providers, he testified before a state legislature that we "are not a profession ... we [the PSC] are in the business of manufacturing chiropractors." Mixer chiropractors demonstrated similarly split personalities, aligning themselves with the "drugless" schools and associations as an alternative to the excessive drugging and surgery associated with allopathic medicine, while participating on the fringes of practice utilized by physicians and surgeons. Chiropractors in California, Oregon, Illinois, and other broad scope states used minor surgery, proctology, eye, ear, nose & throat procedures, electrotherapy, and other procedures. While those doing so probably never exceeded 20 percent of the nation's chiropractors, this constituted a significant minority.

Coupled with this issue was the fact that chiropractors in the profession's earliest years were but a footnote in the galaxy of alternative therapies. Flexner declined to even visit chiropractic schools, dismissing the profession with a curt reference to "chiropractics" (sic) in his chapter on medical sects.[6]

CHIROPRACTIC AND THE CONTEMPORARY ALTERNATIVE HEALTH MOVEMENT

Scorned by the academic and political wings of the medical establishment, early chiropractors incrementally built a grassroots movement one patient at a time. Over several stormy decades, the profession attracted tens of millions of supporters and gathered political strength from this far-flung constituency. In addition to securing its own place in the health care system, chiropractic emerged as a crucial linchpin in the natural health movement that in the closing years of the twentieth century is growing at an unprecedented pace.

A landmark event in the recognition of the alternative movement was the 1993 publication in *The New England Journal of Medicine*[24] of Harvard physician David Eisenberg's study on the prevalence, costs, and patterns of use of a wide array of health alternatives. This study has been widely quoted for its finding that one-third of American adults use alternative therapies, and for its startling disclosure that the number of visits to alternative practitioners in the United States exceeds the number of visits to conventional general practitioners.[24]

Less widely noted is the fact that Eisenberg's statistics were heavily dependent on chiropractic utilization figures, which accounted for a substantial majority of visits to alternative practitioners. (Eisenberg defined alternative therapies as those methods not generally taught in medical schools or generally provided in hospitals, a definition that currently includes chiropractic.) Chiropractic is widely perceived, both inside and outside the alternative health community, as the alternative (after osteopathy) that has moved closest to mainstream status. The question of whether to consider chiropractic "alternative" remains controversial among chiropractors who wish to avoid the marginalization currently implied in this designation.[25] Chiropractic has clearly been in the alternative camp throughout much of its past but in recent years has attained many professional characteristics of mainstream status such as licensure, insurance reimbursement, a significant research base, and a well-developed educational system. The question of "alternative versus mainstream" will likely remain unresolved until chiropractic's professional status is unquestioned.

BUILDING THE FUTURE ON THE FOUNDATION OF THE PAST

The alternative schools of practice in this century have responded to similar social forces to those that provided encouragement and then disapproval to the nineteenth century sectarians. The political climate, legislative trends, the rise of a strong, sophisticated medical community, and educational reform have been sea change factors in the marketplace of healing. Chiropractic has survived despite its own civil wars.

Its pioneers sought a place in the healing arts, not quite understanding all these social forces. The Palmers and their contemporaries were of a different time, yet their concepts have weathered an entire century. Understanding that history, as Santayana suggests, may provide an image of the future that shows how to avoid reliving the mistakes of the past.

Terminology

alternative medicine
botanic medicine
Flexner Report
Grahamism
heroic medicine
homeopathy
hydropathy
metaphysical healing
mixers
Popular Health Movement
straights

Review Questions

1. Who was the Pulitzer Prize-winning author of a study of the social history of American medicine?

2. What was the Popular Health Movement?

3. Name three alternative schools of medicine in the late 19th century.

4. What "sectarian" medical association was formed before the American Medical Association?

5. Who was Abraham Flexner and what was the Flexner Report?

6. How did B.J. Palmer define "purist" chiropractic?

7. Name some early chiropractic "mixers."

8. In what decade were the last naturopathic degrees offered by chiropractic schools?

9. What was the significance of the Wilk decision?

10. How was Alma Arnold distinctive in the early years of chiropractic?

Concept Questions

1. During the nineteenth century, following the French Revolution and the democratic experience in America, a new toleration for dissent arose in science and medicine, as well as in political and economic theory. Show how this relationship evolved into new concepts about disease and health, as well as the challenges to the "regular" or orthodox school of medicine.

2. Name some of the medical and religious philosophers who influenced healing and alternative medicine during the early and mid-nineteenth century, and describe the "spiritualizing" of non-traditional healing, with particular emphasis on the manipulative protest schools, osteopathy and chiropractic.

3. Andrew Taylor Still, the founder of osteopathy, and Daniel David Palmer, the founder of chiropractic, were contemporaries who shared similar backgrounds and concepts in their philosophy of alternative medicine. List these, and develop your own assessment of how they complemented each other and influenced health care in the past century.

References

1. Starr P: The Social Transformation of American Medicine. Basic Books, New York, 1982

2. Ehrenreich B, English D: For Her Own Good. Anchor Books, New York, 1978

3. Fuller RC: Alternative Medicine and American Religious Life. Oxford University Press, New York, 1989

4. Duffy J: The Healers: A History of American Medicine. University of Illinois Press, Urbana, 1979

5. Kirchfeld F, Boyle W: Nature Doctors: Pioneers in Naturopathic Medicine. Medicine Biologica, Portland, OR, 1994

6. Flexner S: Medical Education in the United States and Canada. Times-Arno Press, New York, 1972

7. Brantingham JW: Still and Palmer: the impact of the first osteopath and the first chiropractor. Chiro Hist 6:1, 1986

8. Gaucher-Peslherbe PG: Chiropractic: Early Concepts in Their Historical Setting. National College Books, Lombard, IL, 1993

9. Gibbons RW: Physician-chiropractors: medical presence in the evolution of chiropractic. Bull Hist Med 55:2, 1981

10. Gevitz N: The DOs: Osteopathic Medicine in America. Johns Hopkins University Press, Baltimore, 1982

11. Gibbons RW: B.J. Palmer (1881–1961) in Who's Who in Chiropractic, Vol. 2. Who's Who in Chiropractic Publishing, Littleton, CO, 1980

12. Wardwell W: Chiropractic: History and Evolution of a New Profession. CV Mosby, Chicago, 1992

13. Gibbons RW: The evolution of chiropractic: medical and social protest in America. p. 17. In Haldeman S (ed): Modern Developments in the Principles and Practice of Chiropractic. Appleton & Lange, E Norwalk, CT, 1980

14. Gibbons RW: Chiropractic in America: the historical conflicts of cultism and science. J Pop Culture 11:3, 1977

15. Gibbons RW: Skeletons in the medical closet: pioneer osteopathic and chiropractic schools in western Pennsylvania. Pittsburgh Hist 76:1, 1993

16. Keating JC: Heat by nerves and not by blood: the first major reduction in chiropractic theory, 1903. Chiro Hist 15:2, 1995

17. Backbone: A Journal of Natural Living 1:2, 1904

18. McAndrews JF, Cleveland CS III: The anti-trust suit. p. 227. In Peterson D, Wiese G (eds): Chiropractic: An Illustrated History. CV Mosby, St. Louis, 1995

19. Gibbons RW: The Search for Alma Arnold. Chiro Hist 16:2 1996

20. Arnold A: The Triangle of Health. Alfred A. Knopf, Inc., New York, 1918

21. Strauss JB: Refined By Fire: The Evolution of Straight Chiropractic. Foundation for the Advancement of Chiropractic Education, Levittown, PA, 1994

22. Carver College of Chiropractic, Oklahoma City, OK Catalogues, 1923, 1941, 1958, 1960. In Logan College Archives, St. Louis.

23. Gibbons RW: Forgotten parameters of practice, the chiropractic obstetrician. Chiro Hist 2:1, 1982

24. Eisenberg DM, Kessler RC, Foster C et al: Unconventional medicine in the United States: prevalence, costs, and patterns of use. N Engl J Med 328:246, 1993

25. Anderson RA: Chiropractic: Alternative or Mainstream? In Lawrence D (ed): Advances in Chiropractic. CV Mosby, St. Louis, 1996

2
Education and Accreditation

A Century of Progress

Herbert Vear

---

*C*hiropractic education began when founder Daniel David Palmer first explained his chiropractic theories to friends and family. It has evolved over the past century from small tutorials to trade schools of variable status, gradually reaching its current position as a fully professional system of higher education, with well-credentialed faculty and a curriculum meeting rigorous educational standards of recognized accrediting agencies.

IN THE BEGINNING: 1895

Chiropractic was discovered by chance in 1895 by the alert and fertile mind of D.D. Palmer,[1] who soon recognized a scientific basis for it, stating, "I founded Chiropractic on Osteology, Neurology and Functions — bones, nerves and the manifestations of impulses." The founder's earlier excursions into magnetic healing had embraced spiritualism and vitalism, which led him to include "innate intelligence" among chiropractic principles, and eventually brought metaphysics and theosophy into chiropractic teachings.[2] Conflict was inevitable because of the inherent tension between these paradigms.

The term "innate intelligence" was selected to express the superiority, individuality, and intuitive power this entity was said to possess. Palmer first introduced this concept to the growing profession in 1904. Donahue writes[3]: "Historically, it is important to note that the concept of innate intelligence was originated and developed by D.D. Palmer although it is more often associated with his son, B.J." The controversies created by the Palmer concept "innate" not only divided the profession for decades but contributed to widespread prolonged criticism and disapproval of chiropractic, including isolation from the education communities of science and medicine. The isolation of chiropractic education lasted for six decades until the 1975 approval of the Council on Chiropractic Education (CCE) as the accrediting agency for chiropractic by the U.S. Department of Education. Further detail on this subject is available in the journal *Chiropractic History* and other scholarly works by Wardwell,[4] Keating,[5] and Peterson.[6]

STATE OF TURN OF THE CENTURY SCIENCE: 1895–1900

Education has been crucial to the growth, development, and maturation of the chiropractic profession. Its importance has often been underestimated, as strong and vocal dogmatists have taken center stage. Gibbons writes[7]:

The story of chiropractic education, then, assumes a greater depth when viewed in the context of the changing political, medical, social and economic landscape of North America in the twentieth century. Born in a reform period of turn of the century America, chiropractic training struggled to maintain identity when proprietary institutions were dominant and the first ventures into large foundation subsidization of medical education was being implemented.

The discovery of chiropractic in 1895, the development of its perceived scientific basis, and the educational process that followed must be interpreted within the context of scientific knowledge available at the time. For example, nutrition, a field of therapeutics utilized for millennia, had no scientific base until 1901 with the recognition of an anti-beriberi factor, which was not finally isolated until 1926. All we know of scientific nutrition begins at that point. This was also the era of Louis Pasteur and Robert Koch and the birth of microbiology. To quote Hall,[8] "Scientists have a tendency to seize on any plausible theory and hang onto it tenaciously, and scientists of that day were profoundly influenced by the work of Pasteur, who had shown that diseases are caused by microbes; ergo all diseases are caused by microbes." Later developments have demonstrated the fallacy of reductionist reasoning that attributes all disease to one cause, whether it be a microbe or a subluxation.

Neurophysiology at the turn of the century asserted that the nervous system was the only controller of function. Hormones had not yet been discovered. Knowledge of central nervous system function was largely theoretical, as was the idea that the nervous system was subject to interference.[9]

Moreover, medical education was in a haphazard state, as vividly described in the influential Flexner Report.[10] Flexner revealed an enormous overproduction of uneducated and ill-trained medical practitioners. He reported the existence of a large number of commercial schools sustained by advertising, that medical schools were a profitable business, that admission was given to academically unqualified students, and that medical schools were isolated from teaching hospitals. It was in this milieu that chiropractic education began. Gibbons posits a unique classification for what he considers the four main periods of educational activity in chiropractic[7]:

the Tutorial Period (1897–1905), Classical Period (1905–1924), Proprietary Period (1924–1960), and Professional Period (1960–present).

THE TUTORIAL PERIOD: 1897–1905

In *The Chiropractor's Adjustor*, D.D. Palmer states that he opened Palmer's School of Magnetic Cure in 1897, although it is not named as such in his textbook. In the same citation he reports that one student attended in 1898; three in 1899; two in 1900; five in 1901 and four in 1902. Bartlett Joshua Palmer, the founder's only son, received his diploma from his father in 1902 at the age of 20. The Palmer School of Magnetic Cure was incorporated on July 10, 1896. Several months later Rev. Samuel Weed suggested the name "chiropractic" for the new profession.

Although the term "chiropractic" appears on the first diplomas issued by D.D. Palmer in 1902, its use was not incorporated by the school until May 1907. The Palmer School and Infirmary of Chiropractic was unofficially referred to as the Palmer School of Chiropractic as early as 1905, although this was not reflected in the institution's papers of incorporation until 1921. Weisse[11] asks several relevant questions: "Why didn't Palmer use the term 'Chiropractic' in his 1896 school title? Was the Palmer School of Cure (1897–1902) ever incorporated? Did Palmer ever incorporate the Palmer Infirmary and Chiropractic Institute (1902–1904)?" It remains a mystery.

The content and quality of education at the early Palmer School are unknown. The course was up to 3 months in duration and consisted of observing Palmer's techniques and then applying these procedures to patients. Oakley Smith, an 1899 Palmer graduate, wrote in 1932 that Palmer provided no instruction, no blackboards, no textbooks or notes, and that observing Palmer giving treatments was all he got for his money. Wardwell[4] describes Smith's further observations in detail. Gibbons[7] provides a slightly different version of Palmer's early instruction (1897–1902) by suggesting that some instruction in science subjects could have been provided by other students, five of whom were medical graduates. However, he emphasizes the informal, almost casual way in which pioneer chiropractic instruction was imparted. It could be that D.D. Palmer was intimidated by the medical knowledge of his early students and avoided controversy by teaching only that in which he perceived himself to be an expert.

The first great pedagogue in chiropractic was Solon M. Langworthy, a 1901 graduate of the Palmer Institute. Rehm[12] suggests that Langworthy was highly educated, that "his earlier achievements give currency to separate accounts that he had a graduate medical education prior to studying under D.D. Palmer. His writings suggest a classical medical experience." Although he founded the American School of Chiropractic in Cedar Rapids, Iowa in 1903 and the (first) American Chiropractic Association in 1905, his accomplishments are largely unknown by members of today's profession. Nevertheless, he was responsible for initiating the first standards for chiropractic education and the first scientific concepts of chiropractic. Gibbons[13] writes:

Consider the Langworthy achievements, largely forgotten today: he was the first to establish a systemized curriculum of chiropractic lectures and clinical work; the first to establish a two year course; the first to publish a regular journal; a coauthor and publisher of the first textbook. He helped to initiate and gain passage of the first chiropractic legislation in the United States and to research a theory which would gain the first serious consideration in the medical community about the validity of spinal therapeutics.

During 1903–1906, Langworthy theorized about the manner in which the vertebral column influences health. Lerner[14] claims that Langworthy was the first to use the term "subluxation" in a chiropractic sense; the first to recognize the significance of the intervertebral foramina; the first to suggest the brain as the source of nerve energy; the first chiropractic reference to erect posture and gravity in human biomechanics; and the first to claim supremacy of nerves versus the osteopathic claim for blood.

In 1905, Langworthy was joined on the faculty by Palmer School graduates Oakley G. Smith and Minora C. Paxson. Langworthy, Smith, and Paxson opened the door to what is now the norm in chiropractic education and practice. They collaborated in writing *Modernized Chiropractic*,[15] the first chiropractic textbook. This text played a major role in attorney Tom Morris's successful 1907 defense of Shegatora Morikubo, a Wisconsin chiropractor charged with practicing medicine without a license. Significantly, B.J. Palmer and the Universal Chiropractors Association financially supported the defense of Shegatora, and as part of their support also embraced the scientific concepts published in *Modernized Chiropractic*. Palmer, who had vociferously criticized Langworthy's work on numerous prior occasions,[16] later adopted Langworthy's vertebral concepts, a credit to his growing maturity.

The Tutorial Period, with few schools and few graduates,[17] was significant for the beginning of the future "straight" and "mixer" conflict, which lasted several decades and drained the intellectual and financial resources of the embryo profession. Even today, this controversy continues to embarrass and confound the profession. The straight-mixer debacle grew out of the "straight" belief that spinal adjustment is the only treatment necessary for correcting spinal subluxation, which is the sole cause of disease. "Mixers" subscribe to a multifactorial theory of disease causation, and use other natural therapeutic modalities to treat patients. The Tutorial Period brought a recognition of the importance of research and scholarship. During this period, there were 15 graduates of the Palmer School. It is estimated that five of these went on to found or join new chiropractic colleges, which changed the educational face of the profession.

THE CLASSICAL PERIOD: 1905–1924

During the Classical Period, chiropractic education and practice spread to at least 26 additional states and 2 Canadian provinces, and Ferguson and Weisse[17] estimate that the number of schools increased from 17 in 1906 to 64 in 1924. Enrollment grew exponentially, although there was a decline during World War I. Precise figures are unavailable, except for the Palmer School.

Most new colleges closed soon after opening, leaving little or no documentation of the number of students or graduates. All colleges were proprietary and dependent on the energy and dedication of the founder. Langworthy's American School of Chiropractic and Nature Cure, despite strong faculty, scholarship and leadership closed in 1918 with little fanfare. Oakley Smith, the prime author of *Modernized Chiropractic*, published in 1906, left the American School in 1907 and moved to Chicago to found a new college and profession, naprapathy, which survived into the 1980s.

Minora Paxson, who may have been a midwife or nurse before studying chiropractic at Palmer, went on to become the first chiropractic educator to teach obstetrics and gynecology.[13] Her short biography in *Modernized Chiropractic*[15] states, "Dr. Paxson is the first chiropractor to apply for and pass an examination before a State Board (Illinois) and receive a license to practice Obstetrics in accordance with the principles of Chiropractic. She likewise was granted the first certificate (Illinois) licensing the treatment of disease by Chiropractic." Based on the publication date of the textbook, Minora Paxson may well have been the first licensed chiropractor in the world.[12]

Although the specific reasons for the failure of individual schools are unknown, it is likely that that lack of students, unqualified faculty, inadequate facilities, and limited financial support contributed to the demise of most failed institutions. It was a time of private ownership of schools, with school owners expecting substantial financial rewards.

Many schools were founded in this era out of dissatisfaction with the philosophy, technique, and educational methods of the Palmer model. The major schools founded by dissident Palmer faculty were Lincoln College in Indianapolis, founded by James Firth; National College, founded by John Howard; and Universal College, founded by Joy Loban. Contemporary schools founded in the Classical Era that trace their origins to non-Palmer graduates include Logan Chiropractic College, Los Angeles Chiropractic College, Canadian Memorial Chiropractic College, and the Cleveland Chiropractic Colleges of Kansas City and Los Angeles.

Table 2-1 lists several graduates of early Palmer schools who opened their own institutions. The list includes D.D. Palmer, who opened several schools on the West Coast, all of which failed. The Pacific

Table 2-1. Chiropractic Schools Formed by D. D. Palmer and Early Graduates

Palmer School of Magnetic Cure: 1896 Palmer School of Cure: 1897–1902 Palmer Infirmary and Chiropractic Institute: 1902–1904 Palmer School and Infirmary of Chiropractic: 1904–1921 Palmer School of Chiropractic: 1921–1961	
Graduate	**School**
Solon Langworthy (1901) Oakley Smith (1899) Minora Paxson (1899)	American School of Chiropractic and Nature Cure, Cedar Rapids, IA, 1903–1918
John Howard (1905)	National School of Chiropractic, Davenport, IA, 1906
Joy M. Loban (1908)	Universal Chiropractic College, Davenport, IA, 1910
Charles Parker (1905)	Parker School of Chiropractic, Ottumwa, IA, 1905
D.D. Palmer A.A. Gregory	Palmer–Gregory College, Oklahoma City, OK, 1906
D.D. Palmer	Portland School of Chiropractic, 1903
D.D. Palmer J. LaValley	Pacific Chiropractic College, Portland, OR, 1907
D.D. Palmer	Circa 1911–1912, he opened a number of schools in CA; all failed
J. Firth (1910) H. Vedder (1912) S. Burich (1913) A. Hendricks (1920)	Lincoln Chiropractic College, Indianapolis, IN, 1926

Chiropractic College (1907), although started with the elder Palmer, owes its survival to John LaValley. Western States Chiropractic College traces its origin to this school.

John Howard and the National School of Chiropractic

After Solon Langworthy, the second Palmer graduate to start a new school was John A. Howard, a medical doctor and a native of Utah. B.J. Palmer and John Howard had serious disagreement over the teaching of anatomy and dissection,[18] which caused Howard to open the National School of Chiropractic in Davenport, Iowa, in 1906. He received written encouragement from D.D. Palmer to open a new school, no doubt to embarrass and antagonize his estranged son B.J. In 1908, Howard moved the school to Chicago, "to secure the clinical, laboratory, dissection, hospital and other (educational) facilities that were lacking in a small town."[19] He continued to strengthen the course of study and quality of faculty, hiring medical physician William Charles Schulze in 1910.

In 1916 Howard sold his interest in the National School to Schulze, who remained president until 1936. New faculty hired by Schulze included another medical doctor, Arthur Forster, in 1912. In 1915, Forster wrote one of the first scientifically based textbooks for chiropractic education and practice, *Principles and Practice of Spinal Adjustment*, which was revised several times and is probably the first chiropractic textbook to be translated into three foreign languages. The significance of this text is that it was based on the orthodox biological sciences rather than speculative philosophy. In later years, Janse, Houser, and Wells would revise this text and publish it under the title *Chiropractic Principles and Technic* in 1939 and 1947. Published by the National College, the textbook was a standard for most colleges until the 1960s.

Joy M. Loban and the Universal School of Chiropractic

The story of Joy M. Loban is exciting though short. He graduated from the Palmer School before D.D. Palmer left for Oklahoma in 1908.[6] For 2 years, B.J. Palmer and Joy Loban enjoyed a unique relationship exemplified by Palmer's 1908 dedication to Loban in the fourth edition of *The Science of Chiropractic*[20]:

One small wiry, sincere and conscientious man, whose whole object is the uplifting of this philosophy … he is more than an acquaintance or friend, but a companion such as gives backbone to my research and to me personally and professionally.

Palmer saw Loban as a "philosopher of chiropractic," appointed him to the first Chair of Chiropractic Philosophy, and apparently viewed him as his eventual successor at the Palmer School. However, in April 1910 Loban is said to have led 40 to 50 students out of B.J.'s class and down Davenport's Brady Street to form the new Universal Chiropractic College, where he became Dean and President. Reasons for this sudden turn of events are not clear. Rehm suggests that Loban objected to Palmer's introduction of x-ray and that there were other philosophical differences.[12] Loban had visions for chiropractic education that could not be realized under the stringent control of B.J. Palmer.

Loban left Universal College about 1914 and became Dean of the Washington School of Chiropractic in Washington, DC, for 2 years before relocating to Pittsburgh and becoming Dean of the Pittsburgh College of Chiropractic. In 1918, Universal College merged with Pittsburgh College, retaining the name Universal Chiropractic College. In 1922, Universal College became the first to offer a 4-year course totaling 32 months.[4] Hugh B. Logan and his son Vinton F. Logan, graduates of the Universal College, formed the Logan College of Chiropractic in 1935. Logan College was a nonprofit institution that offered a 4-year course from the beginning. Swiss researcher Fred Illi, another Universal graduate, produced in-depth research on the sacrum and pelvis including the first radiographic research studies of that anatomic area. Illi's pioneering study of biomechanics remains one of the great bodies of work produced by the chiropractic profession.[21] Universal College was a quality institution that fell victim to the Depression and World War II, merging with Lincoln College in 1944 (Table 2-2).

The Neurocalometer Debacle

Gibbons[7] views the Classical Period as a "mini-Golden Age" that ended with the neurocalometer (NCM) crisis in 1924. He writes of this watershed event, "The neurocalometer debacle of 1924 had an impact that was significant enough to change the whole course of

Table 2-2. Affiliation, Amalgamation, and Merging of Principal Schools

College	Consolidated with
National College 1906, moved to Chicago 1908	Merged with University of Natural Healing Arts, 1965; Chiropractic Institute of New York, 1968; Lincoln College of Chiropractic, 1971
Universal College 1910, moved to Pittsburgh 1918	Amalgamated with Pittsburg School, 1919; merged with Lincoln College, 1944, which merged with National, 1971
Carver-Denny College 1906; became Carver College 1908	Merged with Logan College of Chiropractic, 1958
Ratledge College of Chiropractic 1911; Ratledge a graduate of Carver-Denny, 1907	Purchased by Cleveland Chiropractic College, LA, 1955

chiropractic education and politics for the rest of the century." The NCM was the invention of Dossa D. Evins, a 1922 graduate of Palmer School (PSC) and an electrical engineer. His instrument was designed to measure skin heat differentials on both sides of the spine,[4,5] and it was implied that the NCM would locate subluxations and the cause of disease.

B.J. Palmer was quick to recognize the financial potential of the NCM and patented the device. At the August 1924 Lyceum in Davenport, Palmer introduced this new invention and extolled beyond reason its clinical capabilities, to the vocal approval of his audience. Then he stunned this same audience by announcing that the NCM was not for sale but would be leased for the then-astronomical fee of $3,500 and $5/month thereafter. The audience immediately split into supporters and dissenters, a schism soon duplicated across the country. This resulted in an immediate loss of support for Palmer and PSC. Facsimile copies of the NCM were soon being manufactured and sold at far more reasonable prices.

Part of Palmer's strategy was to demand that every faculty member support his NCM program or leave the faculty.[22] Much to Palmer's surprise and disappointment, three senior faculty, James Firth, Steve Burich, and Harry Vedder, decided to resign. B.J. Palmer's influence on the profession never again reached its pre-1924 level.

THE PROPRIETARY PERIOD: 1924–1960

Gibbons[7] names this period "Proprietary," a term meaning privately owned but not necessarily for profit. Lincoln, Logan, and Western States were among the early proprietary nonprofit colleges. Gibbons writes:

The Proprietary Period is so designated because the character of school ownership in this 36-year phase was one similar to that which existed in medical education prior to 1910 ... isolated from the mainstream of education and science, the owners and faculties of chiropractic schools resided in a world in which external hostility and internal controversies were commonplace.

The chiropractic profession, only three decades old at this point, lacked the maturity and discipline of older professions and the empathy of society at large. If there was a time in history when chiropractic was most likely to have failed, it was during the first half of this period. Intense rivalry within the political ranks of chiropractic overflowed into education. The impact of the economic depression and World War II added to the uncertainty, although many of the changes wrought by these global events eventually proved beneficial.

The Founding of Lincoln College

Lincoln College opened its doors in August 1926, founded by dissident Palmer faculty members James Firth, Harry Vedder, and Stephen Burich, who left PSC in the wake of major disagreements with B.J. Palmer over the content and quality of education at PSC. These arguments stemmed from the NCM crisis of 1924 and Palmer's dictatorial position on academic freedom. Joined by Arthur

Hendricks, another former Palmer faculty member, the Lincoln founders became known as the "Big Four."[4,12,23]

Vedder was the first president of Lincoln College, followed by Firth in 1940. Burich left the faculty of Lincoln in 1945 due to poor health, but remained as college secretary until his death in 1946. Hendricks became the third president of Lincoln in 1954 upon Firth's retirement and served until his death in 1962. These four chiropractic educators and scholars wrote five major clinical textbooks which were used by students in many colleges for many years.[22]

The Depression and World War II were not kind to Lincoln and the high standards adopted from its inception, which included mandatory admission standards, a 4-year course of study, and emphasis on the life sciences. In 1971 the college merged with National College of Chiropractic where its traditions continue to be upheld.

Lincoln graduates Rudy Mueller, Ronald Watkins, and Ronald Levardsen, had a major impact on the early development of Canadian Memorial Chiropractic College, joining the new institution in 1946–1947. Mueller became dean, Watkins the first clinic director, and Levardsen a teacher in clinical sciences.

Decline in the Number of Colleges

Ferguson and Wiese[17] estimate that there were 82 schools in 1925, which declined to 22 by 1960. Aside from the impact of the Depression and World War II, other events that powerfully influenced the climate of chiropractic education and practice were basic science laws, educational standards, and the passing of many state and provincial practice acts. Although high educational standards were previously instituted by a few individual schools, the broader educational standards movement did not begin until 1935, with the National Chiropractic Association's (NCA) Committee on Education. It took four decades for accreditation to achieve national approval and nearly five decades for world compliance.

Basic Science Laws and Chiropractic Education

Following the great strains of the Depression and war years, the introduction of Basic Science Laws (BSL) into a majority of states caused a deepening crisis. Some chiropractic leaders welcomed this intrusion into education as a means to a positive end, the upgrading and eventual accreditation of chiropractic education. But most chiropractors, including college owners and the profession's political leadership, considered these laws a burdensome intrusion. The first BSLs were passed in Wisconsin and Connecticut in 1925[24] and in 21 other states by 1945. Certainly BSLs were a serious attempt to contain the profession by legislative means. But despite initial concerns BSLs became a driving force for uplifting all facets of chiropractic education.

W.A. Budden, president of Western States College, favored BSLs as a means toward improved education. A strong advocate of high academic standards throughout his academic career, Budden demonstrated his academic commitment by initiating a 32-month, 4-year course of study in 1928. Known as the "cum laude" course, it consisted of 5,620 three-quarter hour periods.[19,25] Gatterman[26] states:

> Dr. Budden was of the opinion that requirements of the basic science exams were not prejudicial to those wanting chiropractic to become one of the learned professions, with educational institutions of equivalent collegiate rating. He felt that those opposing these laws were willing to let the profession degenerate into a trade with their teaching institutions equivalent to trade schools.

Concern for chiropractic basic science education was not confined to chiropractic academics. Among numerous politically minded chiropractors who campaigned for higher educational standards were Claude O. Watkins and John J. Nugent of the NCA. Keating,[26] writes: "Watkins was apparently the first chairman of the NCA Committee on Education and presumably helped to set the direction for John J. Nugent's subsequent efforts as the NCA Director of Education." While Watkins was emphatic about the importance of scientific research data and basing clinical practice upon it, Nugent was a staunch advocate for educational standards and accreditation. It may be that the origins of accreditation for chiropractic education are rooted in the progressive thinking of Budden, Watkins, and Nugent.

Concerns About School Ownership

Proprietary ownership of educational institutions isolates them from mainstream education. For a health discipline, this also entails isolation from science and research opportunities. Chiropractic schools experienced open hostility where there should have been interaction, dogma where there should have been research, and educational confusion where there should have been an accreditation system with established standards.

The shift from profit-making proprietary ownership to public nonprofit status took decades. Although this movement was supported by some college leaders the major thrust came from the political side of the profession, primarily the NCA and its successors. The movement toward accreditation was also significant in moving the process forward.

The literature is not clear as to which colleges first adopted a nonprofit structure. Smallie and Evans[27] state that Logan College of Chiropractic in St. Louis has been nonprofit and tax exempt since 1935. Cleveland College of Chiropractic was nonprofit by 1922. Other colleges that became nonprofit during this period were: Western States Chiropractic College, 1935; National College of Chiropractic, 1941; Northwestern College of Chiropractic, 1941; Canadian Memorial Chiropractic College, 1945; Los Angeles College of Chiropractic, 1947; and Palmer College of Chiropractic, 1961. Blacher[28] writes: "By 1950, 46 of the 51 private school owners had surrendered their equities into 19 colleges under terms negotiated by Nugent. By 1960, the number of chiropractic schools had decreased to 22." The evolution of chiropractic schools from proprietary, for-profit to public, not-for-profit is an important landmark in chiropractic history.

The Great Depression and World War II

Oddly, the debate on chiropractic educational standards began during the Great Depression, a period of severe economic pressure on the schools. This, added to the urgency of the wartime drain on manpower, created a survival mentality among the college leaders. The end of World War II brought renewed optimism to the established colleges and also stimulated the creation of Canadian Memorial Chiropractic College (CMCC) at 1 month after the end of the war. Thousands of war veterans enrolled in universities and colleges, including chiropractic colleges as a spirit of renewal swept North America. As one who was part of this crusade, I think it relevant to note that the early postwar graduates became the political and academic leaders for the next 25 years.

THE PROFESSIONAL PERIOD: 1960–PRESENT

Accreditation

Accreditation of education in most countries is the responsibility of central governments, but in the United States and Canada authority for education rests with the states and provinces. In Canada there are currently no freestanding universities, and accreditation is unofficially granted by government. This does not pose a problem for most postsecondary schools, but it is a problem for CMCC and similar freestanding institutions. If chiropractic graduates plan on returning or emigrating to the United States to practice, it is incumbent upon CMCC and the new School of Chiropractic, University of Quebec, Three Rivers, to be accredited according to American standards. All Canadian provinces require chiropractic practitioners to have graduated from a CCE accredited college, as do most American states. Accreditation is a voluntary nongovernmental evaluation that has evolved to advance regional and national educational goals. Status is granted to educational institutions with a mandate to meet or exceed minimum criteria of educational quality. It is an important pledge as to the quality of education offered by an institution, and is used as a benchmark by government, funding agencies, licensing boards, scholarship commissions, foundations and potential students. Accreditation, although private and voluntary, has become a quasipublic entity with important responsibilities and duties to the public interest.[29]

The Beginnings of Accreditation

The chiropractic accreditation story begins in 1930 with the formation of the NCA, from the membership of the Universal Chiropractic Association and the first American Chiropractic Association.[24] The NCA was dominated by broad scope chiropractic practitioners with concern for higher standards of college education, matriculation requirements, faculty qualifications, and the need for voluntary efforts to improve chiropractic education.

The NCA formed the Committee on Educational Standards (CES) in 1935. Claude O. Watkins of Montana was the first chairman, followed in 1938 by Gordon M. Goodfellow of Los Angeles. During this time, the Council on State Chiropractic Examining Boards (CESCB) was formed to improve chiropractic education for licensure. The two committees merged in 1938 to form a new Committee on Educational Standards (CES)[29,30] renamed in 1947 the Council on Chiropractic Accreditation. During 1939–1940, the new committee undertook an analysis of the curricula of the 37 colleges then in existence. This difficult assignment was a first for chiropractic education. The first CES report, delivered at the 1940 NCA convention,[31] was far from flattering. It listed 10 points (Table 2-3). In 1942 the CES granted provisional accreditation to 12 of 37 colleges.

Table 2-3. 1940 National Chiropractic Education Report

A report submitted to the NCA House of Delegates at its annual convention in 1940 included the following observations:

1. All chiropractic colleges were proprietary institutions.
2. Chiropractic colleges differed in their teachings.
3. A broad spectrum of program length was apparent; they ranged from 18 months to 36 months, with some schools seeking to support curricula of two course lengths.
4. Some schools possessed two charters, one in chiropractic and another in drugless therapy, naturopathy or mechanotherapy.
5. A marked variation of course depth was apparent, especially in the basic science and diagnostic subjects.
6. Individualized concepts were being administered, in an on-campus setting.
7. A general need of laboratory and classroom facilities was evident.
8. Heterogeneity in curriculum composition was evident.
9. The need for coordination among the colleges was noted.
10. Greater emphasis had to be placed on standardization in entrance requirements, faculty selection, and student academic progress.

John J. Nugent

The CES was a part-time responsibility of NCA members and functioned without staff. In 1941, NCA formed a Department of Education (DOE) and hired John J. Nugent to be the first Director of Education, a position he held for 20 years. At the same time the CES organized the colleges into the Council of Educational Institutions (CEI).[28] Based on his work organizing CES and CEI, John J. Nugent may appropriately be considered the father of today's Councils on Chiropractic Education in the United States, Canada, Australia, and Europe. He has been compared to Abraham Flexner, the medical education reformer, whose classic analysis of medicine changed the face of medical education.[10]

Nugent's odyssey began in 1935 with his concern and criticism for the quality of chiropractic education. As Gibbons writes,[32] "The proprietary school abolition issue was clearly the most controversial and the most difficult which Nugent had to face." Other challenging issues included entrance requirements, the 4-year course of study, a standard curriculum and an authoritative accreditation process. In the eye of this storm, Nugent quickly became the chiropractor most hated by the fundamentalist following of B.J. Palmer, who once referred to him as "the Antichrist of chiropractic."[4]

Nugent oversaw development of the first guidelines and recommendations for colleges to use in seeking accredited status. Nugent's original manual continues to evolve as the current Educational Standards for Chiropractic Colleges. He also gave guidance to state boards on using standardized evaluation procedures for licensure. He shepherded the conversion of many colleges to non-proprietary status. He used the power of his office to apply constant pressure on colleges to expand matriculation and graduation standards and academic qualifications for faculty. Nugent retired in August 1961 and has been followed by five successors at the Council on Chiropractic Education. Significantly, all have been professional educators with no chiropractic affiliation.

Council on Chiropractic Education

The Committee on Educational Standards made the progression from a committee of the American Chiropractic Association (ACA), successor to the NCA, to an autonomous national accrediting agency in 1971.[31] I represented the CMCC at CCE meetings starting in January 1970. At this time, the revision of bylaws, preparation of articles of incorporation, and revision of educational standards dominated the Council's activities. In 1971, CCE was incorporated in the state of Wisconsin as an autonomous chiropractic accrediting agency.

The CCE filed an application with the United States Office of Education (USOE, later USDE) in August 1972 and was granted an initial listing as a National Recognized Accrediting Agency. It took 3 more years for CCE to earn full USDE recognition for a 3-year period. Since then CCE has retained its status as a member of the Council of Specialized Accrediting Agencies and recognition by the independent Council on Postsecondary Accreditation (COPA). These accomplishments were earned by the chiropractic profession without any public sector financial subsidies or grants (Table 2-4).

Reciprocity with Foreign Countries

The CCE (USA) has reciprocal agreements with foreign organizations for the accreditation of foreign colleges.[30] The essential criteria for such agreements include; equivalent educational standards to CCE (USA) with consideration of the peculiarities of foreign systems; procedures, policies and rules equivalent to CCE (USA); and that all prescribed costs for reciprocity are sustained by the foreign agency.

Canada was the first foreign country to form and charter its own Council on Chiropractic Education in 1978 with a broad base of professional financial support. A reciprocal agreement was initiated and ratified in June 1982. CMCC was granted full accredited status in October 1982. Similar reciprocal agreements have since been ratified with Australasia and Europe. Reciprocity functions equally among all members of the CCE international family. However, CCE (USA) with most colleges and the

---

Table 2-4. Chiropractic Colleges and Accredited Status

Chiropractic Colleges Holding Accredited Status With the Council on Chiropractic Education (CCE-USA)
  Cleveland Chiropractic College, Kansas City, MO
  Cleveland Chiropractic College, Los Angeles, CA
  Life Chiropractic College, Marietta, GA
  Life Chiropractic College West, San Lorenzo, CA
  Logan College of Chiropractic, Chesterfield, MO
  Los Angeles College of Chiropractic, Whittier, CA
  National College of Chiropractic, Lombard, IL
  New York Chiropractic College, Seneca Falls, NY
  Northwestern College of Chiropractic, Bloomington, MN
  Palmer College of Chiropractic, Davenport, IA
  Palmer College of Chiropractic West, San Jose, CA
  Parker College of Chiropractic, Dallas, TX
  Sherman College of Straight Chiropractic, Spartanburg, SC
  Texas Chiropractic College, Pasadena, TX
  University of Bridgeport, College of Chiropractic, Bridgeport, CT
  Western States Chiropractic College, Portland, OR
Non-U.S. Colleges Holding Accredited Status
  Anglo-European College of Chiropractic, Bournemouth, England
  Canadian Memorial Chiropractic College, Toronto, ON, Canada
  Macquarie University, Centre for Chiropractic, Summerhill, NSW, Australia
  Royal Melbourne Institute of Technology, Chiropractic Unit, Bundoora, Victoria, Australia
Non-U.S. Colleges Seeking Accredited Status
  University of Quebec, School of Chiropractic, Three Rivers, PQ, Canada

need to harmonize national and state educational needs with ongoing changes in United States professional health educational standards, initiates most changes to the standards.

Benefits of Accreditation to the Chiropractic Profession

Accreditation has helped to raise chiropractic educational standards, faculty qualifications, scientific research, scholarship, and matriculation and graduation requirements. In turn, accreditation has forced state and provincial practice acts to reflect societal changes to health care delivery and health care education. As new chiropractic colleges open worldwide, there will be a corresponding expansion of the standards and policies of currently ratified CCEs and adoption of these revised standards by new foreign accrediting agencies as they are formed.

Parallel to the advances in college accreditation has been the development of chiropractic scientific, educational, and historical journals, which are indexed in the world's scientific literature and available for others to monitor the research and scholarship of the profession.

Current Status of the Council on Chiropractic Education

The CCE is now in its 21st year as an accrediting agency under the United States Department of Education and the Council on Postsecondary Accreditation. It is recognized by all states and the District of Columbia and by inference all jurisdictions in Canada, Australasia, and Europe. This is a remarkable achievement for a "bootstrap" profession that has endured decades of organized opposition. At present there are 16 United States colleges with more than 13,000 students being served by CCE. For the first time in history, all United States colleges have common educational standards regardless of differences in philosophy. If the students in colleges accredited by foreign CCEs are included, the world's chiropractic student population is about 15,000. The profession's future looks promising.[33]

AFFILIATION AND IMMERSION OF CHIROPRACTIC EDUCATION IN UNIVERSITIES

Though the United States is predominate in the number of colleges and students, other nations have led the way in university affiliation for chiropractic education. University affiliation provides great advantages for the standards of education, faculty, research, graduate study, academic recognition, interaction with other disciplines, and finances. The first North American chiropractic school within a university environment opened its doors in 1991 at the University of Bridgeport in Bridgeport, Connecticut, a private nonprofit institution. Bridgeport's chiropractic program was granted CCE accredited status in 1995.

The University of Quebec at Three Rivers is the only university-based chiropractic school in Canada. It opened with 45 students in 1993 as the first chiropractic doctorate program in North America in a public university. The number of first-year students was raised to 60 in 1994. The school has submitted documentation to the CCE (CAN) indicating its intention to seek accreditation and recently provided eligibility documentation for that purpose. The new chiropractic building that houses the school of chiropractic's academic facilities and outpatient clinic opened in September 1995 (personal letter from Dr. A.M. Gonthier, Head, Chiropractic Section). At present CMCC in Toronto is negotiating with York University for formal affiliation within five years. Seeking affiliation with an Ontario University has been CMCC policy since 1965.

Australia has two university-based schools of chiropractic. The oldest is the School of Chiropractic and Osteopathy, Royal Melbourne Institute of Technology University in Melbourne. The second is The Centre for Chiropractic, Macquarie University, Sydney. In the United Kingdom, the Anglo-European Chiropractic College, Bournemouth has degree-granting privileges, and is affiliated with the University of Southampton for anatomy and dissection instruction.

An interesting educational development is taking place at the University of Odense in Denmark for Scandinavian students wanting to study chiropractic. In 1994 a 5-year course of study in chiropractic and clinical biomechanics began at the University of Odense with an initial enrollment of 25, which increased to 50 in 1996. Matriculation standards are the same as for medicine. Graduates will receive a masters degree in clinical biomechanics followed by a 1-year internship program for licensure as a chiropractor. This parallels a masters degree in medicine.

In keeping with continental European tradition, the course will be validated/accredited by the Danish Ministry of Health, and therefore the graduates will, under European government treaties, qualify for licensure in any Scandinavian or European Union countries that have registration/licensure of chiropractors. The first graduation will be 1999.

Today chiropractic is practiced in over 65 countries with licensing legislation in all U.S. and Australian states, all Canadian provinces, plus most European countries and the United Kingdom. All jurisdictions share minimum qualifications for entry to practice including at least 2 years of pre-professional education and graduation from an accredited college. Some countries, notably the United States and Canada, require national and/or state and provincial licensing board examinations to be licensed for practice.[34]

THIS IS NOT THE END ...

Chiropractic education and research is no longer marginal. The public has decided that there is a major role for complementary health care in contemporary society. Hopefully the profession will define that role with minimal rancor. In the words of Sir Winston Churchill, "This is not the end, nor is it the beginning of the end, but it is the end of the beginning."

Terminology

accreditation
basic science laws
Council on Chiropractic Education (CCE)
innate intelligence
neurocalometer

Review Questions

1. D.D. Palmer's original scientific basis for chiropractic was founded on osteology, neurology, and function (physiology). Was this a reasonable hypothesis for Palmer to promote, in view of the level of scientific research and knowledge circa 1900?

2. Since a scientific basis for chiropractic was his first choice, why did Palmer adopt a metaphysical explanation as well?

3. How did the adoption of theosophical metaphors influence the unity and acceptance of chiropractic?

4. Between 1903–1906, Solon Langworthy was responsible for developing the first standards for chiropractic education and the scientific concepts that set the profession's agenda for decades to come, but he is largely unknown today. What explains this neglect?

5. Who is believed to have been the first licensed chiropractor?

6. Three colleges were founded by dissident Palmer graduates or faculty members. Which one still survives?

7. Why was the 1924 neurocalometer debacle a major watershed in chiropractic history?

8. Basic science laws were an attempt to contain the expansion of chiropractic practice and education, but they also had positive effects on the profession. Discuss.

9. Describe the origins of chiropractic accreditation.

10. Review the current status of chiropractic accreditation and the impact this United States phenomenon has had on world chiropractic education and research.

Concept Questions

1. What challenges are faced by an educational institution when its founder retires or dies?

2. How did decades of isolation from mainstream education affect the development of chiropractic schools? How did it affect the profession as a whole?

References

1. Palmer DD: The Science Art and Philosophy of Chiropractic. Portland Publishing House, Portland, OR, 1910

2. Keating JC: The embryology of chiropractic thought. Eur J Chiropractic 39:75, 1991

3. Donahue J: Palmer and innate intelligence: development, division, and derision. Chiropractic Hist 6:31, 1986

4. Wardwell WI: Chiropractic History and Evolution of a New Profession. CV Mosby, St. Louis, 1992

5. Keating JC: Toward a Philosophy for the Science of Chiropractic. Stockton Foundation, Stockton, CA, 1992

6. Peterson D, Weise G: Chiropractic: An Illustrated History. CV Mosby, St Louis, 1995

7. Gibbons RW: Rise of the chiropractic establishment, p. 339. In Dzaman F (ed): Who's Who in Chiropractic. 2nd Ed. Who's Who International Publishing, Littleton, CO, 1980

8. Hall RM: Food for Thought. Harper & Row, Hagerstown, MD, 1974

9. Haldeman S, Hammerich K: The evolution of neurology and the concept of chiropractic. p. 44. In Vear HJ (ed): Introduction to Chiropractic Science, Western States Chiropractic College, Portland, OR, 1981

10. Flexner A: Medical Education in the United States and Canada. Carnegie Foundation for the Advancement of Teaching, New York, 1910

11. Weisse G: New questions: why did D.D. not use "chiropractic" in his 1896 charter? Chiropractic Hist 6:63, 1986

12. Rehm WS: Who Was Who in Chiropractic: A Necrology. p. 271. In Dzaman F (ed): Who's Who in Chiropractic. Who's Who International, Littleton, CO, 1980

13. Gibbons RW: Solon Massey Langworthy: keeper of the flame during the lost years of chiropractic. Chiropractic History 11(1):23, 1981

14. Lerner C: Report on the History of Chiropractic. Unpublished manuscript. Palmer College Library, Vol V. Davenport, IA, 1954

15. Langworthy SM, Smith OG, Paxson MC: Textbook of Modernized Chiropractic. American School of Chiropractic. Cedar Rapids, IA, 1906

16. Rehm WS: Legally defensible: chiropractic in the courtroom and after, 1907. Chiropractic Hist 6:51, 1986

17. Ferguson A, Wiese G: How many chiropractic schools? Chiropractic Hist 8:27, 1988

18. Gibbons RW: Chiropractic history turbulence and triumph. p 139. In Dzaman F (ed): Who's Who in Chiropractic. 1st Ed. Who's Who International Publishing, Littleton, CO, 1977

19. Beidman RP: Seeking the rational alternative: the National College of Chiropractic from 1906 to 1982. Chiropractic Hist 6:31, 1986

20. Gibbons RW: Joy Loban and Andrew P. Davis: itinerant healers and schoolmen, 1910–1923. Chiropractic Hist 11:23, 1991

21. Illi FW: The Vertebral Column, Life Line of the Body. National College of Chiropractic, Chicago, 1951

22. Quigley WH: Early days at Palmer lyceums. Part III. DC 7(2):16. Palmer College Library, 1989

23. Stowell CC: Lincoln college and the big four: a chiropractic protest 1926–1962. Chiropractic Hist 3:75, 1983

24. Evans HW: Historical Chiropractic Data. Worldwide Report, Stockton, CA, 1979

25. Gatterman M: Budden: the transition through proprietary education, 1924–1954. Chiropractic Hist 1:21, 1982

26. Keating JC: Claude O. Watkins: pioneer advocate for clinical scientific chiropractic. Chiropractic Hist 2:11, 1987

27. Smallie P, Evans H: Chiropractic Encyclopedia. World Wide Report, Sacramento, CA, 1979

28. Blacher P: The evolution of higher education in chiropractic; a survey 1906–74. Chiropractic Hist 1:37, 1992

29. Council on Chiropractic Education: 1985 Annual Report. Council on Chiropractic Education, Des Moines, IA, 1985

30. Napolitano EG: The struggle for accreditation: a unique history of educational bootstrapping. Chiropractic Hist 1:23, 1981

31. Committee on Educational Standards. Report to the National Chiropractic Convention 1940 on Educational Standards. Annual Report of the Council on Chiropractic Education, Des Moines, IA, 1985

32. Gibbons RW: Chiropractic's Abraham Flexner: the lonely journey of John J. Nugent, 1935–1963. Chiropractic Hist 5:45, 1985

33. Cleveland CS: Reflections on the Council of Chiropractic Education. Dynam Chiropractic 14(7):7, 1996

34. Chapman-Smith D: Chiropractic education and licensure. Chiropractic Rep 8(4):2, 1994

3

Vertebral Subluxation

Carl S. Cleveland III

Vertebral subluxation is at the core of chiropractic theory, and its detection and correction are at the heart of chiropractic practice. In the first century of chiropractic, the description of subluxation has evolved from a simplistic static concept, interpreted as a malpositioned spinal segment (bone out of place), to a dynamic contemporary model presented as a complex biomechanical entity of multiple components. These components include abnormal joint motion or position; muscular and connective tissue changes; and vascular, inflammatory, and biochemical changes. In addition and most significantly, associated neurologic manifestations may result in symptoms either locally or at segmentally innervated anatomic levels far distant from the point of vertebral dysfunction. The neurologic component of the vertebral subluxation complex (VSC) provides chiropractors with the potential to move beyond symptomatic treatment of low back pain and other musculoskeletal ailments and to contribute to patient health, wellness, and enhanced quality of life.

The term *subluxation* comes from the Latin *sub*, meaning "under" or "less than" and *luxation*, which means "dislocation." Steadman's defines the term as 'an incomplete luxation or dislocation; though a relationship is altered, contact between joint surfaces remains.'[1]

Application of this term is fundamental to communication between chiropractors and their patients. For explaining the subluxation to laypersons, a good working definition is "loss of proper motion or position of a vertebral joint which may affect proper nerve function."[2] By contrast, the term may be described technically as the vertebral subluxation complex and presented as a theoretical model of vertebral motion segment dysfunction that incorporates the complex interactions of pathologic changes in nerve, muscle, ligamentous, vascular, and connective tissue.[3] This latter model serves as a basis for communication of chiropractic concepts to the scientific community.

Subluxation has been referred to extensively by classic and contemporary medical practitioners, osteopaths, and chiropractors.[4] These professions differ on definition of the term and interpretation of its clinical significance. In the scientific literature, the term *subluxation* has been applied to gross dislocations with separation of joint surfaces as well as minor misalignment of articulations.[4] In an extensive literature review, Rome[5] has identified more than 296 synonyms (41 used to describe sacroiliac subluxation) and terms for the biomechanic condition known to chiropractors as "subluxation." This lack of uniform terminology has impeded interprofessional discussion.

SUBLUXATION: EARLY HISTORY

The earliest concepts of subluxation predate chiropractic by more than 200 years. Haldeman cites the earliest English definition of subluxation from Randle Holme in 1688,[6] who described it as, "dislocation or putting out of joynt." Haldeman[4] and others[7–9] cite the following 1746 description from Joannes Herricus Hieronymus,[10] who wrote, "subluxation of joints is recognized by lessened motion of the joints, by slight change in position of the articulating bones and pain."

Terrett[11] cites an 1821 description by Edward Harrison: "When any of the vertebrae become displaced or too prominent, the patient experiences inconvenience from a local derangement in the nerves or the part. He, in consequence is tormented with a train of nervous symptoms, which are obscure in their origin as they are stubborn in their nature." Harrison pursed the subject further, writing in 1824 that motion as well as alignment played a defining role in subluxation: "The articulating extremities are only partially separated, not imperfectly disjoined … and … the articular motions are imperfectly performed, because the surfaces of the bones do not fully correspond."

Thomas Brown, writing in the *Glasgow Medical Journal* in 1828, coined the term "spinal irritation."[12] Four years later, *The American Journal of Medical Sciences* began citing reports from European physicians about tenderness of vertebrae corresponding to diseased organs, with such observations taken as confirming a diagnosis of spinal irritation.[12]

Donald Tower[13] quotes physician J.E. Riadore's 1843 *Irritation of the Spinal Nerves*, as follows: "if any organ is deficiently supplied with nervous energy or of blood, its functions immediately, and sooner or later its structure, becomes deranged." Riadore concluded that irritation of nerve roots resulted in disease and advocated treatment by manipulation. These conclusions regarding nerve irritation were published two years prior to the birth of D.D. Palmer.[8]

By 1874, Andrew Taylor Still, a medical physician who founded osteopathy 21 years before Palmer's discovery of chiropractic, developed his own concept and terminology. Still described the "osteopathic lesion" in terms of pressure applied by muscles to blood vessels coursing through and around those muscles, thereby shutting off the life force of the involved tissue.[14]

CHIROPRACTIC SUBLUXATION — EARLY CONCEPTS

In the December 1904 Palmer School of Chiropractic periodical, *The Chiropractor*, presented as "A monthly journal devoted to the interests of chiropractic — 'KI-RO-PRAK-TIK,'"[15] D.D. Palmer states, "Ninety-five percent of all deranged nerves are made by sub-luxations of vertebrae which pinch nerves to some one of the 51 joint articulations of the spinal column. Therefore to relieve the pressure upon these nerves means to restore normal action —hence, normal functions, perfect health." This likely represents the earliest published mention of subluxation in the chiropractic literature. Significantly, the senior Palmer saw at least limited value (5 percent) in the adjustment of non-spinal articulations, stating that nerves related to non-vertebral joints may be "impinged" as opposed to pinched.

According to Gibbons,[16] *Modernized Chiropractic*,[17] by Langworthy, Smith, and Paxson, published in 1906 was the first chiropractic textbook to use the term *subluxation* and to relate it to the intervertebral foramen. It was also the first to assert the supremacy of the nerves in relation to health and disease, in contrast to the osteopathic concept of supremacy of the blood. In chiropractic's early years, this citation often served as legal defense in arguing the distinction between the practice of chiropractic and that of osteopathy and medicine. In addition, chiropractic's focus on the importance of the nervous system and its emphasis on the correction of vertebral subluxation became key factors in the defense of chiropractors and in early attempts by the profession to gain separate licensure.

Langworthy and colleagues also were the first to characterize subluxation as a *fixation* and to describe the *field of motion* of a vertebra. This view of subluxation as a dysfunctional state of vertebral motion gradually fell into disuse until 1938, when the dynamic concept of subluxation was reintroduced with the motion palpation research of the Belgian chiropractors Gillet and Lichens.[18]

The Founder's Definition

In 1910, D.D. Palmer discussed subluxation in his text, *Science, Art and Philosophy of Chiropractic*,[19] as follows:

A vertebra is said to be displaced or a luxation when the joint surfaces are entirely separated. Subluxation is a partial or incomplete separation; one in which the articulation surfaces remain in partial contact. This later condition is so often referred to and known by chiropractors as sub-luxation. The relationship existing between bones and nerves are so nicely adjusted that any one of the 200 bones, more especially those of the vertebral column, cannot be displaced ever so little without impinging upon adjacent nerves. Pressure on nerves excites, agitates, creates an excess of molecular vibration, whose effects, when local are known as inflammation, when general, as fever. A subluxation does not restrain or liberate vital energy. Vital energy is expressed in functional activity. A subluxation may impinge against nerves, the transmitting channel may increase or decrease the momentum of impulses, not energy.

The Younger Palmer's Definition

By the early 1930s, B.J. Palmer had developed a concept of subluxation distinct from that of his father. The younger Palmer represented subluxation as a displaced upper cervical vertebra that created nerve impingement, resulting in interference with the transmission of vital nerve energy.[20] In his 1934 textbook, *The Subluxation Specific—The Adjustment Specific*, B.J. maintained that the only subluxation of significance was that of the atlas vertebra in relation to occiput or axis: "I reaffirm that no amount of 'adjusting' upon any, many or all vertebrae below occiput, atlas, or axis, could or would directly ADJUST THE SPECIFIC three-direction torqued subluxation causing any, many or all sickness in a body. Any vertebra below atlas or axis MAY BE misaligned but CANNOT BE SUBLUXATED"[20] (emphasis in original text).

B.J. Palmer's delineation between simple misalignment and true subluxation is significant. Misalignment of a vertebra was described as no more than a compensation to the major subluxation. Thus, in a span of 30 years, the Palmer School con-

cept of subluxation and adjustment evolved from the founder's 1904 description of an entity affecting any of the joints of the body, but primarily the spinal column, to the younger Palmer's insistence on exclusive adjustment of the full spinal column only, and later to his idea that subluxation was an entity limited only to the atlas vertebra in relation to the occiput and axis. This later concept, known as the "Hole in One Technique (HIO)," was developed in the early 1930s. For two decades Palmer College taught no adjusting methods except upper cervical specific technique. Not until 1956 did the school reintroduce instruction in adjusting techniques for the full spine (Himes HM, "Policy Talk," unpublished letter, January 4, 1956).

Stephenson's Definition

According to Lantz,[21] the definition of subluxation most widely quoted by early chiropractors was from R.W. Stephenson's 1927 *Chiropractic Text Book*, which states: "A subluxation is a condition of a vertebra that has lost its proper juxtaposition with the one above or the one below, or both; to an extent less that a luxation; which impinges nerves and interferes with the transmission of mental impulses."[22] Stephenson, a 1921 Palmer School graduate, insisted that nerve interference must exist to qualify the condition as a subluxation.

CONTEMPORARY DEFINITIONS

Contemporary definitions describe the subluxation as central to the principles of chiropractic science. Examples of policy statements regarding subluxation are as follows.

American Chiropractic Association

The Indexed Synopsis of American Chiropractic Association (ACA) Policies[23] describes subluxation as, "A motion segment, in which alignment, movement integrity, and/or physiological function are altered although contact between joint surfaces remain intact."

The ACA has also adopted the consensus definitions agreed on by the nominal and Delphi panels of the Consortium for Chiropractic Research (CCR)[23,24]:

Subluxation is an aberrant relationship between two adjacent articular structures that may have functional or pathological sequelae, causing an alteration in the biomechanical and/or neurophysiological reflections of these articular structures, the proximal structures, and/or body systems that may be directly or indirectly affected by them.

The ACA-endorsed CCR definition for *subluxation complex* is, "A theoretical model of motion segment dysfunction (subluxation) which incorporates the complex interaction of pathological changes in nerve, muscle, ligamentous, vascular and connective tissues."[23]

International Chiropractors Association

The International Chiropractors Association (ICA) Policy Statements[25] related to subluxation include the following:

Of primary concern to chiropractic are abnormalities of structure or function of the vertebral column known clinically as the vertebral subluxation complex. The subluxation complex includes any alteration of the biomechanical and physiological dynamics of contiguous spinal structures which can cause neuronal disturbances. ... Directly or indirectly, all bodily function is controlled by the nervous system, consequently a central theme of chiropractic theories on health is the premise that abnormal bodily function may be caused by interference with nerve transmission and expression due to pressure, strain or tension upon the spinal cord, spinal nerves, or peripheral nerves as a result of displacement of spinal segments or other skeletal structures (subluxation).

The vertebral subluxation syndrome and/or complex and its component parts is any alteration of the biomechanical and physiological dynamics of the contiguous structures which can cause neuronal disturbances.[26]

The science of chiropractic deals with the relationship between the articulations of the skeleton and the nervous system and the role of this relationship in the restoration and maintenance of health. Of primary concern to chiropractic are abnormalities of structure or function of the vertebral column known clinically as the vertebral subluxation complex. The subluxation complex includes any alteration of the biomechanical and physiological dynamics of contiguous spinal structures which can cause neuronal disturbances.

According to the ICA Official Policy Handbook[25]:

Chiropractic is based on the premises that the relationship between structure and function in the human body is a significant health factor and that such relationships between the spinal column and nervous system are the most significant, since the normal transmission and expression of nerve energy is essential to the restoration and maintenance of health.

State Statutes

The concept of subluxation is specifically in many U.S. state statutes defining the practice of chiropractic. After extensive review, Hendrickson[27] concluded that most state chiropractic statutes either directly or implicitly identify chiropractic with subluxation or the elements of subluxation complex, and specify the doctor of chiropractic's responsibility for adjustment of the spine and adjacent tissues for the purpose of eliminating nerve interference. Eleven states specifically identify "subluxation" in their chiropractic practice statutes: Alaska, Arizona, Florida, Kentucky, Maine, Massachusetts, Michigan, New York, Texas, Washington, and Wisconsin.

Medicare Definition

The U.S. federal government recognizes the detection and correction of subluxation as the primary function of the doctor of chiropractic. The Medicare Act,[28] in defining *physician*, states:

The term "physician," when used in connection with the performance of any function or action, means ... (4) a chiropractor who is licensed as such by the State ... and who meets uniform minimum standards ... only with respect to treatment by means of manual manipulation of the spine (to correct a subluxation demonstrated by X-ray to exist) which he is legally authorized to perform by the State of jurisdiction in which such treatment is provided.

World Health Organization Classification

The World Health Organization (WHO), a multilateral health care agency of the United Nations, has accepted subluxation as a listing in the International Classification of Diseases[29] referring to it as "M99.1 Subluxation complex (vertebral)." WHO also recognizes the classification "M99.0 Segmental and somatic dysfunction," a subtle variation.

Consortium for Chiropractic Research

The 1993 consensus definition of the nominal and Delphi panels of the CCR[24] refers to subluxation as follows:

A motion segment in which alignment, movement integrity, and/or physiologic function are altered although contact between the joint surfaces remains intact.

VERTEBRAL SUBLUXATION COMPLEX

As noted in the ACA and ICA definitions cited above, the contemporary concept of subluxation has been expanded beyond a joint phenomenon affecting nerve function to also include the role of muscular, connective, vascular, and biochemic components as part of a complex. This subluxation complex has been defined by Gatterman[7] as "a theoretical model of motion segment dysfunction (subluxation) that incorporates the complex interaction of pathologic change in nerve, muscle, ligamentous, vascular and connective tissues."

Although Janse and colleagues,[30,31] Illi,[32] Gillet and Lichens,[18] and Holmwood[33] provided an early foundation, it was Faye,[34] who beginning in 1967 popularized the concept of the subluxation complex and organized a five-component model. Dishman[35] characterized the concept as "the chiropractic subluxation complex," providing additional rationale for Faye's model. Lantz[9,21] modified the original five components of the VSC model by postulating three more components: connective tissue pathology, vascular abnormalities, and the inflammatory response.

Faye Model of Vertebral Subluxation Complex

Building on the work of Gillet and Liekens[18] as well as earlier pioneers Smith, Langworthy, and Paxson,[17] Faye[34] moved beyond the static "bone out of place" or "displaced vertebra" theory of subluxation, placing primary emphasis on dynamic vertebral joint motion. Basic movements of spinal segments include rotation about the longitudinal axis, right or left lateral flexion, anterior flexion, posterior extension, and long-axis distention. Factors inhibiting movement in one or more of these directions may cause abnormal translation and rotation, contributing to biomechanic and subsequent physiologic dysfunction and pathologic expressions.

Schafer and Faye[34] defined the term *fixation* as referring to any physical, functional, or psychic mechanism that produces a loss of segmental mobility within its normal physiologic range of motion. As an example, ankylosis of a joint would be considered a 100 percent fixation. These authors state that clinically most fixations are in the 20 to 80 percent range of normal mobility. According to Schafer and Faye, once the chiropractor has identified the hypomobility, adjustive procedures are used to mobilize the fixation. The therapeutic objective is to deliver a dynamic thrust employing a specific contact and line of drive with the intention of freeing restricted vertebral joint motion altering specific symptomatology.

The Faye model[34] of the vertebral subluxation complex presents subluxation as a complex clinical entity comprising one or more of the following components: neuropathophysiology, kinesiopathology, myopathology, histopathology, and a biochemical component. A central element of this concept is that subluxation results in pathophysiology, which can then lead to frank pathologic changes. Moreover, correction of a subluxation is considered to lead to the restoration of normal physiologic processes, thus allowing the reversal of reversible pathologic changes (Fig. 3-1).

Components of the Faye Model

Neuropathophysiologic Component

Biomechanical insult to nerve tissue may be manifested in three forms, individually or in combination, to include:

1. Irritation to nerve receptors or nerve tissue resulting in facilitation of nerve cells located in: (a)the anterior horn manifesting as hypertonicity or spasm of muscles; (b) lateral horn cell irrita-

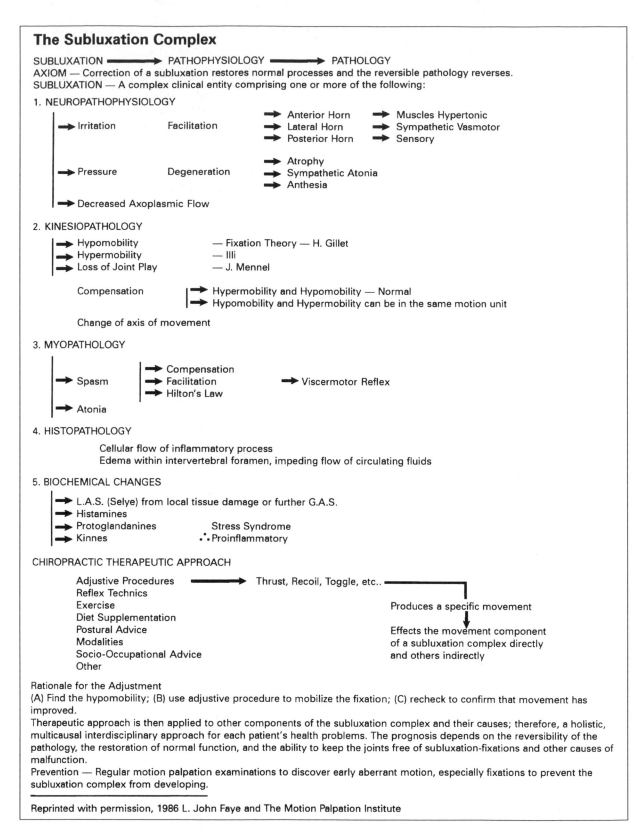

The Subluxation Complex

SUBLUXATION ⟶ PATHOPHYSIOLOGY ⟶ PATHOLOGY

AXIOM — Correction of a subluxation restores normal processes and the reversible pathology reverses.

SUBLUXATION — A complex clinical entity comprising one or more of the following:

1. NEUROPATHOPHYSIOLOGY

Irritation   Facilitation
- Anterior Horn → Muscles Hypertonic
- Lateral Horn → Sympathetic Vasmotor
- Posterior Horn → Sensory

Pressure   Degeneration
- Atrophy
- Sympathetic Atonia
- Anthesia

Decreased Axoplasmic Flow

2. KINESIOPATHOLOGY

- Hypomobility — Fixation Theory — H. Gillet
- Hypermobility — Illi
- Loss of Joint Play — J. Mennel

Compensation
- Hypermobility and Hypomobility — Normal
- Hypomobility and Hypermobility can be in the same motion unit

Change of axis of movement

3. MYOPATHOLOGY

Spasm
- Compensation
- Facilitation → Viscermotor Reflex
- Hilton's Law

Atonia

4. HISTOPATHOLOGY

Cellular flow of inflammatory process

Edema within intervertebral foramen, impeding flow of circulating fluids

5. BIOCHEMICAL CHANGES

- L.A.S. (Selye) from local tissue damage or further G.A.S.
- Histamines
- Protoglandanines   Stress Syndrome
- Kinnes   ∴ Proinflammatory

CHIROPRACTIC THERAPEUTIC APPROACH

Adjustive Procedures ⟶ Thrust, Recoil, Toggle, etc..
Reflex Technics
Exercise
Diet Supplementation
Postural Advice
Modalities
Socio-Occupational Advice
Other

Produces a specific movement

Effects the movement component of a subluxation complex directly and others indirectly

Rationale for the Adjustment

(A) Find the hypomobility; (B) use adjustive procedure to mobilize the fixation; (C) recheck to confirm that movement has improved.

Therapeutic approach is then applied to other components of the subluxation complex and their causes; therefore, a holistic, multicausal interdisciplinary approach for each patient's health problems. The prognosis depends on the reversibility of the pathology, the restoration of normal function, and the ability to keep the joints free of subluxation-fixations and other causes of malfunction.

Prevention — Regular motion palpation examinations to discover early aberrant motion, especially fixations to prevent the subluxation complex from developing.

Reprinted with permission, 1986 L. John Faye and The Motion Palpation Institute

Figure 3-1. Faye model of subluxation complex. (From Schafer and Faye,[34] with permission.)

tion manifesting as vasomotor changes to include hypersympathicotonic vasoconstriction; and
(c) irritation to the posterior horn manifesting as sensory changes.

2. Compression (pressure) to neural elements resulting in degeneration manifesting as muscular atrophy, anesthesia, and sympathetic atonia to include hyposympathicotonic vasodilation and vascular stasis.

3. Decreased axoplasmic transport affecting delivery of macromolecules via the axon to end organs innervated by the nerve. Impediments to this microcellular transport mechanism may alter the development, growth, and maintenance of cells or structures dependent on this trophic (growth) influence via the nerve.

Kinesiopathologic Component

The kinesiopathologic component is described as hypomobility, diminished or absent joint play, or compensatory segmental kinematic hypermobility. Lack of appropriate joint motion is proposed to be associated with a variety of mechanoreceptive reflex functions that include proprioception and nociception. In addition, an early manifestation of a chronically fixated vertebral articulation is shortening of ligaments as an adaptation to limited range of motion.

Myopathologic Component

The myopathologic component may include spasm or hypertonicity of muscles as a result of compensation, facilitation, and/or Hilton's Law. [John Hilton, a 19th century English surgeon, stated that the nerve supplying a joint also supplies the muscles which move the joint and the skin covering the articular insertion of those muscles.[1]]

Histopathologic Component

The histopathologic component relates to inflammation including pain, heat, and swelling. It can result from trauma, hypermobile irritation, or occur as part of the repair process. It includes osseous tissue changes in the joint which may be expressed according to the clinical principles of Weigert's law and Wolff's law. Carl Weigert, a nineteenth century German pathologist, stated that loss or destruction of a part or element is likely to result in compensatory replacement and overproduction of tissue

during the process of regeneration and/or repair, as in the formation of callus when a fractured bone heals. Weigert's law is also known as the over production theory.[1] Julius Wolff, a German anatomist of the same era, stated that every change in the form and the function of a bone, or in its function alone, is followed by certain definite changes in its internal architecture and secondary alterations in its external conformation.[1]

Biochemical Component

Hormonal and chemical effects or imbalance related to the preinflammatory stress syndrome, and the production of histamine, prostaglandin, and bradykinin as a result of trauma or fixation of the spinal articulation are proposed to affect nociceptive impulses resulting in aberrant (differing from the normal) somatic afferent input into the segmental spinal cord.[36]

Primary Therapeutic Approach

The primary therapeutic approach related to the Faye model of VSC is a specific dynamic adjustive thrust (e.g., toggle recoil, impulse) to either directly or indirectly release sites of fixation. In addition, supportive procedures designed to enhance the healing process, including reflex techniques, exercise, rehabilitation, adjunctive physiotherapy, biofeedback, and lifestyle counseling regarding posture, diet, and stress reduction, may be incorporated in clinical management of the patient.[34]

Lantz Model of Vertebral Subluxation Complex

Lantz[9] provides a more structured organization for the VSC model by describing a hierarchy of organization and a pattern of interrelatedness of the various components. In addition to the components proposed by Faye, Lantz adds:

- Connective tissue pathology
- Vascular abnormalities
- Inflammatory response

In an update to this nine-component model,[3] reference to the suffix, *pathology* has been changed in favor of more generic terminology. Thus, *neurologic component* is used in place of neuropathology, *kinesio-*

logic component replaces kinesiopathology, and the *myologic component* is substituted for myopathology. The three foundational principles—anatomy, physiology and biochemistry—form the basis for understanding the other six components in the Lantz model (Fig. 3-2).

A common denominator between the Faye and Lantz models is the focus on restricted motion of the manipulable subluxation. Such restriction or immobilization of the joint causes some degree of degenerative change in the musculoskeletal system and connective tissue that may adversely affect nerve system function. The early introduction of motion via adjustment or manipulation, mobilization, trac-tion, and continuous passive motion may overcome these harmful effects.[38]

Kinesiologic Component

The kinesiologic component is represented at the apex of the Lantz VSC model, emphasizing the importance of motion and its interrelationship with other components. Positioned beneath the kinesio-logic component, but interconnected on the same level are the neurologic, myologic, vascular, and connective tissue components. Lantz states, "Movement is affected by muscles (myologic component); guided, limited and stabilized by connective tissue; and controlled largely by the nervous system. The

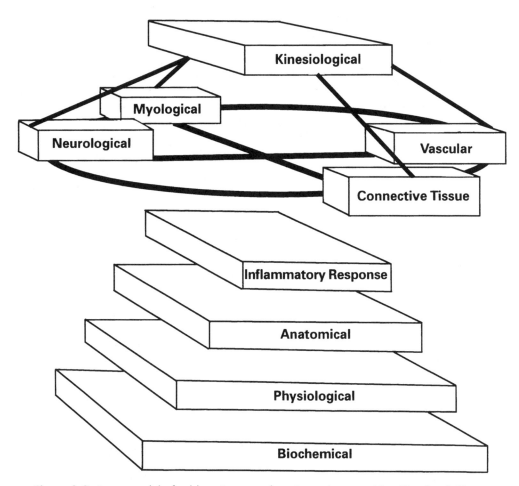

Figure 3-2. Lantz model of subluxation complex. Artwork created by Cleveland Chiro-practic College. (Adapted from Lantz,[37] with permission.)

vascular system serves the essential nutritive and cleansing role for all tissues and is the conduit for the immediate stages of the inflammatory response (at least in vascularized tissues). These constitute the tissue-level components of the VSC and each works in coordination with the others to permit and sustain proper movement. Interference with any single component affects all others." The neurologic component, as described by Lantz, includes the nerve roots, dorsal root ganglia, spinal nerve, recurrent meningeal nerve, and the articular neurology to include mechanoreceptors and nociceptors and related spinal reflex pathways.

Connective Tissue Component

Lantz's connective tissue component describes the impact of joint immobilization and connective tissue changes. This component includes bone, the intervertebral discs, articular cartilage, interspinous ligaments, and related supportive tissue elements. With connective tissue immobilization, synovial fluid undergoes fibrofatty consolidation, progressing to more adherent fibrous tissue and matrix development for the deposition of bone salts in the final stages of ankylosis.[39] In the immobilized joint, articular cartilage shrinks due to loss of proteoglycans.[40] This shrinkage leads to softening of cartilage, thus rendering the articulation more susceptible to damage by minor trauma.[41]

In the immobilized joint, adhesions form between adjacent connective tissue structures.[39] This may occur between the nerve root sleeve and adjacent capsular and osseous structures in the intervertebral foramen, between tendons and articular capsules, or between other connective tissue structures. Forced motion creates a physical disruption of the adhesions breaking intermolecular cross-linkages.[42]

Vascular Component

The vascular component may also be affected by abnormal spinal biomechanics. Each motion segment is supplied by a segmental artery passing through the intervertebral canal into the spinal canal. Through branching, this provides blood supply to the dorsal and ventral nerve roots. Each canal contains a segmental vein that drains the spinal canal and vertebral column. These blood vessels are susceptible to the same mechanical insults as nerve

roots and may be compressed. Lantz[37] proposes that immobilization may lead to localized venous stasis, creating a negative relative pressure at the area of immobilization, and that lack of proper venous drainage may lead to inflammatory states.

Inflammatory Component

Immobilization of a joint leads to an inflammatory response.[43] The inflammatory process may affect surrounding tissues and affect nerve function as implied in the concept of chemical radiculitis.[44] This may represent one example of how degeneration of spinal joints affects the neurologic component of the VSC. Inflamed nerves are hyperexcitable, and exhibit behavior different from normal nerve function.[45] The dorsal root ganglia (DRG) of normal nerves respond to mechanical stimulation by discharge of action potentials, which stops on cessation of the stimulation. In an inflamed DRG, the action potential discharge continues long after the mechanical stimulus has ceased.[44]

Although some investigators consider the inflammatory component part of the vascular component of VSC, others such as Faye[46] and Dishman[35] discuss inflammation under the histopathology component of the five-part Faye VSC model. In addition, given the chemical nature of inflammation and tissue repair, inflammation cannot be considered independent of the VSC biochemistry component.

The model of the VSC represents the current state of the art concept of subluxation, and provides a context bridging the basic science and clinical aspects of spinal function, dysfunction, and degeneration. This model offers a framework for discussion of the varied approaches to spinal manipulative therapy, the specific chiropractic vertebral adjustment, and adjunctive or rehabilitative management of the spine. Use of this model in interaction with other health care providers may enhance interprofessional cooperation between chiropractors and others in co-management and inter-referral of patients.

ASSOCIATION OF CHIROPRACTIC COLLEGES POSITION STATEMENTS

On July 1, 1996, presidents of all North American chiropractic colleges, as members of the Association of Chiropractic Colleges (ACC), seeking to clarify professional common ground and define chiropractic's role within the health care delivery system, generated a series of consensus position statements.[47] This was the first time in the 100-year history of chiropractic education that all college presidents, representing schools with diverse institutional missions, have reached unanimous consensus on common core definitions fundamental to the principles of chiropractic (Fig. 3-3).

ACC Consensus Definitions:

On chiropractic:

Chiropractic is a health-care discipline which emphasizes the inherent recuperative powers of the body to heal itself without the use of drugs or surgery.

The practice of chiropractic focuses on the relationship between structure (primarily of the spine) and function (as coordinated by the nervous system) and how that relationship affects the preservation and restoration of health.

Doctors of Chiropractic recognize the value and responsibility of working in cooperation with other health care practitioners when in the best interest of the patient.

The ACC continues to foster a unique, distinct chiropractic profession that serves as a health care discipline for all. The ACC advocates a profession that generates, develops, and utilizes the highest level of evidence possible in the provision of effective, prudent and cost-conscious patient evaluation and care.

On subluxation:

A subluxation is a complex of functional, structural, and/or pathological articular changes that compromise neural integrity and may influence organ system function and general health.

A subluxation is evaluated, diagnosed and managed through the use of chiropractic procedures

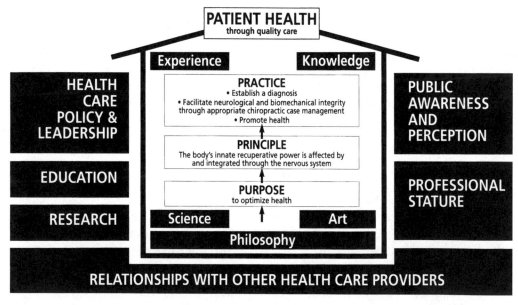

Figure 3-3. Association of Chiropractic Colleges Chiropractic Paradigm.

based on the best available rational and empirical evidence.

The preservation and restoration of health is enhanced through the correction of the subluxation.

DEFINITIONS RELATED TO SUBLUXATION AND CLINICAL PROCEDURES

Other definitions related to subluxation and its management as presented by Gatterman[7] include the following:

Manipulable subluxation: A subluxation in which altered alignment, movement, or function can be improved by manual thrust procedures.

Subluxation syndrome: An aggregate of signs and symptoms that relate to pathophysiology or dysfunction of spinal and pelvic motion segment or to peripheral joints.

Motion segment: A functional unit made up of two adjacent articulating surfaces and the connecting tissues binding to them to each other.

Spinal motion segment: Two adjacent vertebrae and the connecting tissues binding them to each other.

Manual therapy: Procedures by which the hands directly contact the body to treat the articulations or soft tissues.

Mobilization: Movement applied singularly or repetitively within or at the physiologic range of joint motion, without imparting a thrust or impulse, with the goal or restoring joint mobility.

Manipulation: A manual procedure that involves a directed thrust to move a joint past the physiologic range of motion without exceeding the anatomic limit.

Adjustment: Any chiropractic therapeutic procedure that uses controlled force, leverage, direction, amplitude, and velocity directed at specific joints or anatomic regions.

EARLY STUDIES OF EFFECTS OF SPINAL MECHANICAL DERANGEMENT

Basic science laboratory investigation into the relationship between altered spinal structure and tis-
sues or organ dysfunction may be traced back to the first part of the 20th century in medical and osteopathic literature, and as early as 1950 for the chiropractic profession.

Louisa Burns: Experimental Osteopathic Lesions in Animals

Early investigation of spinal reflexes by osteopath Louisa Burns[48] from 1907 onward focused on effects of the osteopathic lesion.[49-52] Research at the A.T. Still Research Institute in Chicago conducted by Burns[52] and colleagues in 1948 investigated the pathogenesis of visceral disease following vertebral lesion. To study certain nervous reflexes and lesion-induced disturbances in distant visceral tissue, Burns produced experimental lesions in a variety of animals, including rabbits, guinea pigs, cats, dogs and goats. To induce a spinal lesion the experimenter would twist and traction a spinal segment. Burns et al.[52] describe that "when the limit of normal motion is reached, slight sudden additional pressure in the same plane is exerted, forcing the vertebra just beyond its normal range of movement and causing a slight strain of the tissue." The term *lesion* is defined as "a mechanical maladjustment of some sort which operates as one of the primary causes of disease." Early stages of the lesion demonstrated impairment of visceral circulation along with changes in smooth muscle function and glandular secretory function. Lesioned articular structures demonstrated changes in synovial fluid and later fibrotic changes. Later stages of the lesion involved circulatory congestion, denervation related changes and segmentally organized somato-autonomic reflex dysfunction, resulting in disturbed regulation of the viscera.

Henry Winsor: Spinal Curvatures and Visceral Disorders

In 1922, using cadavers from the University of Pennsylvania, medical physician Henry K. Winsor,[53] conducted necropsies to determine whether a connection existed between minor curvatures of the spine and diseased organs. Fifty bodies were examined. The anterior thoracic and abdominal wall was removed, the organs removed and examined, and the anterior surfaces of the vertebral bodies were cleared for ease of examination for curvature. Forty-nine of the fifty cadavers showed minor curvatures. Winsor reported that:

In fifty cadavers with diseases in 139 organs, there was found curve of the vertebrae, belonging to the same sympathetic segments as the diseased organs 128 times, leaving an apparent discrepancy of ten, in which the vertebrae in the curve belonged to an adjacent segment to that which should supply the diseased organs with sympathetic filaments. However, the nerve filaments entering the cord or leaving it travel or have traveled up or down the cord for a few segments, accounting for all the apparent discrepancies.

Tabulation of Winsor's observations (Table 3-1) provides the following examples:

1. Heart and pericardium disease was observed in 20 cases of the 50 cadavers. Minor spinal curvatures were identified in the upper five dorsal segments in 18 of the cases. Two cases involved neighboring segment C7 and D1.
2. Stomach disease was identified in 9 cases with 8 of the 9 demonstrating curvature in dorsal segments 5 to 9. In one case, curvature was found in a neighboring segment.
3. Kidney disease was observed in 17 cases. Curvature was observed at dorsal segments 10 to 12 in 14 cases. One case demonstrated curvature at neighboring dorsal segments 5 to 9 and "few" at lumbar segments L1 and L2.

Winsor took these observations as "evidences of the association, in the dissected cadavers, of the visceral disease with vertebral deformities of the same sympathetic segments."

Carl Cleveland, Jr: Experimental Subluxation Effects in Rabbits

During the early 1950s, Carl S. Cleveland, Jr.,[54,55] in a pilot study investigated the effects of subluxation on the domestic rabbit. Misalignment of the intervertebral joint was produced by application of a spinal subluxation splint consisting of three adjustable metal pin clamps supported by a common suprastructure frame. With minimal surgical incision the pin clamps were attached to the base of

spinous processes of three contingous vertebrae. Subluxation was produced by tightening Allen screws on the splint frame, thereby drawing the middle vertebra to the posterior and then laterally to produce misalignment. This procedure was accomplished under fluoroscopic assistance and verified by radiographs. Physiologic outcomes such as heart rate, blood pressure, and urinalysis were evaluated. Postmortem pathologic analysis was conducted on various organs and tissues. Findings included two cases of 12th thoracic subluxation with subsequent kidney abnormalities. Other experimental subjects demonstrated "heart diseases, valvular leakages, paralysis, arrhythmias, vasomotor paralysis, dropsy, kidney conditions, and the formation of tumors." Vernon[56] cites this study as an innovative first attempt by chiropractic investigators to employ an animal model of spinal subluxation.

RETROSPECTIVE

The forceful dynamic thrust as part of the application of spinal manipulation dates from the time of ancient Greece[12,57] as identified by Withington's 1959 English translation of the writings of Hippocrates, circa 400 BC. Hippocrates recommended that with the patient lying prone on a wooden bed, combined extension and pressure should be exerted on the patient's spine, and:

The physician, or an assistant who is strong and not untrained, should put the palm of hand on the hump, and the palm of the other hand on that, to reduce it forcibly, taking into consideration whether the reduction should naturally be made straight downwards or towards the head or towards the hip.

References in this ancient writing to positioning of the hands and whether to direct the force straight downward or toward the head or the hip are strikingly similar to the fundamental components of toggle type dynamic thrusts and angle of drive (direction of thrust) found in contemporary chiropractic technique texts.

The concept of spinal biomechanical dysfunction described and treated as the "hump" some 20 centuries earlier by Hippocrates, reappeared in the medical literature some 300 years ago as the term

Table 3-1 Winsor's Correlation of Spinal Curvatures and Diseased Organs in Cadavers

Visceral Disturbances		Vertebral Curvatures				Sympathetic Connections Between Vertebrae and Diseased Organ	Check System
		Same Sympathetic Segment as Visceral Trouble		Neighboring Segment to Discera			
Thymus diseased	2	C7 & D1	1	None	0	Inf. cervical ganglia	2
		D2.3.4	1				
Pleurae adherent	21	Upper dorsal	19	Lower dorsal	2	Upper dorsal ganglia	19 } 21
						Lower dorsal ganglia	2
Lung diseases	26	Upper dorsal	26	Lower dorsal	0	Upper dorsal ganglia	26–26
Heart and peri- cardium cases	20	Upper five dorsal	18	C7 and D1	2	Upper dorsal ganglia	18 } 20
						Inf. cervical ganglia	2
Stomach diseases	9	Dorsal 5–9	8		1	Greater splanchnic (Dorsal 5–9)	8
Liver diseases	13	Dorsal 5–9	12		1	Greater splanchnic (Dorsal 5–9)	12
Cholelithiasis cases	5	Dorsal 5–9	5		0	Greater splanchnic (Dorsal 5–9)	5
							5
Pancreas cases	5	Dorsal 5–9	3		0	Greater splanchnic (Dorsal 5–9)	3
Splenic affections	11	Dorsal 5–9	10	Dorsal 10,11,12	1	Greater splanchnic (Dorsal 5–9)	
						Lesser and least Splanchnic	10 } 10
							1 } 11
Inguinal diseases	2	Dorsal 12	2		0	Somatic nerve Ilio-inguinal	2
Kidney diseases	17	Dorsal 10, 11 & 12	14	Dorsal 5–9	1	Least, lesser and greater splanchnic	
				Lumbar 1 and 2	few	Upper lumbar ganglia	17
Prostate and bladder diseases	8	Lumbar 1,2,3	7	Dorsal 12	1	Upper lumbar ganglia	7
				Sacral curve	1	Last dorsal and sacral few	8
Uterus and adnexa	2	Lumbar Lordosis	2	0		Lumbar and sacral ganglia	2
Visceral diseases	139	Vertebral curve of same smyp. seg. as disease		Vertebral curve of adjacent segment	10	Vertebral curve of segments not related to	
	139	site	128			diseased site 1–5	138

subluxation.[6] Historical literature[10–13] records that spinal biomechanical dysfunction and its treatment by manipulation, represented an area of substantive interest in the early 19th century medical community. This later fell into disuse in North America as that profession moved toward the chemically focused allopathic model of patient care. This abandonment of manipulation by conventional medicine provided chiropractors the opportunity to progress with little competition from non-DC manual therapy practitioners, and thus to become the most skilled practitioners of the spinal adjustment and manipulative procedures.

Maintaining this leadership role in conservative management of spinal function will depend on the chiropractic profession's ability to advance knowledge through research and clinical outcome assessment, especially regarding the effectiveness of chiropractic procedures in the restoration and preservation of health. The model of the vertebral subluxation complex provides a common context bridging the basic science and clinical aspects of spinal function, dysfunction, and degeneration and may serve to enhance interprofessional cooperation between doctors of chiropractic and other health care providers participating in co-management and inter-referral of patients.

Terminology

adjustment
articulation
atrophy
atonia
biomechanics
degeneration
dislocation
Faye model
fixation
hypomobility
hypermobility
intervertebral foramen
Lantz model
manipulable subluxation
manipulation
manual therapy
Medicare
motion segment
mobilization
spinal motion segment
subluxation
subluxation syndrome
trophic nerve function
World Health Organization

Review Questions

1. What is the earliest known English definition of subluxation? In what year was it proposed?

2. What was D.D. Palmer's view of subluxation?

3. How did B.J. Palmer redefine subluxation?

4. What are the similarities and differences between Andrew Taylor Still's osteopathic concepts and the chiropractic concepts of Daniel David Palmer?

5. What role did unique chiropractic nomenclature such as the term "subluxation" play in the struggle for separate licensure?

6. Which early chiropractors were the first to characterize subluxation as a "fixation" and to describe the "field of motion" of a vertebra?

7. Which two Belgian chiropractors developed the concepts of motion palpation?

8. In what ways are contemporary definitions of subluxation similar to, and different from, early definitions of the Palmers, Stephenson, and Langworthy?

9. What are the major characteristics of the Faye model of vertebral subluxation complex?

10. What additional concepts are incorporated in the Lantz model?

Concept Questions

1. Why did it take until 1996 for the presidents of all North American chiropractic colleges to reach unanimous consensus on common core definitions fundamental to the principles of chiropractic? What intra-professional divisions kept this from occurring earlier?

2. Is subluxation the cause of all or almost all human ailments? What evidence supports your answer?

References

1. Steadman's Medical Dictionary. 26th Ed. Williams & Wilkins, Baltimore, 1995

2. Cleveland CS III: Chiropractic 811. Lecture Notes. Cleveland Chiropractic College, Kansas City, 1995

3. Gatterman MI: Foundations of Chiropractic—Subluxation. CV Mosby, St. Louis, 1995

4. Haldeman SC: The pathophysiology of the spinal subluxation. p. 217. In Goldstein M (ed): The Research Status of Spinal Manipulative Therapy. Monog No. 15. HEW/NINCDS, Bethesda, 1975

5. Rome PL: Usage of chiropractic terminology in the literature: 296 ways to say "subluxation": complex issues of the vertebral subluxation. Chiro Tech 8(2):49, 1996

6. Holme R: Academy of Armory, Printed in Chester by author, 1688. Reprinted by the Scholar Press Limited, Menston, England, 1972

7. Gatterman MI: What's in a word? p. 6. In Gatterman MI (ed): Foundations of Chiropractic—Subluxation. CV Mosby, St. Louis, 1995

8. Leach RA: The Chiropractic Theories—Principles and Clinical Applications. 3rd Ed. Williams & Wilkins, Baltimore, 1994

9. Lantz CA: The vertebral subluxation complex. ICA Int Rev Chiro 45:37, 1989

10. Hieronymus JH: De luxationibus et subluxationibus. Thesis, Jena, 1746

11. Terrett A: The search for the subluxation: an investigation of medical literature to 1985. Assoc Hist Chiro 7:29, 1987

12. Lomax E: Manipulative therapy: a historical perspective from ancient times to the modern era. p. 11. In Goldstein M (ed): The Research Status of Spinal Manipulative Therapy. Monog No. 15, HEW/NINCDS, Bethesda, 1975

13. Tower D: Chairman's summary: evolution and development of the concepts of manipulative therapy. p. 59. In Goldstein M (ed): The Research Status of Spinal Manipulative Therapy. Monog No. 15, HEW/NINCDS, Bethesda, 1975

14. Wardwell WI: Before the Palmers: an overview of chiropractic's antecedents. Chiro Hist 7(2):27, 1987

15. Palmer DD: The Chiropractor 1(1):8, 1904

16. Gibbons RW: Solon Massey Langworthy: keeper of the flame during the "lost years" of chiropractic. Chiro Hist 1:15, 1981

17. Smith O, Langworthy SM, Paxson M: Modernized Chiropractic. American School of Chiropractic. Cedar Rapids, IA, 1906

18. Gillet H, Lichens M: Belgian Chiropractic Research Notes. Motion Palpation Institute, Huntington Beach, CA, 1981

19. Palmer DD: The Science, Art and Philosophy of Chiropractic. Portland Printing House, Portland, 1910

20. Palmer BJ: The Subluxation Specific—The Adjustment Specific. Palmer School of Chiropractic, Davenport, IA, 1934

21. Lantz CA: A review of the evolution of chiropractic concepts of subluxation. Top Clin Chiro 2(2):1, 1995

22. Stephenson RW: Chiropractic Text Book. Palmer School of Chiropractic, Davenport, IA, 1948

23. American Chiropractic Association: Indexed Synopsis of Policies on Public Health and Related Matters. American Chiropractic Association, Arlington, VA, 1995–1996

24. Gatterman M, Hansen D: The development of chiropractic nomenclature through consensus. J Manipul Physiol Ther 17:302, 1994

25. International Chiropractors Association: Membership Referral Directory, ICA Policy Statements. International Chiropractors Association, Arlington, VA, 1996

26. ICA: Minutes of Midyear Board of Directors Meeting, Universal City, CA, January 21–24, 1988. International Chiropractors Association, Arlington, VA, 1988

27. Hendrickson RM: The Legal Establishment of Chiropractic. International Chiropractors Association, Arlington, VA, 1992

28. Medicare Act, the United States Code Annotated, Title 42, The Public Health and Welfare, Section 10/395x, under (r) Physician, 1974

29. World Health Organization: International Classification of Diseases. 10th Ed. World Health Organization, Geneva, 1992

30. Janse J, Houser RH, Wells BF: Chiropractic principles and technic—for use by students and practitioners. 2nd Ed. National College of Chiropractic, Chicago, 1947

31. Janse J, Hildebrandt RW (eds): Principles and Practice of Chiropractic—An Anthology National College of Chiropractic, Chicago, 1976

32. Illi FW: The Vertebral Column: Life Line of the Body. National College of Chiropractic, Chicago, 1951

33. Homewood AE: The Neurodynamics of the Vertebral Subluxation. 3rd Ed. Valkyrie Press, St. Petersburg, FL, 1981

34. Schafer RC, Faye LJ: Motion Palpation and Chiropractic Technic: Principles of Dynamic Chiropractic. The Motion Palpation Institute, Huntington Beach, CA, 1989

35. Dishman R: Review of the literature supporting a scientific basis for the chiropractic subluxation complex. J Manipul Physiol Ther 8:163, 1988

36. Seaman DR: Chiropractic and Pain Control. 3rd Ed. DRS Systems, Hendersonville, NC, 1995

37. Lantz CA: The vertebral subluxation complex. p. 149. In Gatterman MI (ed): Foundations of chiropractic—subluxation. CV Mosby, St. Louis, 1995

38. Videman T: Connective tissue and immobilization. Clin Orthop 221:26, 1987

39. Evans EB, Eggers GWN, Butler JK, Blumel J: Experimental immobilization and remobilization of rat knee. J Bone Joint Surg 42A:737, 1960

40. Troyer H: The effect of short-term immobilization on the rabbit knee in joint cartilage. Clin Orthop 107:249, 1975

41. Palmoski MJ, Colyer RA, Brandt KD: Joint motion in the absence of normal loading does not maintain normal articular cartilage. Arthritis Rheum 23:325, 1980

42. Woo SL-Y, Matthew JV, Akeson WH et al: Connective tissue response to immobility: Correlative study of biomechanical and biochemical measurements of normal and immobilized rabbit knees. Arthritis Rheum 18:257, 1975

43. Davis D: Respiratory manifestations of dorsal spine radiculitis simulating cardiac asthma. Ann Intern Med 32:954, 1950

44. Marshall LL, Thethewie ER, Curtain CC: Chemical radiculitis: a clinical, physiological and immunological study. Clin Orthop 129:61, 1977

45. Howe JF, Loeser JD, Calvin WH: Mechanosensitivity of dorsal root ganglia and chronically injured axons: a physiological basis for radicular pain of nerve root compression. Pain 3:25, 1977

46. Faye LJ: Motion palpation of the spine. Motion Palpation Institute, Huntington Beach, CA, 1983

47. Association of Chiropractic Colleges. Minutes. Chicago, July 1, 1996

48. Burns LA: Viscero-somatic and somato-visceral spinal reflexes. J Am Osteopath Assoc 7:51, 1907

50. Burns LA: Effects of upper cervical and upper thoracic lesions. J Am Osteopath Assoc 22:266, 1923

51. Burns LA: Laboratory proofs of the osteopathic lesion. J Am Osteopath Assoc 31:123, 1931

52. Burns L, Chandler L, Rice R: Pathogenesis of Visceral Diseases Following Vertebral Lesions. American Osteopathic Association, Chicago, 1948

53. Winsor HK: Sympathetic segmental disturbances. II. Medical Times 49:267, 1922

54. Cleveland CS Jr: Researching the Subluxation on the Domestic Rabbit. Cleveland Chiropractic College Monograph, Kansas City, 1961

55. Cleveland CS Jr: Researching the subluxation on the domestic rabbit. Science Rev Chir 1(4):5, 1965

56. Vernon H: Basic scientific evidence for chiropractic subluxation. p. 35. In Gatterman M (ed): Foundations of Chiropractic—Subluxation. CV Mosby, St. Louis, 1995

57. Cleveland CS III: The high-velocity thrust adjustment. p. 459. In Haldeman S (ed): Principles and Practice of Chiropractic. Appleton & Lange, E Norwalk, CT, 1992

4
Neurobiologic Relations

Carl S. Cleveland III

The conceptual model of vertebral subluxation proposes that spinal biomechanical derangement causes some form of "nerve interference." According to Vernon,[1] "this has come to be understood as either (1) some element of compression of the spinal nerves in the environs of the intervertebral foramen or (2) ... initiation of pain in the spinal joints ... capable of creating secondary aberrant reflex effects such as increases in motorneuron or sympathetic neural activity."

A variety of hypotheses have been advanced to explain the association of vertebral subluxation complex (VSC) with neuronal disturbance and related dysfunction and symptoms.

NERVE COMPRESSION HYPOTHESIS

From the beginnings of the chiropractic profession, the theory that nerves can become compressed through impingement from intersegmental spinal biomechanical derangements has been accorded biomechanical, functional, and clinical significance,[2–10] and has even been proposed as a primary cause of disease.[2–10] Chiropractic authors emphasize the importance of the intervertebral foramen (IVF) and its anatomic contents—the spinal nerve, nerve roots, recurrent meningeal (sinuvertebral) nerves, blood vessels, lymphatics, and connective tissue—and devote much attention to changes resulting from compression of the elements within the IVF.[2–7,9–15]

Although contemporary research[16–21] has demonstrated that other mechanisms of spinal biomechanical derangement may be responsible for inducing neuronal disturbances, the clinical significance of nerve compression should not be discounted.[10] Cramer[11] attributes much of the importance of the IVF to the fact that it provides an osteoligamentous boundary between the central nervous system and the peripheral nervous system.

The question is: to what extent are spinal nerves, nerve roots, and dorsal root ganglia vulnerable to compression or irritation by abnormal biomechanics affecting the IVF? The anatomy of the lumbar and thoracic spine suggests that sufficient room exists for spinal nerves to pass unimpeded through IVFs in these areas. However, the anatomic relationship of the spinal nerve to the cervical intervertebral foramen is significantly different.

Anatomy of the Cervical Intervertebral Foramen

Orthopedic surgeons DePalma and Rothman[12] describe the cervical spine intervertebral foramina as small ovoid canals with vertical diameters approximately 10 mm in height, with the anteroposterior diameter about one-half the size of the vertical diameter. These workers state that, "the nerve roots and mixed spinal nerves completely fill the anteroposterior diameter of the intervertebral foramina.

The upper one quarter of the canal is filled with areolar tissue and small veins" and "small arteries arising from the vertebra." DePalma and Rothman continue, "any space taking lesion which pinches the anteroposterior diameter of the intervertebral foramen might be expected to cause some compression of the nervous tissue elements traversing this limited space." By contrast, these authors describe the normal lumbar IVF as 5 to 6 times the diameter of the spinal nerve, permitting relatively great freedom from constriction.

In describing the boundaries of the cervical IVF, Jackson,[13] an orthopedist, states that,

The posterior walls of the canals are formed by the adjacent posterior articular processes, but primarily by the superior articulating process of the distal vertebrae. The anterior walls are formed by the lateral portion of the bodies of the adjacent vertebrae and the margins of the intervening interbody articulations. The anterior walls are of great significance from a mechanical standpoint, in as much as the nerve roots pass directly over and are in intimate contact with the margins of the lateral interbody joints. The gliding motion which occurs between these joints whenever the head and neck are turned or moved in any direction subjects the nerve roots to irritation if there is any mechanical derangement present.

Parallel to the conclusions of Rothman and DePalma, Jackson concludes:

The nerve roots lie on the floor of the canals and fill their anteroposterior diameter completely. The upper one-eighth to one-fourth of the foramina, or the canals, is filled with areolar and fatty tissues and small veins. Small spinal arteries which are branches from the vertebral artery pass back through the intervertebral foramina to enter the vertebral canal. Minute branches from the nerve trunks, which are known as the recurrent meningeal nerve, pass back through the intervertebral foramina anterior to the nerve roots.

Jackson notes that ventral nerve root fibers are in intimate contact with the margins of the lateral interbody joints. The posterior fibers, or posterior nerve roots, are in intimate contact with the posterior superior articular processes of the adjacent distal vertebrae. Jackson explains, "because of their close proximity to the anterior and posterior walls of the intervertebral foramina the cervical nerve roots are extremely vulnerable to compression or to irritation from any mechanical derangement or inflammatory condition in or about the foramina. Such irritation or compression may cause pain and/or sensory and motor disturbances anywhere along the segmental distribution of the nerves." Jackson uses the term *cervical syndrome* to describe the group of symptoms and clinical findings resulting from irritation or compression of the cervical nerve roots in or about the IVF.[13]

Crelin's Efforts to Disprove Nerve Compression

In a 1974 article frequently quoted by opponents of chiropractic, Crelin,[22] an anatomist, argued that nerve roots pass through "spacious intervertebral foramina" and that therefore exertion of pressure on a spinal nerve does not occur. However, a review of the study's methodology, coupled with current research, demonstrates that Crelin's conclusion is in error concerning the effects of joint subluxation.[23]

Seeking to "prove" that the theory of spinal nerve impingement is "impossible," Crelin[24] obtained vertebral columns from six individuals. Three were from full-term infants, the others from adults ages 35, 73, and 76 years. The vertebral column of each was excised within 3 to 6 hours after death. The skull was disarticulated from the first cervical vertebra and the fifth lumbar vertebra was disarticulated from the sacrum. Each spinal nerve was transected 8 cm after emerging from the IVF. Deep paraspinal musculature, ligaments, and joint capsules were left intact.

Two metal vices were clamped to a platform supporting the vertebral column while it was subjected to compressive forces. Five vertebral segments of the newborn column and 3 of the adult columns were suspended between the vises. A Dillon force gauge was used to measure force of compression applied to the vertebra. A range of maximum compression forces, including twisting and flexion, were applied. The osseous boundary of the foramen did not come in contact with the nerve and Crelin reported that there was never less than 1.5 mm of space completely surrounding the cervical nerves, 3 mm around the thoracics, and 4 mm surrounding the lumbar nerves. Crelin explained that all spinal nerves emerging from their IVFs were exposed prior to testing and that gentle teasing with small forceps removed the flimsy areolar tissue surrounding the nerves to expose the border of the "spacious vertebral foramina."

However, this very tissue removed by Crelin contains important connective tissue elements that may be compressible[25] or when irritated may release chemicals having an adverse effect on nerve function[26–30] Some critics of the nerve compression theory have neglected to recognize that spinal biomechanical derangements do not involve "hard bone on soft nerve." Instead, the key issue is the potential for altered interforaminal mechanics to affect vascular and connective tissue support structures as well as the important neural components within the IVF.

Contemporary information describes the IVF as an extended interpedicular zone,[31] often containing transforaminal ligaments.[32–36] These anatomical factors, combined with current understanding of spinal nerve root sensitivity to pressure[37–39] and irritation[25–30] render Crelin's conclusions unsupportable.[23]

The Interpedicular Zone

Giles[31] maintains that the IVF should no longer be conceptualized as a two-dimensional hole, but rather as a canal or tunnel through which the spinal nerve and other related structures pass. He maintains that "neural and associated vascular structures within the important interpedicular zone may well be compromised due to vertebral joint subluxation. This may result in chronic compression," adding, "The precise significance clinically … is yet to be determined."

Giles took nine randomly chosen sections of adult lumbosacral spinal tissue and examined them histologically for measurement of the L4–L5 and L5–S1 IVF canals. The zone between the pedicles of adjacent vertebrae was found to have a horizontal length of 8.2 to 12.2 mm. At a minimum the distance between the nerve structures and the side of the IVF canal was 0.4 to 0.8 mm for both the L4–5 and L5–S1 segments. Giles concludes that the Crelin study was "meaningless as a basis for consideration of the possible physiologic and/or pathophysiologic functions of spinal nerves beyond the intervertebral canal as he did not examine the important interpedicular zone" that contains the spinal nerve root and ganglion, but rather examined only "the relatively insignificant lateral border."

Transforaminal Ligaments— A Key Anatomic Structure

As described by Golub and Silverman,[32] transforaminal ligaments (TFL) are ligamentous bands crossing the IVF at any spinal level (Fig. 4-1). In dissections of fifteen lumbar spines representing 150 IVFs, Bachop and Hilgendorf[33] found varying numbers of TFLs. Bakkum[34] determined that TFLs, once considered an abnormality, are normal and greatly reduce the functional compartment or space available for the spinal nerve. In Bakkum's study, four adult lumbosacral spines without visible pathology or degenerative changes were examined, yielding the following results: 35 of the 49 IVFs examined (71 percent) had at least one TFL. More than one quarter (27 percent) had 2 TFLs, and 8 percent had 3 or 4.

In the presence of TFLs, the superior to inferior dimension (height) of the functional compartment containing the ventral ramus of the spinal nerve was "significantly decreased." The average height reduction was approximately one-third (31.5 percent). In 12 percent of cases, the reduction was at least 50 percent in the IVF containing a TFL, with one case being reduced by over two-thirds (67.8 percent).

According to Bachop and Janse,[35] the higher the TFL is situated in the foramen, the less space remains for the spinal vessels. This can conceivably lead to ischemia or venous congestion. On the other hand, the lower the TFL is located, the greater the possibility of sensory and/or motor deficits. In a study of accessory ligaments of the IVF, Amonoo-Kuoffi et al.[36] conclude that the spinal nerve, segmental veins and arteries, and the recurrent meningeal nerve are held in place through the openings between the accessory ligaments within the IVF. In IVFs in which multiple TFLs are present, these nerves and vessels are literally threaded through a lattice created by the TFLs.

Hadley on Subluxation and the Intervertebral Foramen

Hadley,[25] a medical radiologist, states that the importance of the IVF lies in the fact that except for the first and second cervical nerves, each peripheral nerve must pass through one of these openings. In the cervical region there is:

a close five-way interrelationship between the foramen, the nerve root which passes through it, the

Ventral and dorsal nerve roots
within the dural root sleeve

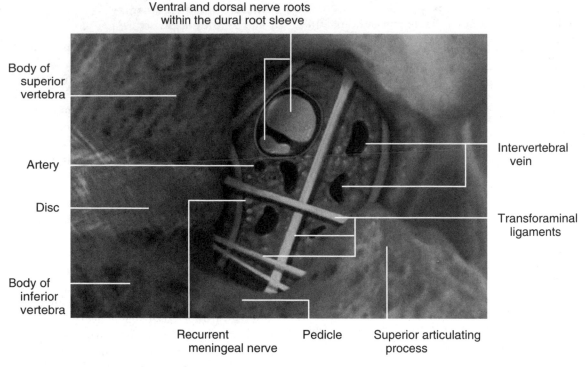

Body of
superior
vertebra

Artery

Disc

Body of
inferior
vertebra

Recurrent
meningeal nerve

Pedicle

Superior articulating
process

Intervertebral
vein

Transforaminal
ligaments

Figure 4-1. The lumbar intevertebral foramen (IVF). Notice the structures that normally traverse the IVF. The most common locations of the transforaminal ligaments are also shown. (From Cramer,[113] with permission.)

vertebral artery contacting the root in front, the covertebral joint anteriorly and the posterior cervical articulation in back.

He also notes that arthrotic and degenerative changes involving these structures may become an important factor resulting in foraminal encroachment and that,

bulging disc substance, exostoses or subluxation of a posterior joint may produce pressure upon the root.

Hadley goes on to state that,

Subluxation (partial displacement) of the vertebral bodies ... may present radiographically one or more of the following features:

1. Shift of the corresponding spinous process toward the side of the subluxation with the patient and film exactly centered

2. Slight increase in the size of the corresponding intervertebral foramen
3. Encroachment of the opposite foramen
4. Displacement of the articular surfaces upon each other
5. Because of the inclined plane of the posterior articulation, the side of the vertebra is elevated as it is carried forward. For that reason the disc appears thicker on the side of the unilateral subluxation.[25]

Regarding cervical encroachment, Hadley[25] observes that, in addition to local and referred pain, patients can suffer from bizarre symptoms called "chronic cervical syndrome," described as paroxysmal deep or superficial pain in parts of the head, face, ear, throat, or sinuses; sensory disturbances in the pharnyx; vertigo; and tinnitus, with diminished hearing. Vasomotor disturbances include sweating, flushing, lacrimation, and salivation. Hadley adds, "spontaneous subluxation at the C1–C2 level either unilateral or bilateral, is usually a sequel to an inflammatory process of the throat."

JOINT RESTRICTION AND THROAT INFLAMMATION

Hadley's observation of "spontaneous subluxation"[25] associated with inflammation of the throat raises interesting questions from a chiropractic perspective. Is this inflammatory process truly a viscerosomatic reflex response? Or are these symptoms a result of somatovisceral manifestations leading to lowered tissue resistance in the throat that contribute to the inflammation?

In a study of 76 children with chronic tonsillitis, Czech physician and manual medicine specialist Lewit[40] observed, "The most striking and constant clinical finding was movement restriction at the craniocervical junction, in the great majority between occiput and atlas (70 cases or 92 percent)." Lewit concluded, "tonsillitis goes hand in hand with movement restriction ... mainly between occiput and atlas, with little tendency to spontaneous recovery," adding, "our experience suggests that blockage (movement restriction) at this level increases the susceptibility to recurrent tonsillitis."

Commenting on the thoracic region, Hadley[25] states, "Since the thoracic roots are relatively small, compression of these structures does not occur in the foramina of this region." Regarding the lumbar region, Hadley affirms that the spinal nerve occupies about one-fifth to one-fourth the diameter of the normal foramen, and that the remainder of the space is taken up by blood and lymphatic vessels, areolar and fatty tissue which together constitute a "compressible safety cushion space which allows the physiological encroachment to occur without nerve compression." Moreover, "any abnormal constriction in the size of a normal IVF if not actually causing nerve root pressure, nevertheless decreases the reserve safety cushion space surrounding that nerve and may predispose to pressure."

Effects of Degeneration

In a study of the kinematics of the lumbar IVF under normal physiologic spinal motions, Panjabi et al.[41] maintain that in cases of spinal degeneration, normal physiologic motion "may be enough to compromise the space around the nerve root to such a degree that very little safety margin is left." These investigators further state that, "with age and degeneration, the nerve loses its flexibility and develops adhesions with the IVF walls. It may not easily slip away from the compressing forces. The result may be a chronic threat of compression and mechanical irritation leading to inflammation of the nerve root." Discussing the research of Sunderland,[37] Panjabi agrees that in contrast to the thicker connective tissue covering of the peripheral nerve, the anatomical and mechanical weakness of the spinal nerve root more easily causes interneural fibrosis and adhesions to the surrounding IVF tissues.

Muscular Influences on Nerves

Korr,[42] a physiologist and osteopathic researcher, observes that much of the pathway taken by nerves as they emerge from the cord is through skeletal muscle. The contractile forces of this muscle along with associated chemical changes exert profound influences on the metabolism and excitability of neurons. In such an environment, neurons are subject to considerable mechanical insult (compression and torsion) as well as chemical influences. Nerve sheaths, which are extensions of the meninges surrounding the spinal cord, extend distally along the spinal nerve roots providing a root sleeve allowing the nerves to slide smoothly in and out without friction during a wide range of vertebral column movement. Over time, however, slight mechanical stresses may produce adhesions, constrictions, and angulations. From a chiropractic perspective, this vulnerability of nerve trunks represents effects associated with the myologic component of the VSC, and also relates to its inflammatory and biochemical components.

Vascular and Sympathetic Influences

Vascular structures pass through the IVF and provide blood supply to both the bony vertebral column and the spinal cord.[38] Ischemia of the nerve cells within the dorsal root ganglia may lead to progressive loss of sensory function, including proprioception. Edematous pressure, from even slight congestion of venous drainage may effect nerve conduction.[38] Such relationships are associated with the vascular and neurological components of VSC.

Sympathetic ganglia in the highly mobile neck area and the cervical chain of ganglia positioned against the vertebral column, are subject to stress imposed by motion. This may exert profound influence on the physiology of sympathetic nerve cells.[38] Furthermore, the mechanical disturbances or somatic insults described above by Korr exert slight forces resulting in slight tissue changes within the IVF and in paraspinal structures. This may adversely affect nerve function. It is further proposed that disorders of muscle tension, tissue texture, and visceral and circulatory function are reflected at the body surface as observable diagnostic elements.[38,39]

Neurophysiologic Effects of Nerve Compression

Spinal nerve roots, as compared to peripheral nerves, have a less abundant protective epineurium, no branching fasciculi, and poor lymphatic drainage.[43–45] These facts imply that the nerve root is more susceptible to injury by mechanical forces.[46] Panjabi et al.[41] state that "the nerve root is constrained in the intervertebral foramen and may be easily compressed or mechanically irritated under adverse conditions of degeneration and movement." In consideration of the effects on nerve function by subluxation or spinal biomechanical impairment, questions arise regarding possible pathophysiological mechanism associated with compression or mechanical irritation of nerves.

In a study to determine the susceptibility of spinal nerve roots to compression, Sharpless[47] concluded, "pressure of only 10 mm Hg produced a significant conduction block, the potential falling to 60 percent of its initial value in 30 minutes. After such a small compressive force is removed, nearly complete recovery occurs in 15 to 30 minutes. With higher levels of pressure, we have observed incomplete recovery after many hours of recording." Rydevik[48] determined that, "Venous blood flow to spinal roots was blocked with 5 to 10 mm Hg pressure. The resultant retrograde venous stasis due to venous congestion is suggested as a significant cause of nerve root compression. Impairment of nutrient flow to spinal nerves is present with similar low pressure." Konno et al.[49] reported that compression of cauda equina nerve roots decreased action potentials with as little as 10 mm Hg of pressure. Hause[50] proposed a mechanism of progression, where mechanical changes lead to circulatory changes, after which inflammatogenic agents produce chemical radiculitis. This, in turn, leads to disturbed flow of cerebrospinal fluid, with defective fibrinolysis and subsequent cellular changes. In addition, the influence of the sympathetic system may result in synaptic sensitization of the central and peripheral nerves, creating a "vicious circle" resulting in radicular pain. Hause also proposes that compressed nerve roots can exist without causing pain.

Compression of spinal nerves has traditionally been proposed by chiropractors as a mechanism associated with spinal subluxation.[2–9,37] Although the neural compression theory leaves many unanswered questions and contemporary research demonstrates that alternate mechanisms induce neural disturbances, the potential clinical significance of nerve compression should not be discarded.[10]

SPINAL REFLEX HYPOTHESES

It is a basic chiropractic hypothesis that abnormal spinal biomechanics and muscle dysfunction have effects, via the nervous system, throughout the body and that the chiropractic adjustment is applied not only to restore range of motion and alignment but also to cause and/or relieve reflex effects in the nervous system. In this respect the chiropractor functions not only as an engineer (correcting joint function) but also as a telecommunications specialist (influencing spinal reflexes and nerve function).[23]

Except for skilled movements, body motions are largely reflexive. Examples include heartbeat, respiratory movements, digestive activity, and postural adjustments. Reflexive responses to stimuli include muscular contraction and glandular secretion. These spinal reflexes, which are beyond voluntary control, are purposeful and exist to regulate physiologic function. Reflex arcs consist of a stimulus-activated receptor, transmission over an afferent pathway to an integration center, transmission over an efferent pathway to the effector, and induction of a reflex response[51] (Fig. 4-2). These reflexes can, however, be altered by joint subluxation or biomechanical impairment. Korr[17,18,52–54] conducted much of the basic clinical research demonstrating that prolonged nerve excitability, sustained hyperactivity of afferent receptors, and reflex response was associated with movement restriction in the spine. This association has been termed "facilitation," the "facilitated segment," or the "facilitated lesion."

Spinal adjustment, manipulation, mobilization, and pressure point therapy are proposed by Korr[42] to influence spinal reflexes in the following ways:

1. *Directly*, as a reflex therapy, through introducing a stimulus that produces a reflex response that interferes with and modifies current established reflex activity.
2. *Indirectly*, by removing spinal joint and muscle dysfunction that produces abnormal levels of spinal reflex activity, producing the facilitated lesion at a given spinal segment.

A more technical summary is provided by Akio Sato,[51] a medical physician and researcher, who states: "Manipulation performed by chiropractors excites somatic afferent fibers in the musculoskeletal structures of the spine. These afferent excitations may, in turn, provoke reflex responses affecting skeletal muscle, autonomic, hormonal, and immunologic functions. An understanding of spinal reflex physiology is, therefore, fundamental to comprehending the effects of manipulation."

Varieties of Spinal Reflexes

Three major types of spinal reflexes—somatosomatic, somatovisceral, and viscerosomatic—are referred to extensively in chiropractic, osteopathic, and medical literature. The order in which the root words are combined indicates the origin of the reflex and the site of its effect, respectively. For example, *somatovisceral* denotes that the initial stimulus or insult to the nervous system was a somatic receptor as in a spinal joint, and that the efferent reflexive manifestation or response is expressed in a visceral tissue or organ.

SOMATOSOMATIC REFLEX HYPOTHESIS

In Greek, *soma* means "body." In the somatosomatic reflex hypothesis, stimulus at one level of the soma or musculoskeletal system produces reflex activity in the nervous system, which then manifests elsewhere in the musculoskeletal system. The knee-jerk reflex is an example of a somatosomatic reflex. A light tap on the patellar ligament activates stretch receptors located within that ligament and in the tendon of the quadriceps muscle which inserts on the patella. Impulses are conducted by sensory (afferent) neurons to the central nervous system, specifically at the intersegmental L3 and L4 levels, where these neurons synapse with motor neurons in the gray matter of the spinal cord. Without conscious involvement of the brain, impulses are then conducted by motor (efferent) neurons back to the quadriceps muscle. The muscle contracts in response to the impulses traveling along its motor nerve.

In this example, a stimulus was applied to a receptor in a somatic structure, eliciting a response in another somatic structure. Similarly, stimuli to receptors in spinal structures, whether from abnormal joint or muscle tension or from chiropractic adjustment[55] or manipulative treatment[19,20,56] to

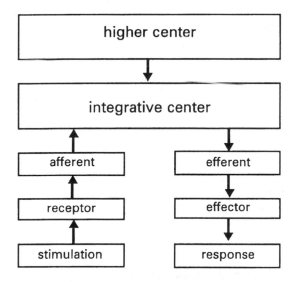

Diagram of a reflex

Figure 4-2. Diagram of a reflex. (From Sato,[51] with permission.)

relieve it, causes various spinal reflex responses in the musculoskeletal system.

It has been suggested by Wyke[19-20] that spinal manipulation stretches mechanoreceptors in the joint capsule and that this stimulus has an inhibitory effect, mediated through spinal cord interneurons, on nociceptive activity. This proposed mechanism is an adaptation of Wall's "gate control theory."[57]

A subcomponent of the somatosomatic reflex model, referred to as the proprioceptive insult hypothesis[15,58,59] suggests that receptors in the highly innervated soft tissue in and around joints may become irritated, leading to reflex modifications in postural tone and neural integration of postural activities. The proprioceptive insult hypothesis has been described in chiropractic writings[16,60,61] as undue irritation and stimulation of sensory receptors (including proprioceptors) located in the articular structures and in the parasegmental ligaments. This irritation may result when structures are under stress from derangement of the intervertebral motor units caused by subluxation. Janse[15] proposes that the afferent barrage of impulses into the nervous system may disturb equilibrium, create somatosomatic reflexes, and cause aberrant somatovisceral and somatopsychic reflexes.

Reflex muscle spasm is another example of a somatosomatic reflex.[62] This has been associated with the facilitated segment, in which muscle spasm may result from and contribute to proprioceptive irritation. It is proposed[62] that the spinal cord segments in the vicinity of a spinal fixation have a lower threshold for firing, and therefore are neurologically hyperexcitable. Korr refers to this as the "facilitated lesion."[63,64]

SOMATOVISCERAL REFLEX HYPOTHESIS

The Latin meaning of *viscera* is "internal organ." In this concept, a stimulus to nerves or receptors related to spinal structures produces reflexive responses influencing function in the visceral organs such as those in the digestive, cardiovascular, or respiratory systems.[23] Alternate terms for this form of spinal reflex are "somatosympathetic" and "somatoautonomic."

In a review of vertebrovisceral relations in a variety of cases, Lewit[40] cites an example where changes in spinal function (blockage or hypomobility) are linked to tachycardia so that when mobility of the spinal column is normalized, heart rhythm also becomes normal and remains so as long as there is no relapse in spinal column dysfunction. Lewit states that "although direct evidence of disturbed motor function causing organic heart disease is lacking, it would seem reasonable to grant it the role of a possible risk factor." Lewit uses the term *blockage* to describe spinal movement restriction, noting that the characteristic pattern of spinal hypomobility in ischemic heart disease is "blockage affecting the thoracic spine from T3 to T5, most frequently between T4 and T5, movement restriction being most noticeable to the left, and at the cervicothoracic junction." It is historically relevant that as early as the 1920s chiropractic authors such as Vedder[65] and Firth[66] recommended adjustment of "Heart Place," identified as the second and third dorsal vertebral segments, for the treatment of tachycardia.

Somatovisceral Pilot Studies: Hypertension, Dysmenorrhea, and Infantile Colic

In a 1988 randomized controlled trial involving 21 hypertensive patients, Yates et al.[67] observed significant decreases in systolic and diastolic blood pressure in the chiropractic adjustment group, while there was no significant change noted in the placebo and control groups. Adjustive procedures were applied to the T1–T5 spinal levels. In a study of 45 subjects, including experimental and "sham" manipulation control groups, Kokjohn et al.[68] concluded that spinal manipulative therapy may be an effective and safe nonpharmacologic alternative for relieving the pain and distress of primary dysmenorrhea. In a prospective study of 316 cases of infantile colic treated by chiropractors, Klougart et al.[69] found satisfactory results in 94 percent of cases receiving chiropractic care. (See Ch. 11 for more detailed discussion of these and other chiropractic research studies on visceral disorders.)

Pikalov Study on Duodenal Ulcers

Going beyond the consideration of visceral dysfunction and observing the effects of spinal adjustment or manipulation on structural visceral pathology, in a 1994 study, Pikalov and Vyatcheslav[70] demonstrated improved remission rates of actual pathology in patients with observable duodenal ulcer. The statistically significant results suggest that spinal somatic dysfunction predisposes the duodenum to disease and is a cause of the true visceral disease and pathology. Andrei Pikalov, who conducted this study, is a medical physician and physiology researcher, formerly of the Medical Research Institute at the Russian Ministry of Internal Affairs in Moscow and now a member of the research faculty of Cleveland Chiropractic College, Kansas City.

In this study, 35 adults attending the Gastroenterological Department at Moscow Central Hospital with acute, uncomplicated duodenal ulcer confirmed by endoscopic examination were examined for vertebral subluxation. Twenty-three demonstrated characteristics of subluxation, that is, displacement, spinous process tenderness, restricted motion, contracture, and painful paravertebral muscles. Spinal segments T9–12 were the most frequently affected. This again coincides with the writings of chiropractors Vedder[65] and Firth,[66] who in 1920 associated duodenal ulcer with subluxation of T9.

In the Pikalov study, patients were assigned to either a standard medical management group or a spinal manipulation group. Patients in the medical group received standard drug therapy and dietary regime over 4 to 7 weeks. For the other group, a course of spinal manipulation up to 14 treatments over a 3-week period was undertaken along with the standard dietary regime. Remission or healing took an average of 16.4 days in the manipulation group, approximately 9 days or 40 percent faster than the 25.7-day average in the medical group. The principal outcome, confirmed by endoscopic examination, was full clinical remission of the ulcer in terms of smooth healing of the lining of duodenum (epithelialization) or healing by scar formation (cicatrization). Pain resolved in 3.8 days on average in the manipulation group. The investigators speculate that possible mechanisms to explain their results include "normalization of the action of the autonomic nervous system which influences both cellular metabolism and the vasomotor dynamics of the stomach and duodenum" and "stimulation of the endogenous opiate system."

These patients did not have simulated or pseudo-ulcer (visceral disease simulation is discussed later in this chapter), but actually exhibited endoscopically observable duodenal ulcers, confirmed by photographs. The manipulation applied to relieve somatic or spinal dysfunction not only relieved the pain but apparently provided a healing effect significantly superior to standard drug therapy.

VISCEROSOMATIC REFLEX HYPOTHESIS

The viscerosomatic reflex is, logically, the opposite of the somatovisceral reflex. Respiratory or digestive dysfunction such as asthma or colic, may cause reflex disturbances in the spine leading to muscle tension and joint subluxation or dysfunction.[23] Margaret Wislowska[71] of the Institute of Clinical Medicine in Warsaw, in a study on the contribution of pain to rotation of vertebrae in the etiology and pathogenesis of lateral spinal curvature, determined that irritation of the nervous system resulting in pain in the abdominal cavity may reflexively cause symptomatic rotation of the lumbar vertebrae. In this study, 30 patients with radiographically confirmed nephrolithiasis (kidney stone) were examined; 15 with calculi in the right kidney, 15 with calculi in the left kidney. Radiographs were made during acute paroxysms of nephrolithiasis. In most cases rotation of lumbar vertebrae was observed. For comparison, 15 patients with other kidney diseases were also examined. Angles of vertebral rotation were observed in anteroposterior radiographs by measuring the relationship of the pedicle to the lateral edge of the vertebral body. Wislowska states, "in 70 percent of the patients with nephrolithiasis studied there is rotation of vertebrae towards the affected kidney." A proposed mechanism is that a viscerosomatic reflex (via visceral afferent nerves) in the kidney resulted in the muscle contraction (via somatic efferents) at segmental spinal levels correlated with sympathetic segmental innervation of the affected organ (kidney).

Based on a controlled study, Danish gastroenterologists Jorgensen and Fossgreen[72] concluded that a high correlation exists between back pain and functional gastrointestinal pain. A "functional ailment" is described as having "symptoms that are persistent, painful, and real," but where "no underlying organic problem can be found." Researchers examined the patients' spines segmentally, testing for tenderness, skin sensibility, and range of motion; 75 percent of the patients with back pain showed physical abnormalities during back examination, especially skin sensibility. Most of the spinal abnormalities were localized to the thoracic and thoracolumbar segments, "the same segments that innervate the upper gastrointestinal tract." According to Jorgensen and Fossgreen, "This suggests the existence of a connection between abdominal pain and back pain."

Jorgensen and Fossgreen suggest two possible pathophysiologic mechanisms: (1) stimulation of receptors in trigger areas of the abdomen, via nerve communication to the spinal cord, causing corresponding changes in the back (viscerosomatic reflex), or (2) irritation of nerve roots at the intervertebral foramina leading to changes in the gut (somatovisceral reflex). One may also speculate that given the "functional" nature of these clinical observations, the vertebral column is causing symptoms that are mistaken for visceral disease.

Joint Dysafferentation

The intervertebral motion segment is richly supplied with mechanoreceptive and nociceptive structures.[73–77] For this reason it has been proposed that spinal biomechanic dysfunction may result in the alteration of normal nociception and/or mechanoreception. Kent[78] proposes that, "aberrated afferent input to the central nervous system may lead to dysponesis. To use the contemporary jargon of the computer industry, 'garbage in–garbage out.'" A similar concept once known by the outdated term, "spillover hypothesis," has been used within the chiropractic profession to imply that aberrant sensory input (i.e., undue irritation of receptors) upon reaching the segmental spinal cord level may "spill over" and evoke an aberrant efferent response.

Seaman[79] proposes that restoration of afferent input is the probable mechanism by which the chiropractic adjustment affords symptom relief and health improvement. He asserts that joint restriction or dysfunction reduces large diameter afferent nerve fiber input from the mechanoreceptors in the articular capsule and from intrinsic muscles (intertransversarii and rotatores) of the spine, resulting in functional deafferentation.

Wyke[20] demonstrates that the results obtained from spinal manipulation are reflexogenic and dependent on adequate stimulation of articular mechanoreceptors. Also addressing reflexogenic effects, Seaman[55] states that "nociceptive reflexes promote the development of various components of subluxation complex." Seaman's concept of "joint dysafferentation" describes abnormal afferent input as a result of joint restriction, involving a functional decrease in the activity of large diameter mechanoreceptor afferent fibers and a simultaneous functional increase in activity of nociceptive afferent nerve fibers. Slosberg[80] has used the phrase "altered articular input" to describe this condition.

Along these lines, Lewit[40] states that "changes of mechanical function alone do not cause clinical symptoms (pain). They constitute, however, the nociceptive stimulus which produces reflex changes in the segment (muscle spasm, hyperalgesic zones, etc.). If these are of sufficient intensity to pass the pain threshold, pain is felt. The most likely nociceptive stimulus is increased tension."

Seaman's Explanation of Subluxation and Adjustment

Seaman[81] proposes that nociceptors are irritated by mechanical insult (trauma or injury, including joint restriction) and chemical irritants (toxins) (Fig. 4-3). He further proposes that the associated nociceptive axons (A-delta and C fibers) enter the spinal cord, conveying signals that excite interneurons originating in the dorsal horn, producing autonomic symptoms and pain, and also exciting visceral afferent neurons (producing sympathetic vasoconstriction) and somatic efferent neurons (producing reflex muscle spasm). The potential end result is local tissue vasoconstriction and muscle spasm which play a role in reducing joint mobility. Local nociceptors may be further irritated by this muscle spasm and sympathetic discharge into the area of injury, creating even greater spasm and vasoconstriction. Seaman states, "As the joint in question becomes more hypomobile, it is likely that the various pathologic components of subluxation complex (histopathology, inflammation, etc.) will become more pronounced and further irritate local nociceptors." (See Ch. 12 for further details on nociception.)

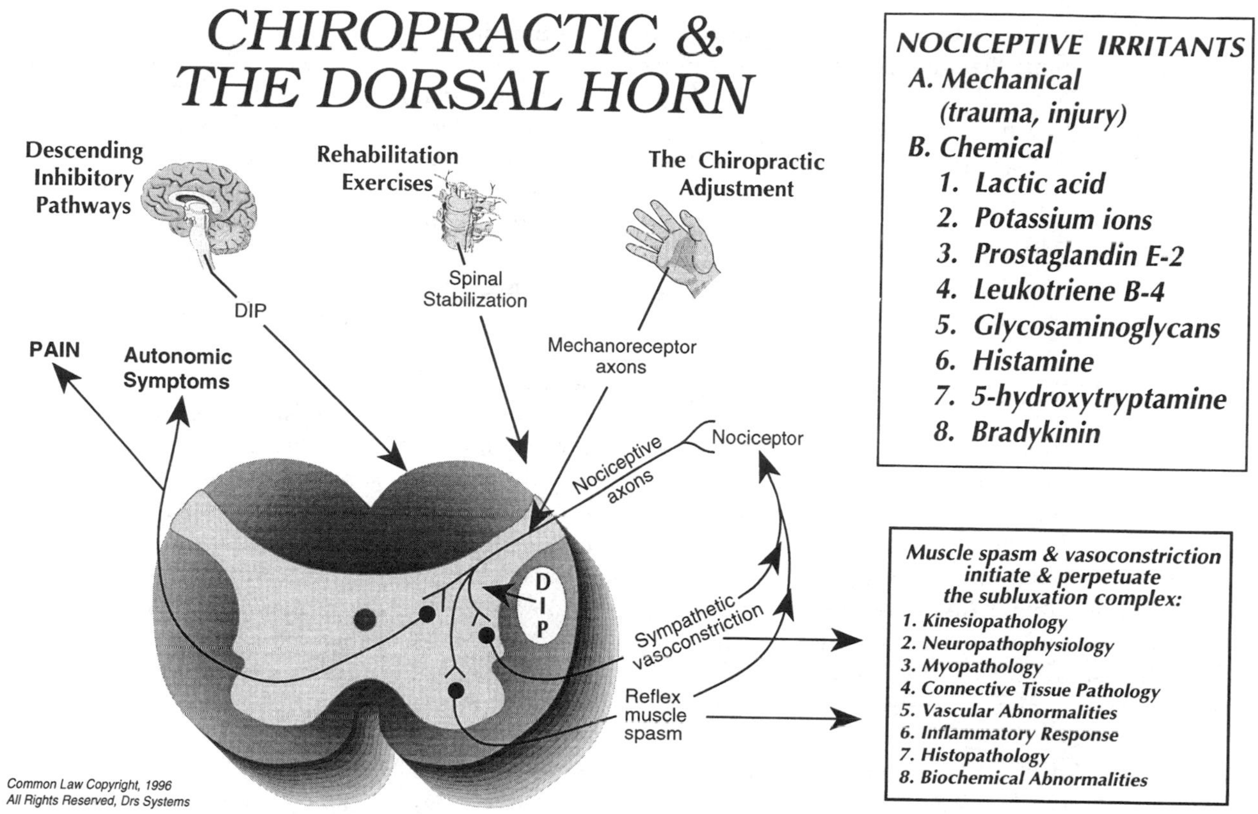

CHIROPRACTIC & THE DORSAL HORN

Descending Inhibitory Pathways

Rehabilitation Exercises

Spinal Stabilization

The Chiropractic Adjustment

DIP

PAIN

Autonomic Symptoms

Mechanoreceptor axons

Nociceptive axons

Nociceptor

D I P

Sympathetic vasoconstriction

Reflex muscle spasm

Common Law Copyright, 1996
All Rights Reserved, Drs Systems

NOCICEPTIVE IRRITANTS
A. *Mechanical*
   (trauma, injury)
B. *Chemical*
   1. *Lactic acid*
   2. *Potassium ions*
   3. *Prostaglandin E-2*
   4. *Leukotriene B-4*
   5. *Glycosaminoglycans*
   6. *Histamine*
   7. *5-hydroxytryptamine*
   8. *Bradykinin*

Muscle spasm & vasoconstriction
initiate & perpetuate
the subluxation complex:
1. *Kinesiopathology*
2. *Neuropathophysiology*
3. *Myopathology*
4. *Connective Tissue Pathology*
5. *Vascular Abnormalities*
6. *Inflammatory Response*
7. *Histopathology*
8. *Biochemical Abnormalities*

Figure 4-3. Chiropractic and the dorsal horn. (From Seaman,[81] with permission.)

Seaman[81] states that, "The adjustment serves to reduce the kinesiopathological component of the subluxation complex and as a result, most likely reduces mechanical and chemical irritation of articular nociceptors. Thus, the restoration of joint motion, with consequently reduced mechanical and chemical irritation, appears to be the direct effect that the adjustment has on the subluxation complex." As Seaman further describes the process:

The reflex effects of mechanoreceptor stimulation include the inhibition of pain, relaxation of spasmed muscles, and reduction of vasoconstriction. Thus, the adjustment appears to inhibit muscle spasm and vasoconstriction, which are known to cause general mechanical and chemical irritation of extra-articular

nociceptors ... The adjustment directly reduces mechanical and chemical irritation of articular tissues by restoring motion to restricted joints. The adjustment indirectly reduces mechanical and chemical irritation of extra-articular tissue by causing a reflex inhibition of muscle spasm and vasoconstriction. The adjustment also stimulates afferent input which drives propriospinal pathways, spinocerebellar tracts and the dorsal column system.

Descending inhibitory pathways, according to Seaman,[81] can influence the pathogenesis of the subluxation complex, as descending fibers from higher centers of the nervous system stimulate the same inhibitory interneurons as does the chiropractic adjustment. Seaman further proposes that positive emotions can influence neural pathways such that pain and sympathetic hyperactivity (vasoconstriction) are inhibited. Conversely, he presents the possibility that negative emotions and depression can have the opposite effect on these neurons, in a contemporary re-statement of D.D. Palmer's idea that "autosuggestion" is one possible cause of subluxation. If these assumptions are correct, therapies such as stress management and biofeedback may have a role in case management of the subluxation complex.[81]

SOMATIC VISCERAL DISEASE SIMULATION

Somatic dysfunction or vertebral subluxation can often simulate, or mimic, the symptoms of visceral disease. Such mimicry may mislead the diagnostician because the clinical patterns of signs and symptoms for somatic and visceral etiologies may be indistinguishable from one another. Alternate names applied to this concept include: pseudo-visceral disease, organ disease mimicry, somatic visceral disease mimicry syndromes, and somatic simulation syndromes.

Nanzel and Szlazak[82] challenge the somatovisceral theory which claims that somatic dysfunction is capable of causing true visceral disease. They present instead the idea of "visceral disease simulation" to explain patients with apparent visceral disease that responds dramatically to a spinal manipulative thrust. Numerous authors[2–9,39,40,65–69,83–86] have proposed theories regarding a vertebrogenic or vertebroviscera relationship associated with the dramatic changes in visceral symptoms following vertebral joint adjustment or spinal manipulation. A central premise of the various theories of somatovisceral disease is "that the patients involved in these rather 'miraculous' clinical situations were really suffering from true visceral disease."[82]

After an extensive literature review, Nansel and Szlazak[82] propose that somatic pain, combined with the complex patterns of symptoms and signs, often is "virtually identical to and, therefore, easily mistaken for those induced by primary visceral disease." Such "pseudo" or "simulated" visceral disease syndromes may often result in misdiagnoses. These somatic visceral disease mimicry syndromes, as proposed, may account for perceived miraculous "cures" of presumed visceral disease in response to spinal manipulation.

Somatically induced visceral disease was described in the 1930s work of Lewis and Kellgren,[87] in which hypertonic saline was injected into deep somatic paraspinal structures. This resulted in diffuse, regional pain referral patterns identical to those characteristic of certain internal organ disease. This noxious stimulation of somatic tissues often evoked a variety of associated somatic and autonomic reflexes, including hyperalgesia, reflex muscle spasm, increased heart rate and blood pressure.

The explanation for visceral disease mimicry, according to Nansel and Szlazak, is that phylogenitically primitive visceral afferent nerves transmit nociceptive information from internal organs, and that equally primitive somatic afferents are involved in transmission of nociceptive information from deep connective tissue (e.g., bone, joint capsules, ligaments, tendons, fascia muscles). These two afferent pathways, "converge on common pools of interneurons within the spinal cord and brainstem." With somatic afferent and visceral afferent signals subsequently transmitted into common central nervous system pathways, afferent neuronal convergence within the spinal cord may lead to clinical manifestations which are difficult to identify as being of visceral or somatic origin. That is, facilitation of the common neuronal pool by either visceral or somatic inputs results in common sets of somatic, autonomic, and neuroendocrine responses leading to indistinguishable sets of signs and symptoms (Fig. 4-4).

Melzack and Wall[88] and Milne et al[89] have shown that nociceptive stimuli from all structures in a segment converge to cells in the lamina V of the basal spinal nucleus of the spinal cord. This also applies to pain signals from receptors in the zygopophyseal joints as well as pain receptors in the walls of blood vessels. Lewit[40] therefore proposes that the locomotor system (spinal column), "can readily simulate visceral pain, and vice versa, and that this constitutes an important aspect to be taken into account in differential diagnosis."

An illustrated synopsis of segmentally related pain referral patterns observed by various investigators is presented in Figure 4-5.[82] From a historical perspective, these pain patterns are in part similar (at least with respect to cutaneous pain distribution) to early chiropractic observations[2,9] from "nerve tracing," an early chiropractic palpation procedure.[9] In nerve tracing, the chiropractor palpated along the

SIMULATED VISCERAL DISEASE MODEL

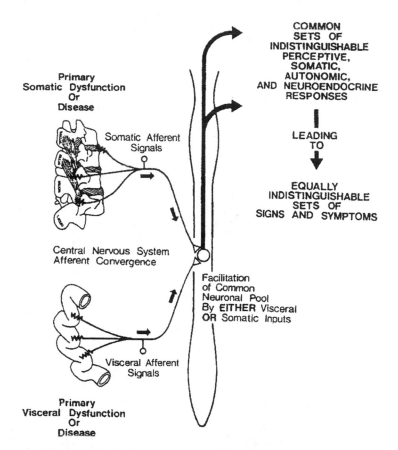

Figure 4-4. Schematic depiction of the basic neurologic mechanism by which dysfunction confined to purely somatic structures is capable of producing signs and symptoms that are identical to those typically associated with primary dysfunction involving various internal organs. It is now well-established that afferent fibers that transmit nociceptive information from deep somatic structures converge on the same central neuronal pools as do the independent afferent fibers that transmit noxious stimuli from regionally related visceral structures. It presents a challenge for the diagnostician that subsequent relaying of either of these two sources of afferent information by this convergent pool of neurons into other common central pathways can often result in overt patterns of signs and symptoms that may be virtually indistinguishable with respect to their somatic versus visceral etiologies. The fact that somatic dysfunction can often mimic, or simulate, the symptoms of visceral disease (and be easily mistaken for it), is supported by an impressive amount of experimental and clinical scientific data. (From Nansel and Szlazak,[82] with permission.)

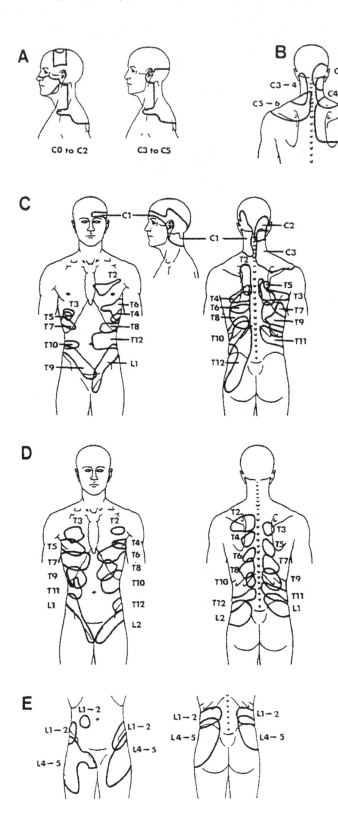

Figure 4-5. Segmentally related referred pain patterns observed over the years by a number of independent investigators immediately after the experimental noxious stimulation over purely somatic paraspinal structures. The illustrations shown above are composite representations of results obtained by **(A)** Campbell and Parsons;[115] **(B)** Dwyer et al;[117] **(C)** Feinstein et al;[118] **(D)** Kellgren;[114] and **(E & F)** McCall et al.[116] Interestingly, the intensity, distribution and affective characteristics of the pain perceptions induced in these normal experimental subjects were often found to be astonishingly similar to those typically exhibited by patients known to be suffering from a variety of primary internal organ diseases or conditions. The diffuse pain referral patterns elicited in these subjects were also often accompanied by a number of additional secondary regional and/or global reflex-based signs and symptoms that were also virtually identical to (and therefore easily mistaken for) those commonly observed in patients harboring true primary visceral disease (see Fig. 4-4). Over the last 50 years, a significant amount of both experimental and clinical information has accumulated in the scientific literature concerning somatic pain syndromes and basic neuronal mechanisms that may often conspire to create overt patterns of signs and symptoms that mimic or simulate those classically associated with a number of regionally related primary visceral disorders. (From Nansel and Szlazak,[82] with permission.)

path of tenderness over "impinged nerves" efferently or afferently (e.g., from the spinal tissues to the site of symptoms and vice versa). Nerve tracing, the tracing of tenderness from a point of emergence from the spine to a point at the periphery was an outgrowth of the Meric system.[90] (See Ch. 11 for further discussion of the Meric system.) Early chiropractic writings[9] considered such tenderness the "cry of nature" or "innate intelligence" indicating that a nerve was affected. The early practitioners considered nerve tracing to be not only a valuable clinical tool, but "very convincing to the patient, for the patient is the only one who can distinguish

between nerves that are tender or affected and those that are not.[9]

Nansel and Szlazak[82] take the position that primary dysfunction of somatic structures of the spinal column cannot cause regionally or segmentally related visceral (internal organ) disease, and that no clinical evidence supports the notion of a regionally or segmentally induced "somato-visceral disease" connection. Furthermore, they assert that the autonomic nervous system does not seem capable of inducing frank tissue disease in any organ it innervates. A well-referenced list developed by these investigators (Table 4-1) presents a correlation of

Table 4-1. Some Somatically Induced Symptoms and the Visceral Disorders That They Simulate or Mimic

Signs and Symptoms	Simulated Visceral Disorders
Referred head, face, eye, ear, sinus, mouth, dental, throat pain and/or hyperesthesias and/or dysesthesias	Pseudomigraine and cluster headache, pseudo–temporal arteritis, pseudo–trigeminal neuralgias, pseudo-Menier's, pseudo–otitis media, pseudoptosis, pseudosinusitis or rhinitis, pseudopharyngitis, pseudolaryngitis, pseudo–cranial nerve involvement
Narrowing of the palpebral fissure	
Vertigo/dizziness, blurred vision, light or sound intolerance, tinnitus, diminished/muffled hearing, difficulty swallowing, sense of object in throat, hoarseness, dysphonia	
Erythemia, sweating, nausea, vomiting, sinus congestion, and runny nose (coryza)	
Referred chest, breast, shoulder, arm pain and/or hyperesthesias, and/or dysesthesias	Pseudo–cardiac angina, pseudo–breast disease, pseudo asthma, pseudo pleurisy
Difficulty breathing/dyspnea	
Sweating, pallor, cardiac palpitations and arrhythmias, anomalous resting and/or treadmill electrocardiographic findings	
Abdominal pain and/or hyperesthesias and/or dysesthesias and/or cramping, pyrosis, intestinal colic, epigastric discomfort after meals (dyspepsia)	Pseudo–peptic ulcer, pseudo–duodenal ulcer, pseudo–gastric ulcer, pseudocholelithiasis, pseudocholycystitis, pseudoappendicitis, pseudoabdominal/intestinal disorders
Food intolerance, irritable bowel	
Sense of abdominal fullness (bloating)	
Hyperperistalsis of intestines (borborygmus)	
Nausea, vomiting, belching, flatulence, constipation, diarrhea	
Urinary urgency/irritable bladder, renal, loin, urethral, pelvic, perineal/ groin/rectal pain and/or hyperesthesias and/or dysesthesias, urge for defecation, dysmenorrhea, dyspareunia, dysuria	Pseudorenal and urinary tract disorders, pseudoendometriosis, pseudosalpingitis, pseudo–pelvic inflammatory disease, pseudo–pelvic disorders
Stress incontinence	

(From Nansel and Szlazak,[82] with permission)

regionally related patterns of signs and symptoms that often result from primary somatic dysfunction, together with a collection of primary visceral conditions that such patterns of signs and symptoms have been shown to mimic or simulate.

Nansel and Szlazak[82] affirm that afferent nociceptive signals generated from dysfunctional deep somatic structures can often result in the referred pain patterns, along with a number of equally misleading autonomic reflex responses. These reflex responses have been shown to simulate (rather than cause) true visceral disease because of their convergence on the same pools of central nervous system neurons that also receive afferent input from regionally related internal organs.

The concept of somatic visceral disease simulation provides an alternative explanation for the apparent effectiveness of a variety of somatic therapeutic interventions in patients presumed to be suffering from true visceral disease. Nansel and Szlazak[82] conclude that the existence of these somatic visceral disease mimicry syndromes justifies cooperation between medical physicians and health care providers such as chiropractors who specialize in the evaluation and treatment of primary somatic dysfunction.

DECREASED AXOPLASMIC TRANSPORT

The consequences of vertebral subluxation or spinal biomechanical impairments include pain and other sensory manifestations, as well as motor and autonomic disturbances. Manifestations discussed thus far have related to disturbances in excitation and conduction of nerve impulses. The impulse-based mechanisms underlying these clinical manifestations seem to be initiated through either direct insult to nerves and nerve roots or altered sensory input from affected joints, ligaments, tendons, and muscles.

Another component of neural function, also proposed to be affected by vertebral subluxation and related musculoskeletal problems is axoplasmic transport. This is a nonimpulse mechanism based not on transmission of signals along the surface of the neuronal neurolemma, but rather on the intra-axonal transport and exchange of macromolecular materials. This involves a neurotrophic relationship between neurons and end organs or target cells.[42] Terms such as *end organs*, *target cells*, and *postsynaptic cells* refer to organs supplied or affected by a nerve.

It is now well established[91–98] that macromolecular substances are synthesized in the nerve cell body, packaged by Golgi apparatus, and transported within the axon to the terminal ending of the neuron. They are released at the synapse and then exert a subtle influence to maintain proper vitality and function of the target issues. The axoplasmic transport system may convey material at a rate up to 400 mm/day.[95,96] Chemicals transported by this process are collectively known as trophic substances, and have been found to be essential for the maintenance of proper tissue function and morphology.[91–102]

Within the context of this discussion, *trophic* means "relating to growth." In the neuroscience literature[94] trophic influence on the peripheral nervous system refers to (1) the influence of the nervous system on differentiation and development of structures into mature end organs, and (2) the role of trophic function in maintenance of end organs.

To distinguish trophic function from the neuron's function of conducting nerve impulses to the end organ, Guth's[93,94] definition of trophic function —"those interactions between nerves and other cells which initiate or control molecular modification in the other cell"—is most appropriate. This definition may be restated as follows: trophic function influences the development and maintenance of chemical changes in cells supplied by the nerve.

The nerve impulse is a fast-acting *nerve membrane phenomenon* (120 m/sec), in contrast to the much slower (up to 400 mm/day ±50)[95,96] intracellular or intraneuronal transport mechanism conveying the trophic influence to target end organs.

Swartz[91] describes the complex transport systems that have evolved to carry large molecules formed in the nerve cell body. These chemicals are carried the full length of the axon to the terminals, after which materials from the terminals are returned to the cell body for reprocessing. Two forms of intracellular transport are identified. The slower kind, axoplasmic flow, conveys materials only from the cell body toward the nerve fiber terminals; the faster form, axonal transport, carries materials in both directions.

Studies by Weiss and colleagues in 1948, as described by Swartz[91] first proved experimentally that substances originating in the neuronal cell body move at a steady rate along the axon (Fig. 4-6). The experimental procedure involved surgical constriction of branches of the sciatic nerve in rats, chickens, and monkeys. After several weeks, examination of the region just above (proximal) the constricted axon demonstrated swelling. This suggested that "axoplasm had accumulated behind the blockade." Furthermore, "The portion of the axon beyond (distal) the constriction had degenerated." Weiss removed the constriction, timed the movement of material, and observed that, "the accumulated axoplasm progressed down the regenerating fibers at a constant rate of one or two millimeters a day."[91] Chiropractors may note a similarity between this observation and B.J. Palmer's simplified "foot on hose" analogy, historically presented to the public as a description of the effects of nerve compression (Fig. 4-7).

KORR'S EXPLANATION OF TROPHIC INFLUENCES

Examples of trophic influences on target tissues as adapted from Korr[42] include the following:

1. *Atrophy of denervation.* An example is the atrophy skeletal muscle undergoes after denervation. It appears that the integrity of the connection between the nerve and muscle, rather than the impulses to the muscle, is the critical factor. When observing the effects of removing the

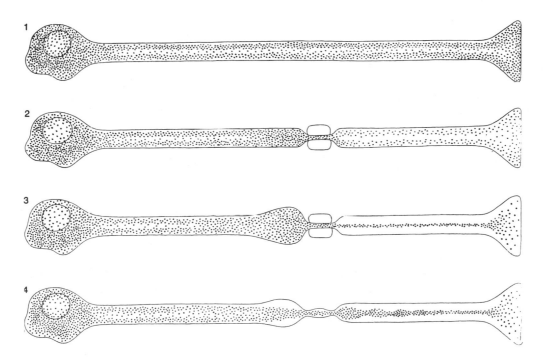

Figure 4-6. Constriction experiments done at the University of Chicago in 1948 by Paul A. Weiss and his colleagues demonstrated that material from the cell body of a neuron moves along the axon at a steady rate. The experiment is depicted here schematically for a single mature nerve fiber (1), with the cell body at the left and the axon leading away from it to the nerve terminal at right. A constricting cuff was applied to the fiber (2). After several weeks the axon was swollen above the constriction (3) and reduced in size below it, showing that the axoplasm (the material from the cell body) had been dammed up by the constriction. It flowed again (4) when the cuff was taken off. (From Swartz,[91] with permission.)

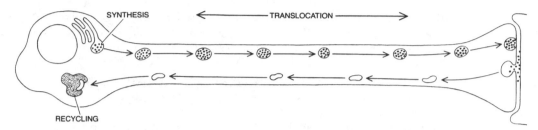

SYNTHESIS ⟵──── TRANSLOCATION ────⟶

RECYCLING

Figure 4-7. Life cycles of vesicles and other membranous organelles involved in the transmission of nerve signals at a synapse (the specialized region of contact between a nerve terminal and another neuron or a muscle cell) begins with their synthesis in the cell body. Organelles move outward along the axon by fast axonal transport. Some of the material is deposited along the axon to maintain the axolemma, the external membrane along which the electrical cells are propagated, and some, including the synaptic vesicles, is delivered to the terminal. The material is then returned to the cell body in retrograde movement, also by fast transport, and there it is either restored or destroyed. (From Swartz,[91] with permission.)

nerve supply from the sensory organ, it is the connectedness between two kinds of cells that has been demonstrated to be the crucial issue. Sensory organs are the initiators of the nerve impulses, not receivers. In the case of gustatory organs (tastebuds), these structures undergo trophic changes or even complete dedifferentiation upon denervation.[97,98] Recovery or restoration of the tastebuds follows soon after reinnervation.[94]

2. *Morphogenetic influences.* In embryonic development complete differentiation and development of muscle requires that nerve supply reach the muscle and that a myoneural junction be established. Hix[99] demonstrated that renal innervation prepares the kidney for response to circulating growth factors. When a pup is deprived of that preparation by denervation in the first few days of postnatal life, kidney development is arrested.

3. *Role of nerve in regeneration:* Certain amphibia are capable of regenerating entire limbs and tails after amputation. Singer[100] demonstrated that regeneration of the amputated forelimb of the newt is prevented by denervation of the fibers coursing towards the amputated stump. Furthermore, only portions of the fibers are required to sustain regeneration and sensory fibers serve this function.

4. *Regulation of genic expression:* Gutman[101] and Guth[102] propose that the nerve that grows into a muscle in the course of embryonic development determines which genes of that muscle's cells will be repressed and which will be expressed. For example, red and white muscles are known to differ morphologically, functionally, and chemically. Their chemical differences include those related to proteins, enzymes, and metabolic pathways.[103] Surgical section of nerves and cross-reinnervation of red and white muscles are followed by a high degree of cross-transformation. Korr[42] interprets this metabolic transformation to be an expression of neurally mediated genetic influence, in which the nerve instructs the muscle what kind of muscle to become.

5. *Nerve-to-muscle transmission:* Another example of neurally influenced genic expression and repression occurs in the transmission from nerve to muscle at the myoneural junction. Receptor molecules for acetylcholine, which is released by the nerve terminals, are normally restricted to the area of the muscle surface where the myoneural junction is located.[42] Cutting the nerve causes the entire surface of muscle cell to become acetylcholine sensitive, in response to removal of the repressive influence of the nerve on the synthesis of the protein receptor molecules in the "extrajunctional areas."[104]

CLINICAL IMPLICATIONS OF AXOPLASMIC TRANSPORT

According to multiple authorities,[91–104] peripheral nerves not only conduct impulses to or from non-neuronal cells and tissues that they innervate, but also exert long-term influences on these end-organs through trophic or neurotrophic influences that are essential for their development, growth, and maintenance.

Korr[42] proposes that:

> Any factor that causes derangement of transport mechanisms in the axon or that chronically alters the quality or quantity of the axonally transported substances could cause the trophic influences to become detrimental. This alteration in turn would produce aberrations of structure, function, and metabolism, thereby contributing to dysfunction and disease.

One such cause is direct mechanical insult such as deformations of nerves and roots, including compression, stretching, angulation and torsion, "that occur commonly and that … disturb the intraaxonal transport mechanisms, intraneural microcirculation." Moreover, "neural structures are especially vulnerable in their passage over highly mobile joints, through bony canals, intervertebral foramina; fascial layers, and tonical contracted muscles."

An additional factor, also biomechanic in origin is, "sustained hyperactivity of peripheral neurons (sensory, motor, and autonomic) related to those portions of the spinal cord associated with intervertebral strain or other types of somatic dysfunction."[105] Korr concludes, "sustained high rates of impulse-discharge place increased energy demands on the affected neurons thus affecting their metabolism and … their synthesis and turnover of proteins and other macromolecules … such intense activity does impair axonal transport, and … trophic interchange with other cells."

NEURODYSTROPHIC HYPOTHESIS

Neurodystrophy is the proposition that neural dysfunction is stressful to viscera and other body structures, which may modify immune responses and alter the trophic function of involved nerves.[106,107] In its most basic form it may be reduced to D.D.

Palmer's assertion that "lowered tissue resistance is the cause of disease."[2] According to the neurodystrophic hypothesis, spinal biochemical insult to nerves may affect intraneural axoplasmic transport mechanisms and in turn affect the quality of neurotrophic influence and molecular (chemical) changes in the cells. This decrease in trophic factors is understood to render innervated structures vulnerable to dysfunction or disease.

CLINICAL CONSIDERATIONS

We have now examined a variety of hypotheses that seek to explain the cause and effect relationship between altered spinal biomechanics and clinical manifestations, dysfunction, and disease. How may these hypotheses be conceptually applied so as to enhance the chiropractor's understanding in a particular clinical situation?

Lewit[40] presents the following explanations of "vertebrovisceral correlations" in his text, *Manipulative Therapy in the Rehabilitation of the Locomotor System:*

1. The vertebral column (locomotor system) is causing or mimicking symptoms that are mistaken for visceral disease.
2. The visceral disease is causing a reflex reaction resulting in the hypomobility or fixation of the corresponding vertebral segment.
3. The visceral disease that reflexively caused restricted segmental mobility has subsided, but the hypomobility remains, causing symptoms simulating visceral disease (as in no. 1).
4. Disturbance of the vertebral locomotor segment is causing visceral disease.

Readers may consult Lewit's text for an expanded presentation on a variety of visceral disorders and their associated segmental spinal relationships.

Keeping Lewit's four choices in mind, consider the following clinical experience presented by Chapman-Smith[23] in *The Chiropractic Report:*

Mr. A.T., a 56-year-old dairy farmer complaining of chest pain that feels like "a tire around my chest", is referred by his family physician to a cardiologist. Examinations including imaging, ECGs, and exercise stress tests, reveal many classic signs and symptoms of myocardial ischemia—deep chest and arm pain, paleness, sweating, cardiac dysrhythmia, and coronary arteriosclerosis.

Mr. A.T. is told he has a heart problem and is treated accordingly. He is advised to stop strenuous physical work and change his occupation. However, the medications prescribed, nitrates, then beta-blockers, are ineffective. Faced with the sale of his farm and anxious to find something that might help, he seeks the advice of a chiropractor.

Chiropractic examination reveals joint subluxation, with restricted joint range of motion and muscle tension in the lower cervical and upper thoracic spine. Palpation of the two top segments in the thoracic spine reproduces the cardiac pain. Radiographs show marked narrowing of the intervertebral foramina at C6/C7.

Following a short course of spinal manipulation, designed to restore normal function to the spinal segments and paraspinal muscles and to relieve irritations of the spinal nerve roots, joint function is normal and pain relieved. Mr. A.T. returns to his normal farm work and lifestyle, and has no further symptoms.

Chapman-Smith adapted this case from one cited by Kunert, a German cardiologist. In his paper, *Functional Disorders of Internal Organs Due to Vertebral Lesions*,[108] Kunert states:

We have records of numerous cases similar to the one described here, in which a definite connection appears to exist between a functional disorder in an internal organ and a spinal lesion … Lesions of the spinal column are perfectly capable of simulating, accentuating, or making a major contribution to (organic) disorders. There can, in fact, be no doubt that the state of the spinal column does have bearing on the functional status of the internal organs.

Chapman-Smith then applies Lewit's vertebrovisceral correlations as possible explanations for Mr. A.T.'s case. He proposes these possibilities:

1. The spinal or somatic problem (subluxation) is simulating or mimicking heart disease.
2. Heart disease and pain have caused a reflex reaction in the spine and paraspinal muscles. The resulting spinal dysfunction (subluxation) then exaggerates or mimics cardiac pain.
3. Heart disease has caused subluxation as in (2), the underlying disease has now subsided, and the spinal lesion gives symptoms simulating continuing heart disease.
4. Spinal subluxation is causing heart disease, maybe through altered somatovisceral reflexes which, either alone or together with other stressors, cause ischemia and disease.

In view of the explanations proposed above regarding patients such as Mr. A.T., it appears necessary that cardiologists and other health practitioners be educated regarding the possible role of subluxation or spinal biomechanical lesion, and its potential role in presumed cardiac pain and other visceral manifestations.

NEUROBIOLOGIC RELATIONS: A REVIEW

Various hypotheses proposing explanation for the apparent effects associated with subluxation and nerve system function have been presented in the chapter. A close interface between spinal biomechanics and nerve function has been established.[40,42,105,109–112] The nervous system has been identified as a major and central mediator of the clinical effects of spinal manipulative therapy, and/or the chiropractic adjustment.[42,105,112] Gutziet, as cited by Lewit,[40] characterizes the spinal column as the "initiator, provoker, multiplier, and localizer" of the pathogenesis of certain diseases. Lewit[40] maintains that any disturbance of function in a single motor segment will have repercussions throughout the body axis and must be compensated, and that once the lesion becomes painful, it is the nervous system that determines how intensely the spinal segment will manifest clinically.

Symptoms resulting from biomechanical impairments of the musculoskeletal system that are responsive to spinal manipulative therapy and/or spinal adjustment encompass sensory manifestations, including pain, as well as motor and autonomic disturbances.[16,40,42,50,52–54,105,109–112] Spinal biomechanic dysfunction (vertebral subluxation) and associated nervous system manifestations appear to be initiated by impulse-based and nonimpulse-based mechanisms.[42]

Impulse-based Neural Mechanisms

Insult to the impulse-based neural mechanisms occurs through:

1. Direct insult to the nerves and nerve roots resulting from compression, torsion, stretching, or angulation due to adhesions[41] or foraminal encroachment.[2–7,9–13,25] Neural structures are vulnerable in their passage over highly mobile joints, intervertebral foramina, fascial layers, and tonically contracted muscles.[25,37,41,42,48,49]

2. Altered sensory input (sustained hyperactivity) from affected muscles, tendons, ligaments, and joints producing aberrant somatosomatic and somatovisceral spinal reflexes.[16,23,42,57,81] Undue irritation to nociceptors in visceral organs is proposed to contribute to aberrant sensory input at intersegmental spinal levels, resulting in abnormal viscerosomatic reflexes and changes in paraspinal musculature that may contribute to spinal joint hypomobility and/or subluxation.[15,42,62,81] Given that somatic afferent and visceral afferent signals converge equally into common central nervous system pathways at intersegmental spinal levels, vertebral subluxation or spinal dysfunction may simulate or mimic symptoms of visceral disease, potentially misleading diagnosticians in all health professions.[83,87]

Nonimpulse-based Neural Mechanisms

Interference with nonimpulse-based neural mechanisms results in decreased axoplasmic transport of neurotrophic factors to the terminal ending of the nerve.[42] Such trophic factors influence chemical changes at the molecular level affecting the development, growth, and maintenance of end organs in tissue supplied by the nerve.[91–105] This mechanism is not based on the transmission of nerve impulses, but on the transport and exchange of macromolecular materials via intra-axonal transport and neurotrophic relationships between neurons and the postsynaptic or target cells.[42,91–93,102,103] The sustained high rates of impulse discharge proposed to result from altered joint function, place increased energy demands on the affected neurons, thus affecting synthesis and turnover of proteins and other macromolecules and impairing axonal transport and trophic interchange with other cells. The intra-axonal transport mechanisms may be affected either by direct deformation of the nerve through mechanical insult, or by altered activity or sustained hyperactivity of sensory receptors. This alteration may in turn produce aberrations of structure, function, and metabolism, thus contributing to dysfunction and disease.

It is difficult to know which hypothesis or combination of hypotheses provides the most plausible explanation in a given clinical situation. What is known is that there is a close interface between spinal biomechanics and nerve function, and that the effects of the vertebral subluxation can best be understood by thorough analysis of the various aspects of this relationship.

Terminology

axoplasmic flow
axoplasmic transport
chronic cervical syndrome
denervation
dysafferentation
dysmenorrhea
dysponesis
end organ
facilitation
functional ailment
interpedicular zone
kinematics
nerve compression hypothesis
nerve interference
nerve sheaths
neurodystrophic hypothesis
mechanoreceptor
morphology
proprioception
reflex arc
sham manipulation
somatosomatic reflex hypothesis
somatovisceral reflex hypothesis
transforaminal ligaments

visceral disease simulation
viscerosomatic reflex hypothesis

Review Questions

1. Discuss the anatomic differences between the intervertebral foramina in the cervical, dorsal, and lumbar regions. How do these differences influence the relevance of the nerve compression hypothesis for these three areas?

2. What was a flaw in Crelin's attempt to refute chiropractic claims regarding spinal nerve pressure?

3. How might the presence of transforaminal ligaments affect the course of a back pain patient's recovery?

4. Discuss the knee jerk reflex as an example of a somatosomatic reflex.

5. Identify two studies that provide clinical support for the assertion that chiropractic adjustments affect somatovisceral reflex responses.

6. What is the significance of Pikalov's study on duodenal ulcers?

7. Discuss Seaman's theory of joint dysafferentation.

8. What are some arguments for and against Nansel and Szlazak's presentation on somatic visceral disease simulation?

9. How does axoplasmic transport differ from nerve impulse transmission?

10. What are Lewit's four explanations of vertebrovisceral correlations?

Concept Questions

1. If a patient's visceral symptoms disappear after a chiropractic adjustment, does this mean that the adjustment cured or relieved a visceral disorder? What other possible explanations exist? What kind of evidence is necessary to justify a claim that chiropractic did in fact bring resolution of a visceral disorder?

2. How might enhanced cooperation between chiropractors and medical physicians benefit patients with visceral symptoms?

References

1. Vernon H: Basic scientific evidence for chiropractic subluxation. p. 35. In Gatterman M (ed): Foundations of Chiropractic—Subluxation. CV Mosby, St. Louis, 1995

2. Palmer DD: The Science, Art and Philosophy of Chiropractic—The Chiropractor's Adjuster. Portland Printing House, Portland, OR, 1910

3. Palmer BJ: The Science of Chiropractic—Its Principles and Philosophies. Vol. I. Palmer School of Chiropractic, Davenport, IA, 1906

4. Beatty HG: Anatomical Adjusting Technique. 2nd Ed. self published, Denver, 1937

5. Firth JN: A Textbook on Chiropractic Symptomatology. Firth Drifill Printing Co., Rock Island, IL, 1914

6. Forster AL: Principles and Practice of Spinal Adjustment for the Use of Students and Practitioners. National School of Chiropractic, Chicago, 1915

7. Loban JM: Technic and Practice of Chiropractic. Universal Chiropractic College, Davenport, IA, 1912

8. Janse J, Houser R, Wells B: Chiropractic Principles and Technic. National College, Chicago, 1947

9. Cleveland CS Sr: Chiropractic Principles and Practice—Outline. Kansas City, 1950

10. Kent C: Models of vertebral subluxation: a review. J Vertebral Subluxation Res 1(1):11, 1996

11. Cramer G, Darby S: Anatomy Related to Spinal Subluxation. p. 18. In Gatterman MI (ed): Foundations of Chiropractic—Subluxation. CV Mosby, St. Louis, 1995

12. DePalma AF, Rothman RF: The Intervertebral Disc. WB Saunders, Philadelphia, 1970

13. Jackson R: The Cervical Syndrome. Charles C Thomas, Springfield, IL, 1976

14. Herbst R (ed): Gonstead Chiropractic Science and Art: The Chiropractic Methodology of Clarence S. Gonstead, D.C. Sci-Chi Publications, Mt. Horeb, WI, undated

15. Janse J: History of the Development of Chiropractic Concepts: Chiropractic Terminology. In Goldstein M (ed): The Research Status of Spinal Manipulative Therapy. Monog No. 15. HEW/NINCDS, Bethesda, 1975

16. Korr IM, Thomas PE, Wright HM: A mobile instrument for recording electrical skin resistance patterns of the human trunk. p. 41. In Korr IM (ed): The Collected Papers of Irvin M. Korr. American Academy of Osteopathy, Colorado Springs, 1979

17. Korr IM: The concept of facilitation and its origins. p. 148. In Korr IM (ed): The Collected Papers of Irvin M. Korr. American Academy of Osteopathy, Colorado Springs, 1979

18. Denslow J, Korr IM, Krems A: Quantitative studies of chronic facilitation in human motoneuron pools.

p. 18. In Korr IM (ed): The Collected Papers of Irvin M. Korr. American Academy of Osteopathy, Colorado Springs, 1979

19. Wyke BD: Articular neurology: a review. Physiotherapy 58:94, 1972

20. Wyke BD: Articular Neurology and Manipulative Therapy. p. 72. In Glasgow EF, Towmey LT, Schull ER et al (eds): Aspects of Manipulative Therapy. 2nd Ed. Churchill Livingstone, Melbourne, 1985

21. Kirkaldy-Willis HK: Managing Low Back Pain. Churchill Livingstone, New York, 1983

22. Crelin ES: A Scientific Test of the Chiropractic Theory. Am Sci 61:574, 1973

23. Chapman-Smith D: Chiropractic research in the centennial year. Part II. Chiropractic Rep 9:1, 1995

24. Plaintiff Exhibit 1483A. Handwritten letter from E.S. Crelin to Ray Sullivan of Connecticut State Medical Society, January 4, 1974. Anti-trust exhibit provided by McAndrews G in *Wilk v. AMA*

25. Hadley LA: Anatomico-Roentgenographic Studies of the Spine. Charles C Thomas, Springfield, IL, 1976

26. Seaman DR: Chiropractic and Pain Control. 3rd Ed. DRS Systems, Hendersonville, NC, 1995

27. Lantz CA: The vertebral subluxation complex. p. 149. In Gatterman MI (ed): Foundations of Chiropractic—Subluxation. CV Mosby, St. Louis, 1995

28. Davis D: Respiratory manifestations of dorsal spine radiculitis simulating cardiac asthma. Ann Intern Med 32:954, 1950

29. Marshall LL, Thethewie ER, Curtain CC: Chemical radiculitis: a clinical, physiological and immunological study. Clin Orthop 129:61, 1977

30. Howe JF, Loeser JD, Calvin WH: Mechanosensitivity of dorsal root ganglia and chronically injured axons: a physiological basis for radicular pain of nerve root compression. Pain 3:25, 1977

31. Giles LFG: A histological investigation of human lower lumbar intervertebral canal (foramen) dimensions. J Manipul Physiol Ther 17:4, 1994

32. Golub B, Silverman B: Transforaminal ligaments of the lumbar spine. J Bone Joint Surg 51:947, 1969

33. Bachop W, Hilgendorf C: Transforaminal ligaments of the human lumbar spine, abstracted. Anat Rec 99(4):14a, 1981

34. Bakkum BW: The effects of transforamental ligaments on the sizes of T11-L5 human intervertebral foramina. J Manipul Physiol Ther 17:517, 1994

35. Bachop W, Janse J: The corporotransverse ligament at the intervertebral foramen, abstracted. Anat Rec 205(3):13a, 1983

36. Amonoo-Kuoffi HS, el-Badawi MG, Fatani JA et al: Ligament associated with lumbar intervertebral foramina. 1. L1 to L4. J Anatomy 156:177, 1988

37. Sunderland S: Meningeal-neural relations in the intervertebral foramen. J Neurosurg 40:756, 1974

38. Korr IM: The Physiological Basis of Osteopathic Medicine. Postgraduate Institute of Osteopathic Medicine and Surgery, New York, 1970

39. Greenman PE: Principles of Manual Medicine. 2nd Ed. Williams & Wilkins, Baltimore, 1996

40. Lewit K: Manipulative Therapy in Rehabilitation of the Locomotor System. 2nd Ed. Butterworth-Heinemann, Oxford, 1991

41. Panjabi M, Takata M, Goel V. Kinematics of the lumbar intervertebral foramen. Spine 8:348, 1983

42. Korr IM. The spinal cord as organizer of disease processes. IV. Axonal transport and neurotrophic function in relation to somatic dysfunction. J Am Osteopath Assoc 80:451, 1981

43. Adams W: The blood supply of nerves. II. The effects of exclusion of its regional sources of supply on the sciatic nerve of the rabbit. J Anat 77:243, 1943

44. Sunderland S: Nerves and Nerve Injuries. Williams & Wilkins, Baltimore, 1968

45. Sunderland S, Bradley K: Stress-strain phenomena in human spinal nerve roots. Brain 84:120, 1961

46. Rydevik B, Lundborg G, Bagge U: Pathoanatomy and pathophysiology of nerve root compression. Spine 9:7, 1984

47. Sharpless SK: Susceptibility of spinal roots to compression block. p. 155. In Goldstein M (ed): The Research Status of Spinal Manipulative Therapy. Monog No. 15. HEW/NINCDS, Bethesda, 1975

48. Rydevik BL: The effects of compression on the physiology of nerve roots. J Manipul Physiol Ther 15:62, 1992

49. Konno S, Olmarker K, Byrod G et al: Intermittent cauda equina compression. Spine 20:1223, 1995

50. Hause M: Pain and the nerve root. Spine 18:2053, 1993

51. Sato A: Spinal Reflex Physiology. p. 87. In Haldeman S (ed): Principles and Practice of Chiropractic. Appleton & Lange, E Norwalk, CT, 1992

52. Korr IM, Goldstein MJ: Abstract: Dermatomal autonomic activity in relation to segmental motor reflex threshold. p. 22. In Korr IM (ed): The Collected Papers of Irvin M. Korr. American Academy of Osteopathy, Colorado Springs, 1979

53. Korr IM, Wright HM, Thomas PE: Effects of experimental myofascial insults on cutaneous patterns of sympathetic activity in man. p. 54. In Korr IM (ed):

The Collected Papers of Irvin M. Korr. American Academy of Osteopathy, Colorado Springs, 1979

54. Korr IM: Sustained sympathicotonia as a factor in disease. p. 77. In Korr IM (ed): The Collected Papers of Irvin M. Korr. American Academy of Osteopathy, Colorado Springs, 1979

55. Seaman DR: The Subluxation Complex: Nutritional Considerations. ACA J Chiro 30:77, 1993

56. Suter E, Herzog W, Conway P, Zhang Y: Reflex responses associated with manipulative treatment of the thoracic spine. J Neuromusculoskel Syst 3:124, 1994

57. Wall PD: The Gate Control Theory of Pain Mechanism: A Re-examination and a Re-statement. Brain 101:1, 1978

58. Mootz R: Theoretic Models of Chiropractic Subluxation. p. 175. In Gatterman MI: Foundations of Chiropractic—Subluxation. CV Mosby, St. Louis, 1995

59. Homewood AE: The Neurodynamics of the Vertebral Subluxation. 3rd Ed. Valkyrie Press, St. Petersburg, FL, 1979

60. Hayes S: The chiropractic subluxation—a new hypothesis for consideration. J Natl Chiro Assoc 27:9, 1957

61. Hviid H: A consideration of contemporary chiropractic theory. J Natl Chiro Assoc 25:17, 1955

62. Korr IM: Proprioceptors and the Behavior of Lesioned Segments. In Stark EH (ed): Publishing Sciences Group, Osteopathic Medicine. Acton, MA, 1975

63. Korr IM (ed): The Neurobiologic Mechanism in Manipulative Therapy. Plenum Press, New York, 1978

64. Korr IM: The Collected Papers of Irvin M. Korr. American Academy of Osteopathy, Colorado Springs, 1979

65. Vedder HE: Analysis Guide. Cleveland College, Kansas City Archives, undated

66. Firth JN: Chiropractic Symptomatology. self published, Davenport, IA, 1925

67. Yates RG, Lamping DL, Abram NL, Wright C: Effects of chiropractic treatment on blood pressure and anxiety: a randomized, controlled trial. J Manipul Physiol Ther 11:484, 1988

68. Kokjohn K, Schmid DM, Triano JJ, Brennan PC: The effect of spinal manipulation on pain and prostaglandin levels in women with primary dysmenorrhea. J Manipul Physiol Ther 15:279, 1992

69. Klougart N, Nilsson N, Jacobsen J: Infantile colic treated by chiropractors: a prospective study of 316 cases. J Manipul Physiol Ther 12:281, 1989

70. Pikalov AA, Vyatcheslav VK: Use of spinal manipulative therapy in the treatment of duodenal ulcer: a pilot study. J Manipul Physiol Ther 17:310, 1994

71. Wislowska M: A study of the contribution of pain to rotation of vertebrae in the etiology and pathogenesis of lateral spinal curvature. J Manual Med 4:161, 1989

72. Jorgensen L, Fossgreen J: Back pain and spinal pathology in patients with functional upper abdominal pain. Scand J Gastroenterol 25:1235, 1990

73. Bogduk N, Tynan W, Wilson A: The nerve supply to the human lumbar interverteral disc. J Anat 132:39, 1981

74. Bogduk N, Twomey L: Clinical Anatomy of the Lumbar Spine. 2nd Ed. Churchill Livingstone, Melbourne, 1991

75. Bogduk N, Windsor M, Inglis A: The human lumbar dorsal rami. J Anat 134:383, 1982

76. Fielding J, Burstein A, Frankel V: The nuchal ligament. Spine 1:3, 1976

77. Bogduk N: The clinical anatomy of the cervical dorsal rami. Spine 7:319, 1982

78. Kent C: Beyond back pain. Calif Chiro Assoc J 21:45, 1996

79. Seaman DR: Chiropractic and Pain Control. DRS Systems, Hendersonville, NC, 1995

80. Slosberg M: Effects of altered afferent articular input on sensation, proprioception, muscle tone and sympathetic reflex response. J Manipul Physiol Ther 11:400, 1988

81. Seaman DR: A physiological explanation of subluxation and its treatment. Calif Chiro Assoc J 21:32, 1996

82. Nanzel D, Szlazak M: Visceral disease simulation. J Manipul Physiol Ther 18:379, 1995

83. Burns LA: Effects of upper cervical and upper thoracic lesions. J Am Osteopath Assoc 22:266, 1923

84. Burns LA: Laboratory proofs of the osteopathic lesion. J Am Osteopath Assoc 31:123, 1931

85. Gregory AA: Spinal Treatment Science and Technique. The Palmer-Gregory College, Oklahoma City, 1912

86. Burns L, Chandler L, Rice R: Pathogenesis of Visceral Diseases Following Vertebral Lesions. The American Osteopathic Association, Chicago, 1948

87. Lewis T, Kellgren JH: Observation relating to referred pain, visceromotor reflexes and other associated phenomena. Clin Sci 4:47, 1939

88. Melzack R, Wall PD: Pain mechanisms. Science 150:974, 1965

89. Milne RJ, Foreman RD, Giesler GJ Jr, Willis WD: Convergence of cutaneous and pelvic visceral nociceptive inputs onto primate spinothalamic neurons. Pain 11:163, 1981

90. Palmer BJ: The Science of Chiropractic. Palmer School of Chiropractic, Davenport, IA, 1920

91. Swartz JH: The transport of substances in nerve cells. Sci Am 242:152, 1980

92. Lubinska L: On the arrest of regeneration of frog peripheral nerves at low temperatures. Acta Biol Exp 16:65, 1952

93. Guth L: Trophic effects of vertebrate neurons. Neurosci Res Prog Bull 7:1, 1969

94. Werner JK: Trophic influence on nerves on the development and maintenance of sensory receptors. Am J Phys Med 53:127, 1974

95. Ochs S, Ranish N: Characteristics of the fast transport in mammalian nerve fibers. J Neurobiol 1:247, 1969

96. Ochs S: A brief review of material transport in nerve fibers. p. 183. In Goldstein M (ed): The research status of spinal manipulative therapy. Monog No. 15. HEW/NINCDS, Bethesda, 1975

97. Zalewski AA: Regeneration of taste buds after reinnervation by peripheral or central fibers of vagal ganglia. Exp Neurol 25:429, 1969

98. Zalewski AA: Combined effects of testosterone and motor, sensory or gustatory nerve reinnervation on the regeneration of tastebuds. Exp Neurol 24:285, 1969

99. Hix EL: An apparent trophic function of renal nerves, abstracted. Fed Proc 21:428, 1962

100. Singer M: Trophic function of the neuron. 6. Other trophic systems; neurotrophic control of limb regeneration in the newt. Ann NY Acad Sci 228:308, 1974

101. Gutman E: Neurotrophic relations. Annu Rev Physiol 38:177, 1976

102. Guth L: "Trophic" influences of nerve on muscle. Physiol Rev 48:645, 1968

103. Guth L: The effects of glossopharyngeal nerve transection on the circumvallate papilla of the rat. Anat Rec 128:715, 1957

104. Fernandez HL, Ramirez BV: Muscle fibrillation induced by blockage of axoplasmic transport in motor nerves. Brain Res 79:385, 1974

105. Korr IM: Discussion. Papers of Sidney Ochs and David E. Pleasure. p. 203. In Goldstein M (ed): The research status of spinal manipulative therapy. Monog No. 15. HEW/NINCDS, Bethesda, 1975

106. Lantz CA: The vertebral subluxation complex. ICA Int Rev Chiro 45:37, 1989

107. Lantz CA: A review of the evolution of chiropractic concepts of subluxation. Top Clin Chiro 2(2):1, 1995

108. Kunert W: Functional disorders of the internal organs due to vertebral lesions. CIBA Symp 13(3):85, 1965

109. Korr IM: The Neurobiologic Mechanisms in Manipulative Therapy. Plenum Press, New York, 1978

110. Korr IM: The spinal cord as organizer of disease processes. Some preliminary perspectives. J Am Osteopath Assoc 76:35, 1976

111. Korr IM: The spinal cord as organizer of disease processes. II. The peripheral autonomic nervous system. J Am Osteopath Assoc 79:82, 1979

112. Korr IM: The spinal cord as organizer of disease processes. III. Hyperactivity of sympathetic innervation as a common factor in disease. J Am Osteopath Assoc 79:232, 1979

113. Cramer G: Clinical anatomy of the lumbar region and sacroiliac joints. In Greenstein G (ed): Clinical Assessment of Neuromusculoskeletal Disorders. Mosby–Year Book, St. Louis, 1996

114. Kellgren JH: On the distribution of pain arising from deep somatic structures with charts of segmental pain areas. Clin Sci 4:35, 1939

115. Campbell DG, Parsons CM: Referred head pain and its concomitants: report of preliminary experimental investigation with implications for the post-traumatic "head" syndrome. J Nerv Ment Dis 99:544, 1944

116. McCall IW, Park WM, O'Brien JP: Induced pain referral from posterior lumbar elements in normal subjects. Spine 4:441, 1979

117. Dwyer A, Aprill C, Bogduk N: Cervical zygapophyseal joint pain patterns. I. A study in normal volunteers. Spine 15:453, 1990

118. Feinstein B, Langton JNK, Jameson RM, Schiller F: Experiments on pain referred from deep somatic tissues. J Bone Joint Surg Am 36:981, 1954

5
Physical Examination and Diagnosis

Henry W. Shull

*P*atient assessment has always been an important facet of chiropractic practice. The lengthy intraprofessional debate over the role of diagnosis has been largely resolved in recent years—it is now broadly agreed that the chiropractor's role must include diagnostic evaluation, to determine the proper course of care and to identify accurately those cases requiring referral to another health practitioner.

Placing diagnosis in its proper context requires understanding a conceptual schism in the healing arts that developed in the mid-19th century concerning the restoration and maintenance of health. Two schools of thought emerged, one arguing the supremacy of host resistance while the other attested the virulence of the pathogen. This difference in worldview has persisted, and represents a fundamental paradigmatic difference between contemporary allopathic medicine and the healing arts now called alternative or complementary.

Neither pole contains the entire truth. Today, we know that it is the balance between resistance and pathogenicity that determines health. The concept of pathogenicity extends beyond the destructive effects of microorganisms. Our experience with acquired immunodeficiency syndrome (AIDS) demonstrates that reduction of host resistance portends near-certain mortality from infection by an otherwise opportunistic pathogen. We also know that extremely virulent pathogens that have been lurking for years in the rain forests of central Africa, when invited into our living rooms, may kill us in a few hours no matter how healthy we think we are. It is the responsibility of the clinician to remain ever mindful of the balance between resistance and pathogenicity, to assess the patient's position on this continuum, and to secure effective management of the health problems presented by the patient.

No chapter-length essay can substitute for the many sound textbooks available for the study of physical diagnosis, orthopedic evaluation, or biomechanics. This chapter is offered instead as a companion text that seeks to recontextualize diagnosis for the student and doctor of chiropractic who intend to practice as responsible portals of entry in an evolving health care system. This responsibility entails the initial delineation of clinical hypotheses to account for the problem the patient presents, the investigation of each of those hypotheses by insightful inquiry, the judicious selection of appropriate examination procedures, and the selection of laboratory studies to confirm the clinical hypothesis that ultimately survives the triage of scrutiny.

BEGINNING THE DIAGNOSTIC PROCESS

Clinical Hypotheses

Patient assessment is initiated at the moment of initial contact. The patient's dress and demeanor cue certain areas of inquiry and the experienced clinician immediately initiates a mental list of hypotheses that could account for the patient's presentation. Rather than seizing on an attractive hypothesis, the clinician's inquiry is designed to support or modify this list of hypotheses. If a hypothesis is correct, corroborative evidence will probably be found in the patient's history; if not, the hypothesis may need to be reconsidered or modified.

After generating a list of reasonable clinical hypotheses that have been corroborated by subjective evidence, the clinician selects examination procedures likely to further narrow the list of remaining hypotheses and clarify the cause of the patient's problem. Again, if a hypothesis is correct, there is a very good chance that a physical finding supporting it will be encountered on performing an appropriate procedure; if not, the list of hypotheses may have to be modified through further subjective and objective investigation. A hypothesis that is supported by objective as well as subjective evidence may be further corroborated by laboratory studies before the diagnosis is made and a therapeutic plan generated.

Subjective Data: the Case History

Just as the reporter seeks to discover the who, what, where, when, why, and how of a news story, or the detective seeks to discover which suspect had motive, method, and opportunity to commit a crime, the clinician seeks to discover the pathophysiologic mechanism responsible for the patient's presentation. This procedure represents an orderly process of subjective and objective inquiry designed to focus on the patient's problem efficiently and effectively.

Information the patient offers is considered subjective because it cannot be verified with the examiner's own senses; what the examiner can detect with his or her own senses is considered objective. A patient would normally not consult a doctor if the problem could be resolved by the patient alone. Patients consult doctors because they are unable to resolve their health problems and need help. Depending on the circumstances, subjective data may not be very accurate. Nevertheless, eliciting subjective data is an important step in the diagnostic process. It is best done in an orderly manner, as follows:

Entrance data constitute information that identifies the patient. The patient's Name, Age, Sex,

Address, Telephone, Employment, etc. is necessary to conduct the business component of a busy practice. Historical data obtained from a third party should be identified as such.

Patient complaints [commonly called Chief Complaints (CC)], identify the problem(s) for which the patient is seeking help. Multiple complaints should be numbered in order of severity. Each complaint should be separately recorded using the patient's own words. The use of quotation marks is helpful. Professional jargon should be avoided.

Present illness (PI) [occasionally called the Present Problem (PP) or History of the Present Illness (HPI)] generates a complete description of each complaint. The PI provides a chronology of the events that ultimately lead the patient to seek your care. An open-ended inquiry (one complaint at a time) is useful, because it allows the patient to include details which might not come to light if the discussion is limited to direct answers to specific questions. An example of an open-ended question is, "Please tell me about this problem you're having."

Listen carefully for each of the following parameters in the patient's response, and follow up with direct questions about those parameters that remain unclear. "*Can you point to where it hurts?*" clarifies information about location that may not have been volunteered in the open-ended response. A picture of the patient's current problems gradually comes into focus and a tentative "list of problems" may be identified. It is wise not to rush. Eliciting a History of Present Illness affords an opportunity to establish strong doctor–patient rapport.

FOCAL POINTS FOR THE PATIENT INTERVIEW

Six elements of inquiry constitute an adequate consultation: date and mode of onset; location, depth, and radiation; quality, frequency, and duration; exacerbation and remission; associated signs and symptoms; and prior care and effect. Sample questions for each element are italicized.

Date and Mode of Onset

When did the problem start? Is it an emergency? Be as specific as possible. Did the problem start minutes, hours, days, weeks, months, years, or decades ago? It is helpful to place the onset of problems in chronological order. "*When did you experience this problem for the very first time?*" How did the problem start? Was the onset spontaneous, as might occur with a fracture or pneumothorax? Inflammations and infections are commonly considered acute, occurring over 1 to 3 days. Subacute disorders are said to occur over 5 to 21 days. Chronic episodic disorders are those that have been present for over six months and only flare up on occasion. Chronic degenerative disorders are dissimilar, in that they exhibit steady and gradual deterioration.

Location, Depth, and Radiation

Identification of the site, together with a knowledge of the clinically significant anatomy, is essential to the analytic process. Problems that emanate from the body wall and limbs are often mechanical in nature. Somatic nociception is mediated by A-delta fibers, so patients can localize somatic problems rather well. Visceral nociception is moderated by type C fibers, which are unmyelinated and operate at a much slower rate. As a consequence, visceral problems cannot be localized as specifically. The appreciation of deep visceral pain is said to be vaguely centralized, only becoming locatable as the soma is affected and A-delta sensory fibers become involved. The course of appendicitis provides a classic example—vague epigastric discomfort localizes as a distinct pain in the right lower quadrant as the problem progresses.

Two inquiries facilitate the differentiation of visceral and somatic disorders. *Can you touch the pain with one finger?* and *Where did the pain start and where is it now?* An inability to accurately localize the problem, coupled with pain that shifts location should alert the examiner to a potential visceral disorder. The patient's perception of depth is of some value in that type C pain, in addition to being vague and of slow onset, is perceived as being deep inside, whereas somatic pain is perceived to be more superficial. Pain that radiates from a somatic origin is usually specific in location. Visceral pain is usually consistent while pain of psychogenic origin is commonly quite variable.

Quality, Frequency, and Duration

Given the diversity among patients, their cultures and sensitivities, the nature of the problem is perhaps the most unreliable element of the Present Illness.

Patient descriptions of severity are notoriously unreliable and should rarely be taken for absolute fact. The stoic will have a very different appreciation of pain than the excitable patient. Nonetheless, the use of certain words or images may be illustrative of the nociceptive mechanism. *How would you describe what you are feeling?* Pain described as "stabbing" should evoke images of sensory fibers while "gnawing" may indicate motor fiber impingement. "Boring" pain may indicate a periosteal mechanism while "aching" commonly indicates a soft tissue origin. Hollow organ colic is commonly described as "cramping," myocardial infarction is said to be "crushing," dissecting aortic aneurysm is "tearing," and use of the term "throbbing" implies a cardiovascular mechanism.

Frequency and duration are somewhat more reliable indicators than quality. Key questions are *How often does the problem occur?* and *When the problem occurs, how long does it last?* Problems of a mechanical or somatic nature are generally constant but vary in intensity and duration. Arthritis and low back strain serve as examples of such conditions. Visceral disorders, being physiologically limited, are commonly intermittent in frequency and duration. Problems of a psychogenic nature usually present with no discernible pattern and are easily diminished when the patient is distracted.

Exacerbation and Remission

The element most helpful in distinguishing the mechanical, visceral, or psychogenic origin of problems is found in the examination procedure itself and best illustrated by the maxim, "Mechanical problems are exacerbated and remissed by mechanical measures." Problems with the body wall and extremities are commonly discoverable by compression, distraction, and torsion, which the components of the relevant orthopedic tests. The several sciatic traction procedures are illustrative of this simple precept.

Exacerbation and remission of visceral disorders, on the other hand, are commonly effected by physiologic rather than mechanical measures. Examples include angina, which is provoked by any measure that increases cardiac workload under circumstances of inadequate coronary perfusion. "*What provokes the problem or makes it worse?*" and "*What relieves it or makes it better?*" are two questions that often prove quite helpful in making a diagnosis.

Associated Signs and Symptoms

These are findings in other systems that become evident when the problem occurs. This association may be indicative of the problem source. Be certain to ask, "*Does anything else happen when the problem occurs?*" As an example, pain at the tip of the right scapula, when associated with an intolerance for fatty foods and digestive difficulty suggests involvement of the biliary system.

Prior Care and Effect

Prior care addresses all that has been done previously for this problem, including consultations, medications, surgeries, and other procedures. "*What have you done about this before now?*" is the relevant question. This information will indicate what others have concluded about the patient's problem. However, it is not advisable to rely on their diagnoses alone. It is also inadvisable to criticize the efforts of other health care providers.

Several good mnemonics exist for the present illness. Each includes all or most of the following parameters: what the problem is, when it started, how it started, where it is located, a description of its nature, what brings it on, what relieves it, what it is associated with, and what has been done for it. An example is OPQRST—onset, provoking, quality, radiation, site, and timing. Regardless of which mnemonic method is adopted, the parameters should be memorized and employed upon each future encounter with a health problem. Figure 5-1 presents a visual perspective of the task.

Past Illness

As opposed to the present illness for which the patient is seeking help, the Past Illness portion of the initial interview is an overall assessment of the patient's personal health before encountering the problems that led him to seek your care. Asking the patient, "*How has your health been in the past?*", elicits information that enables you to compile an inventory of past surgeries, illnesses, and traumas, which should include the approximate date and nature of each event. Hospitalizations and medications should be noted.

Family History

"Consanguinuity and living relationships" is an assessment of the patient's genetic background. Only blood relatives should be investigated, perhaps

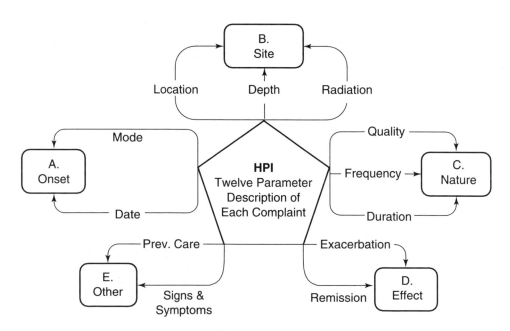

Figure 5-1. Diagnostic flowchart.

with the open-ended question, *"Do any problems run in your family?"* Relatives by marriage are not included. Tendencies toward heart disease, high blood pressure, stroke, cancer, diabetes, gout, kidney disorders, thyroid problems, allergies, or hereditary disorders should be investigated.

Social History

Social history affords an assessment of the patient's life experiences and social relationships. It can include information relevant to the extended or nongenetic family, occupational and environmental matters, or anything else related to daily activities. Exposure to toxins and occupational stresses are examples of conditions that might bear upon the patient's present illness.

Review of Systems

Systems review provides a mechanism to review all symptoms that may have been overlooked in the History of the Present Illness or Past History. By reviewing each system in an organized manner (usually from the head down), additional, unrelated problems may be discovered. A checklist of symptoms is commonly read; the patient is asked to respond "yes" or "no." Affirmative responses warrant additional clarification with direct questions. A summary is included in Table 5-1.

At the end of the interview, the patient should be afforded another opportunity to discuss his health problems. Further, he is allowed "the final say" as the interview is closed. One might ask, *"Have we missed anything?"*

Constructing the Problem List

Construction of the initial problem list begins with the cues observed and the development of clinical hypotheses begun during the initial contact with the patient. Delineation of the problem(s) was initiated upon discovery of the Chief Complaint(s). During the History of the Present Illness, the Past History, the Family History, the Social History, and the Review of Systems, these hypotheses were tested with direct and indirect questions. In the process, each hypothesis was reinforced or modified. The patient's problems, and the reasons for them, became increasingly clear. The Problem List is initiated by simply writing them all down in order of probability and selecting examination procedures that further refine the hypotheses.

PHYSICAL EXAMINATION

Preparatory Thought Process

Having explored the subjective data accessible through the patient history, five fundamental procedures (inspection, palpation, percussion, auscultation, and motion) are available for selective application during the physical examination. Not all procedures will be appropriate for each patient that

Table 5-1. Areas for Questioning, by System

System	Query
General health	Fever, chills, malaise, "fatiguability"
Diet	Restrictions, allergies, vitamins, caffeine, alcohol
Skin, hair, nails	Itching, dryness
Nervous	Irritability, seizures, weakness, paralysis, coordination
Musculoskeletal	Pain, restricted motion, swelling, deformity
Head and neck	Headache, vision, hearing, swallowing
Chest and lungs	Difficulty breathing, cyanosis, cough, hemoptysis
Heart and vessels	Chest pain, irregular beats, limping, blood pressure
Hematology	Bruises, bleeding, inflammation of veins
Gastrointestinal	Abdominal pain, indigestion, constipation, diarrhea, bleeding
Genitourinary	Pain, incontinence, hematuria, dysuria
Endocrine	Temperature change, weight change, hair pattern

is examined and some examination procedures can be used to confirm the findings determined by others. Each is a tool used to confirm or modify the subjective image of the patient's problem by the examiner's own objective means.

Only when subjective and objective data are in accord can a clear image of the patient's problem be entertained with confidence. As the clinician masters these individual assessment tools, a clear understanding of the fundamental purpose of each emerges, and with it the ability to select the specific tools most appropriate to the particular patient.

Inspection

Inspection begins with the initial patient contact and continues through the entire examination. Careful inspection has been called the cornerstone of diagnosis; some assert that more health problems are missed by not looking than are missed by not knowing. Similarly, it has been argued that 60 to 80 percent of a diagnosis is made by inspection alone. Whatever the merit of these arguments, it is safe to say that the experienced clinician will temper the original hypotheses with studied observation prior to the execution of other physical or laboratory procedures.

Inspection is a sensory phenomenon not limited to visual observation alone. Valid examination data may also be obtained by smell, as is the case with an uncontrolled diabetic, or taste, as in patients with cystic fibrosis. Inspection by visual observation obviously requires good lighting in order to actually clearly see the sought-after phenomenon. The frequencies in natural sunlight provide the best medium for visual inspection, especially for the detection of jaundice and cyanosis. Examination conducted under common fluorescent lighting with its limited spectrum often prohibits such detection.

Visual inspection may be conducted in a manner that is direct, oblique, or tangential. Although direct, right angle observation provides the visual means for careful, detailed, and systematic observation of the field, the detection of fine movement using this method can be limited by the examiner's ability to perceive depth. Visual perception of the cardiac apical impulse, for example, is best appreciated by looking across the precordium at a tangent

to the chest rather than looking at the area straight on. The slight pulsation generated by left ventricular contraction driving the tip of the heart against the inside of the chest wall may serve to detect cardiac hypertrophy or mediastinal displacement. An examiner can sometimes better appreciate movement and shadow using peripheral vision and oblique observation as if looking out of the "corner of one's eye."

Given normal osseous structures and intact neuromuscular control mechanisms, the soma should reflect normalcy in both structure and function. Movement should flow, exhibiting the grace that normal articulations exhibit over a full range of motion. To maximize its benefit, visual inspection should include kinematic as well as static observation. As the human body is inherently resilient, observed variations may reflect the natural, homeostatic attempt to restore normalcy by modifying biomechanics to accommodate to the problem. In most cases accommodation is only partially successful; even artful compensations can be detected with controlled and systematic observation.

Shaking Hands With the Patient

In addition to the exercise of civility, shaking the patient's hand for the first time affords an opportunity to observe several systems in an unobtrusive manner. Station and possibly gait may be briefly assessed as contact is made. Integrity of the motor cortex and pyramidal system which facilitates volitional movements of the arm may also be assessed. The intention tremor and dysmetria of cerebellar deficit may become evident as may the resting tremor of extrapyramidal deficit. An ability to extend the arm requires an intact radial nerve and extensor muscles, particularly those forearm extensors that stabilize the wrist while the finger and thumb flexors generate the grip. Inasmuch as demonstrable weakness in any of these muscle groups or articular deficit in the shoulder, wrist, or hand may first become evident during this activity, the handshake provides an unobtrusive opportunity to inspect the integrated function of the upper extremity in a social setting.

Visual and Auditory Inspection

Comparison of the amount of sclera showing on either side of the iris may indicate a clinical need for the further investigation of oculomotion, especially if the patient complains of diplopia. Asymmetric reflection of light can likewise indicate an ocular phoria and the relationship of the eyelid to the iris is indicative of blepharoptosis. An absence of sweating over one side of the forehead is indicative of a cervical sympathetic deficit, and unilateral ptosis of normal facial features is strongly indicative of a motor deficit of the seventh cranial nerve. Patterns of repeated and painful wincing are often indicative of tic doloreaux, an inflammation of the trigeminal nerve although wincing without pain may be indicative of facial nerve irritation or spasm of psychogenic origin. Observation of the patient's inability to articulate lingual consonants (e.g., D, L, and T) is evidence of the need for further assessment of the hypoglossal nerve, the mouth, and the tongue. An observed inability to articulate labial sounds (e.g., B, M, P) warrants similar investigation of the facial nerve and the orbicularis oris. Inspection need not be in-person—these deficits may be perceived in a telephone conversation.

Respiratory Function

Assessment of respiratory function may be expedited by accurately observing that system. Patient compliance with the examiner's request for a rapid and maximum inspiration followed by a forceful expiration through an open mouth allows an initial observation of respiratory function. Rapid inspiration is facilitated by intact phrenic nerves, intact hemidiaphragms, the apposition of the visceral and parietal pleura, open airways, and complaint pulmonary parenchyma. To induce negative intrathoracic pressure rapidly, the sternum and ribs move up and out, increasing the anteroposterior and transverse chest dimensions. Movement of one hemithorax may lag behind the other, indicating a spinal, costal, or pleural deficit that must be explored. Although bilateral phrenic or diaphragmatic deficits are unlikely in the ambulatory patient, the incarceration of a hiatal hernia in an obese and recumbent patient is not.

Airflow into and out of the tracheobronchial tree is normally laminar, except where the airway bifurcates. Partial obstruction or distortion of the tracheobronchial tree generates turbulence on deep and rapid inspiration. As the mortality rate of bronchogenic carcinoma has remained high, the detection of a localized and persistent wheeze warrants immediate investigation.

Aside from the recruitment of the accessory muscles of respiration frequently seen in obstructive and metabolic pulmonary disorders, expiration is normally effected by the elastic component of the parenchyma itself. Energy is stored in these elastic, interalveolar tissues during inspiration; it is this energy that is normally responsible for evacuating the acinar units during expiration. Loss of this elasticity through inflammation, fibrosis, or erosion diminishes the ability to evacuate air from the alveoli, prolongs expiration, and reduces expiratory volume. The patient may be able to get air into the lungs, but he cannot efficiently get it out.

Cardiovascular System

Assessment of venous pressure in the cardiopulmonary circulation is likewise expedited by simple observation. The standing patient is asked to drop his arm to the side of his thigh and allow the veins on the back of his hands to fill. Keeping the elbow fixed in extension, the patient is instructed to abduct the shoulder, bringing the arm up until the veins in the hand abruptly collapse. At the point of collapse, the pressure in the veins of the hand approximates that within the systemic venous return and the right atrium. Flexing the elbow and bringing the hand to the chest allows a rough estimation of venous backpressure; given the principle of the siphon, a hand that contacts the chest above the level of the heart is indicative of the need for a thorough cardiopulmonary examination. The possibility of hemodynamic obstruction or cardiac failure should be entertained. Just as the amplitude of any arterial pulse is a rough indication of the contractile health of the left ventricle, a pulse that collapses above the level of the heart is indicative of increased pressure in the systemic venous return.

Neuromusculoskeletal System

The observation of unequal shoulder height mandates investigation of the neuromuscular mechanisms that maintain natural balance of the spine and shoulder girdle. Paresis or paralysis of a prime mover can functionally distort that natural balance, as can prolonged spasm of its opposite number.

Abnormalities and trauma can structurally distort that balance, abating the grace with which shoulder movements are normally made. The observation of full and active abduction of the extended arms through 180 degrees, from palm against thigh to overhead palmar apposition, will screen shoulder movement. To comply with the request to perform this maneuver, the patient's auditory, cerebration, pyramidal, extrapyramidal, and cerebellar mechanisms must be largely intact, as must the final common pathway, from cord level C5 through the musculocutaneous nerve and the deltoid muscle it innervates. As completion of the procedure requires the maintenance of elbow and wrist extension as well as internal rotation of the forearms, integrity of these neuromuscular mechanisms is screened as well.

Observation of the grace and facility with which the movements are conducted provides a mechanism through which the glenohumeral and scapulothoracic movements may be screened as well as the integrity of the neuromuscular mechanisms responsible for their generation. The patient's compliance with a subsequent request to flex the elbows, clench the fists, and bring them down behind the neck affords further opportunity to screen flexion of the upper extremity, joint mobility, and the neuromuscular mechanisms responsible for external rotation and abduction of the shoulders, flexion of the elbow, flexion of the fingers, and apposition of the thumbs.

Similar screening mechanisms are available to the careful observer with knowledge of clinically significant structure and function and an appreciation of how these elements are integrated in the healthy individual. Observation of the patient's ability to stand with heels together, eyes closed, arms outstretched, and hands supinated, for example, can screen the integrity of the posterior columns, the cerebellum, the vestibular apparatus, and the pyramidal systems. Barring subjective or objective evidence of a deficit in those separate systems, the examiner may appropriately conclude that the patient's ability to perform this screening procedure successfully is incipient evidence of their integrity.

Observation of the patient's gait may provide evidence of cerebellar coordination, pyramidal and extrapyramidal integrity, and neuromuscular

integrity of the major muscles of the lower extremities as well as the weight-bearing elements of the lower spine, pelvis, hips, knees, ankles, and feet. The loss of cortical control in a patient who has suffered a significant cerebrovascular accident allows the normally stronger upper extremity flexors to overpower the weaker extensors, resulting in a classic posture in which the arm is applied to the chest. The reverse obtains in the lower extremity, where extensors are normally stronger than flexors and the gait is modified to swing the paralyzed leg around instead of demonstrating the mechanics of a normal stride. While this example is a spastic paralysis resulting from a serious vascular accident, careful observation of the gait may allow the detection of muscular paresis as well. An inability to effect normal ankle dorsiflexion may be the result of a focal lesion in the motor cortex, a lesion in the final common pathway, a muscular lesion in the anterior leg or a structural problem with the ankle mortise itself.

The ability to walk on tiptoe further screens the major extensors of the lower extremity and the pathways that innervate them. The ability to walk on the heels, arise from a seated position, or don a jacket provide opportunities to screen the neuromusculoskeletal structures and the functions that govern the coordinated performance of these common tasks. Some of these screening procedures are contraindicated when the patient's balance is obviously compromised. In such instances, patient safety mandates the selection of individual examination procedures that do not put the patient at risk. Knowledge of the anatomy, physiology, and the mechanics of assessment will expedite examinations conducted under less than ideal conditions.

While each problem the patient presents must be fully investigated by all appropriate means, it should be fully understood that the performance of examination procedures for the sake of their performance alone is unwarranted in today's health care environment. While there is no shortage of assessment procedures to order or perform, selection of those procedures which offer the best risk-benefit and cost-benefit ratios corroborates clinical competence. Attention to the art of inspection facilitates the selection of appropriate procedures. An enormous amount of information can be had from inspection alone. Most diagnoses are initiated on inspection and modified or substantiated by subsequent physical, imaging, and laboratory procedures.

Palpation

While inspection may be defined as acquisition of information through the art of observation, palpation may be defined as acquisition of information through the art of touch. As the sense of touch has been used to confirm visual information since the beginning of time, it is only reasonable that the art of palpation offers a significant contribution to the confirmation of observed physical findings. An enlarged joint, for example, may be the result of osteoarthritis, rheumatoid arthritis, or previous trauma; the distinction is facilitated by the palpable discovery of the heat, pain, redness, swelling, and loss of function of active inflammation. Mastery of the art of palpation affords the examiner four modes of patient assessment: temperature, vibration, gross distinction, and fine distinction. Each assessment mode is conducted in a different manner.

Temperature

Although a patient's core temperature is commonly assessed with a thermometer, a remarkably good indication of fever can be made by applying the back of the examiner's hand to the patient's forehead. Aside from fever, the palpatory assessment of local skin temperature is a valuable asset in the detection of inflammatory change, infectious or otherwise. Evaluation of the swollen joint referenced above provides a good example.

Detection of a circulation deficit is also facilitated by the art of touch. Because of the body's bilateral nature, each extremity offers a standard of comparison for its opposite. One aspect of this internal standard is the comparable perfusion of tissues as evidenced by the heat and color provided by an intact and unimpeded vasculature. A discrepancy in the palpable temperatures of two essentially identical structures in the human body should alert the examiner to the possibility of a perfusion deficit. The discrepancy may be due to normal anatomic variation, unilateral arterial vasospasm or partial obstruction of the arterial lumen. Further comparison of pulse amplitude, pulse contour, and nutritional status of tissues perfused will facilitate the

differentiation, as will the detection of arterial turbulence on auscultation.

Vibration

The perception of vibration is another assessment tool facilitated by touch. Vibration is detected by two types of mechanoreceptors in the joints—Pacinian corpuscles respond to rapid and minute deformations, whereas those of Meissner respond to vibrations of much lower frequency. Both receptors stimulate large, myelinated, A-beta, sensory fibers, which rapidly transmit this sensitive and phasic modality through the dorsal column, the contralateral medial lemniscus, and thalamus to the sensory cortex. Unlike temperature assessment, vibration is best appreciated when the examiner's own articulations are applied to the area under examination. The metacarpo-phalangeal joints at the base of the fingers, the distal interphalangeal joints, or those in the ulnar surface of the hand provide the best vehicle for the practical assessment of vibration.

The transmission of vibration is affected by the density of the medium through which it passes. A grasp of this relationship facilitates understanding of several common assessment procedures. The use of a tuning fork to initially distinguish conductive from sensorineural or nerve deafness, for instance, uses a comparison between vibration transmitted through the air and through bone. Pallesthesia, the patient's ability to perceive vibration, is commonly assessed by the application of a lower frequency tuning fork applied to the most distal knuckle of the great toe. A patient who can report the presence or absence of vibration in both feet is a patient whose dorsal columns and medial lemnisci are presumably intact. Although the art of palpation is not represented by these examples, each serves to illustrate the inherent clinical utility of the principles of vibration.

Fremitus and Tissue Density

One procedure that uses palpation to assess vibration is the tactile assessment of vocal fremitus, which facilitates detection of pulmonary consolidation when chest radiographs are not available. Fremitus is patient-induced vibration of the chest wall via laryngeal phonation. The patient is commonly asked to repeatedly speak the phrase "ninety-nine," using the lowest voice possible, as the examiner palpates the lateral walls of the chest, the apices, and the upper back using the joints of his fingers. Vibration of the patient's vocal cords, maximized by the low frequency, is transmitted through the tracheobronchial tree, the pulmonary parenchyma, the pleura, and the chest wall where it is perceived by the examiner's finger joints.

A variety of densities naturally occur in the chest, ranging from the air-filled alveoli to the solid bone of the thoracic cage. This variation in density lends value to radiographs in which one structure can be visually distinguished from another. Knowledge of these different densities and their location is prerequisite to the mastery of physical examination and radiography. The character of normal fremitus can be appreciated by placing a hand over one's own sternum, repeating the phrase in the lowest pitch possible, and comparing the vibration to that felt over the lateral chest wall. One notes that air-filled structures transmit vocal vibration less efficiently than do structures that are more solid.

Fremitus is of great value in assessing the pulmonary parenchyma. Departures from normal pulmonary tissue density arise from a variety of conditions in which either parenchymal rarefaction or parenchymal consolidation occurs. Panlobular emphysema, for example, is the histologic result of septal erosion and the subsequent coalescence of alveolar airspace. Tissue density becomes rarefied in the affected lung fields, the transmission of vocal vibration diminishes, and there is less tactile fremitus for the examiner's interphalangeal articulations to perceive. This reduction of tissue density also decreases the normal barrier to the penetration of radiation and causes these areas of the film to turn black in a normally exposed study.

Fremitus can also be reduced by other mechanisms that break the physical connection between the patient's vocal cords and the examiner's palpating fingers. The separate right and left pleurae each consist of a parietal layer, which is adherent to the undersurface of the chest wall and innervated by lightly myelinated, type A-delta sensory fibers that transmit somatic or first pain, and a contiguous visceral layer which is adherent to the surface of the lung itself and is innervated by unmyelinated, type C sensory fibers that transmit visceral or so-called second pain. Assessment of the quality of pain transmit-

ted by these two distinct sensory fiber types can be helpful in the initial differentiation of visceral and somatic disorders.

Between these continuous and contiguous layers of separately innervated pleura lies the potential pleural space, properly considered the crux of pleural function. Each pleural space contains a very small amount of mucoid substance that serves to lubricate the layers as they slide along each other when the chest wall and lungs expand and contract. Loss of this lubrication provokes the chest pain known as pleurisy, a pain that is commonly multisegmental and exacerbated on diaphragmatic excursion. A constant negative pressure is also maintained in each pleural space by the hydrostatic, osmotic, and gaseous gradients normally present between the pleural space and the capillaries in the parietal and visceral layers of the pleura. Preservation of this negative pressure that holds the pleural layers in opposition maintains the potentiality of the pleural space and transmits vibration through the pleurae to be perceived as tactile fremitus. Any phenomenon that violates this potentiality and allows an air gap between the layers will also diminish tactile fremitis. Such conditions are commonly identified by the suffix -thorax.

While fremitus decreases in conditions of parenchymal rarefaction, the opposite obtains in conditions of increased parenchymal density. Tactile appreciation of vocal fremitus is increased in the chest wall overlying the area in which parenchymal consolidation occurs. Fremitus increases as alveoli progressively fill with bacterial exudate in the early stages of a lobar pneumonia. Concurrently, the infected area offers a progressively greater barrier to the penetration of ionizing radiation and demonstrates increased delineation on a properly exposed chest radiograph. When parenchymal density is in question, the assessment of tactile fremitus can facilitate the determination of rarefaction or consolidation as long as the pleurae remain intact.

Firm and Light Palpation

In addition to the assessment of temperature and vibration, the art of palpation is also very important in the investigation of gross anatomical structure and fine tissue texture. The assessment of organ hypertrophy and displacement by firm palpation is a common element in examination of the viscera and gross dislocations of skeletal structure. Lighter palpation is appropriate for the evaluation of more subtle changes in tissue texture, such as that exhibited by the taut and tender fibers accompanying a subluxation or subtle changes in tension discovered during assessment of articular end range.

Pathways Mediating Palpatory Information

Although crude touch and the sense of pressure are commonly held to be mediated through the anterior and lateral spinothalamic tracts of the contralateral cord, it can be argued that the clinician's appreciation of the sensations perceived on gross or deep palpation must also be mediated through the dorsal columns in order to be of clinical value. The spinothalamic tracts which transmit multimodal sensation in addition to crude touch decussate at segment level whereas the essentially unimodal sensation of fine touch ascends in the ipsilateral dorsal column before decussating to the contralateral brainstem via the medial lemniscus. While this contrast in a patient's appreciation of temperature, pain, and pressure versus the sensibilities of vibration, light touch, and position sense is a fundamental principle of neurologic diagnosis, it would seem unreasonable to suggest that this ontologically older system, with its slower, unmyelinated fibers could transmit discrete data that would facilitate the examiner's judgment of pressure intensity.

Abdominal Palpation

Perhaps the most common example of gross palpation is illustrated by examination of the abdomen. Physical assessment of the deeper abdominal organs cannot be considered complete without an estimation of their size and location though the art of palpation. The spleen, for instance, lies along the axis of the left tenth rib and usually cannot be palpated in the normal individual. In splenomegaly, the spleen cannot enlarge upward through the diaphragm nor backward through the left erector spinae. The path of least resistance for an enlarged spleen is along the rib axis, permitting palpation of the mass.

Position, texture, and enlargement of the liver are also assessed by gross palpation. The edge of the normal liver, commonly described as having the con-

sistency of a hot dog, can be felt along the right lower rib cage. Prolonged inflammation of the hepatic parenchyma, as in chronic alcoholism, forces the affected tissue to undergo fibrosis, which changes the feel of the tissue encountered by the examiner's fingers. As is common to all fibrosis, the affected tissue undergoes change in size as well as consistency; the fibers contract over time and the structure shrinks. A small, hard, non-functioning liver is palpated in those patients whose livers have suffered sustained abuse.

A liver border that can be palpated below this costal margin may be the result of hepatic enlargement, inflammation, ptosis, or the restriction in diaphragmatic excursion often seen in panlobular emphysema. The same structures that direct splenic enlargement also restrict enlargement of the liver. Obstruction of the systemic venous return, such as that seen in right heart failure, can rest in a hepatic engorgement that swells the liver down past the costal margin. The parenchymal inflammation of hepatitis, as it exhibits the cardinal signs of calor, dolor, rubor, tumor, and funcio laesa, also enlarges the liver and causes it to protrude past the costal margin. The suspensory ligaments that normally hold the liver in place may become lax, allowing a liver of normal size and consistency to drop past the costal margin. Another example is the small, hardened liver of alcoholic cirrhosis that may have been pushed down by the right hemidiaphragm of a patient displaying the barrel chest configuration caused by the septal erosion contracted while his liver was slowly being destroyed in a smoke-filled pub.

As an exercise in determining why a liver is protruding past the costal margin, the clinician might ask:

1. Are there other signs of dependent edema that would argue for an obstruction of the systemic venous return?
2. Are there signs of local inflammation which would support the diagnosis of a hepatitis?
3. Is there evidence of past trauma in the absence of vascular and inflammatory signs?
4. Are there respiratory findings that advance the contention that the patient suffers from two problems instead of one?

This exercise is a simple example of the diagnostic process. Remember that nothing can be taken by itself—the value of any findings lies in its contribution to the constellation of findings that make the diagnosis.

Palpation of Musculoskeletal Structures

Since the discovery of the discipline in 1895, the ability to discern fine differences in texture through the art of light palpation has remained the hallmark of the competent chiropractor. Manual detection of the taut and tender fibers commonly attendant to the vertebral subluxation was the chiropractor's primary diagnostic technique before the advent of spinal radiography. Palpation remains a crucial clinical skill in contemporary chiropractic, one that must be honed through many hours of practice before competence is achieved.

The modality of light touch is mediated through specialized cutaneous and mechanoreceptors that enjoy abundant distribution over the hairless skin of the fingertips. Included in this distribution are the subdermal Pacinian corpuscles and the more superficial Meissner's corpuscles. All receptors alter transmembrane potential by opening ion channels in order to effect depolarization of the sensory nerve. Mechanoreceptors open these channels by deformation of the receptor membrane itself. The size of the receptor field served by an individual sensory neuron determines the degree to which the one can discriminate between two adjacent points of contact on the skin. Two-point discrimination is greater over the fingertips than any other part of the body.

A single caveat is appropriate to the mastery of light palpation. Cutaneous mechanoreceptors have been further classified as being either rapidly or slowly adaptive to the stimulus they are designed to detect. As long as the mechanical stimulus remains unchanged, the receptor will eventually cease to stimulate the nerve.

Pacinian and Meissner's corpuscles are considered rapidly adaptive; these structures adapt to extinction within a fraction of a second after the stimulus has become static. Since the sensitivity of these end-organs is directly related to the degree to which they are deformed, it behooves the clinician to palpate as lightly as possible in order to avoid extinction of the tools that make such fine distinc-

tion possible. Such sensibility is not available to the heavy hand, whether the examiner is searching for spastic intertransversarii, subtle change in tissue texture, or a feeble pulse.

Percussion

In addition to the assessment of tactile fremitus, in which changes in parenchymal pulmonary density may be confirmed through the transmission of vibration produced by the patient's vocal cords, the examiner may rely on the art of percussion to inject vibration into an area of the body to objectively verify a suspicion derived from subjective or objective data. Over the centuries, routine percussion of an area has been used to: determine the density of underlying tissue, estimate the position and size of an organ, and discover or confirm the presence of inflammation.

Since the advent of radiography in 1895, the clinical rationale for percussion has been increasingly overshadowed by the ability to generate a radiographic image of the area under study. Clinical expediency notwithstanding, the art of percussion remains an efficient, valuable, and cost-effective modality in the hands of an experienced clinician. The value of the procedure is well worth the time necessary for its mastery.

Percussion Technique

Density of the underlying tissue is assessed by noting the tone created when an area of the body is quickly struck with just enough force to set the tissue into vibration and elicit a percussion note. The most common method of inducing this vibration is indirect or mediate percussion. One finger of the examiner's nondominant hand, the pleximeter, is firmly applied to the area under examination. The pleximeter is rapidly struck by one finger of the examiner's dominant hand, the plexor, with enough force to inject a sudden vibration into the tissue that lies up to five centimeters below the skin surface. The unique note elicited provides information about the type of tissue under the area percussed.

Three procedural comments are worthy of mention. First, when percussing the thorax, the pleximeter should be firmly applied to the intercostal spaces in order to transmit vibration directly into pulmonary tissue.

Placement of the pleximeter across adjacent ribs rather than firmly along the interspaces will confound the procedure and elicit a note from the ribs themselves as opposed to the tissue underneath. Second, for the pleximeter to remain an effective tool, the vibration should be transmitted directly into the tissue under study; it should not be dampened by contact with the adjacent fingers of the hand. The third point relates to the generation of the striking motion itself. All striking motion should come from the wrist, none from the elbow; the examiner's elbow should remain largely stationary while the wrist demonstrates a great degree of flexibility. With practice, the art will develop.

Tissue Densities and Percussive Tones

Four fundamental tissue densities (air, water, oil, and bone) are evident throughout the body, each generating a different note when percussed and each offering an increasing barrier to the penetration of ionizing radiation. The lightest of these densities is air, a medium which offers so little obstruction to the penetration of x-ray that the exposed crystals turn black on development of that part of the radiographic film. Air is normally contained in the pulmonary alveoli, the fundus of the stomach, and the lumen of the large and small intestines, while the walls of these structures are composed of a heavier tissue density which is largely water. When percussed, each of these air filled structures emits a distinctly hollow note in contrast to the more solid note emitted by percussion of an organ such as the liver. The borders of a visceral structure can often be ascertained using percussion in much the same way that fluid level within a large cask has been determined since man's early encounters with the grape.

Tissue Densities

As an example of the value of percussion, the air-filled stomach is normally contained within the left upper quadrant of the abdominal cavity rather than the chest. Percussion of the abdomen usually elicits a drum-like note of tympani over the gastric air bubble. As there is no similarly hollow structure in the normal chest, the discovery of a large tympanitic area over the left mid-clavicular line at its junction with the fifth left intercostal space is highly presumptive of hiatal herniation in a patient who is experiencing digestive upset. This normal contrast of air and water densities also makes radiographic studies of these areas valuable. Observed departure from a normal pattern of density contrasts in a radiograph confirms the clinician's conjecture that the esophageal hiatus in the patient's central tendon has enlarged, allowed the gastric fundus to roll up alongside the esophagus, and created the pain of which the patient complains.

In addition to air and water, two other densities exist in the radiographer's lexicon. Just as an oil spill floats on the sea, tissues of oil density are heavier than air but lighter than water. Oil density is present in fatty tissue and produces no unique percussion note of its own. The value of an oil density is limited to radiography, in which breast shadows may be identified on a chest radiograph and the gray epicardial fat pad may be distinguished from the whiter myocardium.

By contrast, the metal density of bone offers diagnostic value in percussion as well as radiography. As bone is the tissue of highest density in the human body, it vibrates with the least resonance. The note evoked by the percussion of bone is said to be flat and lifeless as opposed to the dullness of a water-containing tissue or the tympani of an air density. The periosteum is the part of a bone most sensitive to painful stimuli, a fact helpful in the detection of fracture, which is often very difficult to detect on flat plate radiographs alone. Violation of periosteal integrity is among the several mechanisms that can cause sharp somatic pain mediated by A-delta fibers; bruises of bone, muscle, and joints can also generate severe pain of this nature. The low-frequency, high-amplitude vibration conveyed through the handle of an activated 128 cps tuning fork when applied to the bone in question can be of considerable value in differentiating sprain, strain, and fracture before the application of a controlled and directed physical force.

Use of Percussion to Detect Inflammation

Examiner-induced vibration is not limited to the detection of tissue density or structural disrelationship. The classic cardinal signs of any inflammation, regardless of the mechanism of origin, include calor, dolor, rubor, tumor, and functio laesa. Although not all these signs may be immediately evident to the clinician, this constellation of heat, pain, redness, swelling, and loss of tissue function announces the presence of inflammation.

A diagnosis of infectious hepatitis is often entertained because the patient has become jaundiced. Put simply, jaundice occurs as the result of three separate mechanisms: excessive destruction of red blood cells that overloads the normally functioning liver; the liver's inability to conjugate bile as the result of inflammation; and obstruction of the biliary pathway to the duodenum resulting in hepatic engorgement and stasis. Gently striking the right upper abdominal quadrant with the side of a closed fist will exacerbate the dolor of hepatitis and provide a clue as to which of these mechanisms is responsible for the patient's jaundice. Of course, one cannot jump to a diagnostic conclusion on the single procedure alone; additional assessment procedures are selected in order to confirm, modify, or rule out clinical conjectures generated during the history and modified through subsequent examination.

Patients who present with unilateral paralumbar pain offer another example of the use of fist percussion to detect inflammation. Included among the problems that might account for this presentation are spinal distortion and renal infection. Pain that exacerbates on light fist percussion of the costophrenic angle, especially when accompanied by discomfort on deep palpation of the ipsilateral kidney, argues for the diagnosis of a kidney infection. The palpable detection of heat over the area coupled with the detection of white cells and protein in the urine makes the diagnosis of renal infection virtually unarguable. The assessment of vibration, whether induced by the patient's own vocal cords or the examiner's fingers, is a modality that should not be abandoned in favor of the radiographic image.

Auscultation

The examiner's sense of hearing is clinically extended through the art of auscultation, which includes the practice of stethoscopy. As naturally occurs in rivers, rapid flow through a vessel or airway is fastest at the center of the stream and slowest along the walls of the channel; because one layer glides smoothly over the other, such flow is said to be laminar. Laminar flow is virtually silent. Like rapids in a river, it is only when the normally laminar current is interrupted by a partial obstruction that flow becomes turbulent and generates a vibration that the listening ear appreciates as noise.

Disruption of Laminar Flow

The partial obstruction may be transient in nature, as is the case with a sympathetic failure to maintain patency in the airways of an asthmatic, or it may be permanent, as in bronchogenic carcinoma where the lumen of the patient's airway is partially occluded by progressive tumor growth. The obstruction may be inflammatory, as when the exudates of bronchitis or the pneumonias spill into the lumen of the tracheobronchial tree, or it may be relative as with erosion of the alveolar septa occasioned by the antitrypsin deficiency of panlobular emphysema. The partial obstruction created by atheromatous placquing in walls of large and medium-sized arteries of patients with hyperlipidemia is yet another example.

In each case, partial obstruction of the lumen disrupts laminar flow, generates turbulence at the site, and creates vibration perceptible on auscultation of the area. The magnitude of the vibration generated correlates strongly with the degree to which the lumen is occluded as well as the pressure gradient that drives the medium across the obstruction. High turbulence is generated by a high flow rate. Of course, in cases of complete obstruction the vessel allows no flow at all, laminar or otherwise.

Varieties of Audible Abnormality

By convention, turbulent flow through the channels of the human body has a variety of names depending upon the system in which the turbulence occurs. The newer term for respiratory turbulence in the smaller airways and terminal bronchioles is *crackles*, although many clinicians still use the older term, *rales*. These crackling sounds are frequently compared to the sound of popping the bubble wrap used as packing material. Turbulence generated by the partial obstruction of larger airways is called a *wheeze* or *rhonchus* and is indicative of mucoid inflammation or aspiration of a foreign body. Turbulence generated by a partial obstruction of an artery is called a *bruit* (broo-ee), that which arises in the heart itself is called a *murmur,* and that which arises in the venous system is called a *hum.* An audible bruit, when palpated, is called a *thrill;* and turbulence arising within a diarthrodial articulation is described as *crepitus.* Whatever term is used, the common denominator is the disruption of the normally silent flow of media within a body part and the generation of clinically significant vibration.

Stethoscopy Procedure

The art of stethoscopy requires adroit use of a simple tool. The acoustic stethoscope must be long enough to permit listening without bending over the patient for lengthy periods, but not long enough to coil upon itself and create extraneous noises. The earpieces, or corbels, should comfortably occlude ear canal and adjust to accommodate the angles at which each of the clinician's canals slant in the petrous portion of the temporal bone. Because of the variety of sounds that emanate from the human body, the endpiece should include a bell, a diaphragm, and a mechanism with which only one endpiece can be functional at a time.

The diaphragm is a flat, circular piece, occasionally corrugated, which is best for detecting high frequency sounds such as those generated during left ventricular systole or rapid intestinal peristalsis. The shape of the bell better detects low frequency sounds such as those generated during cardiac diastole, although pressing the bell firmly into the chest can stretch the underlying skin to the point that it mimics the action of a diaphragm. One of the most common errors in stethoscopy is the failure to ensure that the selected endpiece is operative before it is applied to the area. Be certain as well to ensure full contact along the circumference of the endpiece. Lifting the endpiece from the surface introduces extraneous noise into the auscultatory process, as does movement of the endpiece itself.

Auscultation of the Cerebrovascular System

Of premier auscultatory importance to the chiropractor is the patency of the cerebrovascular system, especially the four vessels that supply arterial blood to the circle of Willis and its tributaries. The prudent clinician assesses the patency of these vessels

through historical evidence of transient ischemic attack, cerebration deficit, or familial tendency to stroke before conducting any procedure in which rotation of the cervical spine is attempted. As atheroma most commonly develops where blood flow is least laminar, the detection of bruit in the cervical vasculature is directed to areas of arterial bifurcation such as occurs in the carotid and subclavian arteries. The detection of arterial turbulence at these bifurcations is strongly indicative of cerebral circulation compromise. The generation of a cerebration deficit on prolonged cervical rotation is further evidence against the selection of manipulative procedures that are rotatory in nature.

Motion

The final examination procedure may be termed motion, in that axial and appendicular structures are subjected to a series of common stresses in order to substantiate the existence of a suspected neuromusculoskeletal disorder. A truly awesome variety of these procedures is available for this purpose, each identified by the name of its creator and each composed of the basic elements of compression, distraction, or rotation. The clinician with a working knowledge of musculoskeletal anatomy, a strong grasp of fundamental mechanical principles, and a healthy dollop of common sense should have no difficulty in exploring the musculoskeletal problems that a patient presents. Indeed, the astute clinician may discover a unique variation on an existing theme and thereby add a new name to the lengthy registry of orthopedic tests.

Distraction

The first common principle of motion examination is distraction, wherein a structure is gently separated from its normal articular companion or otherwise stretched along its longitudinal axis. Classic examples of this procedure are the several ways that a sciatic nerve can be tractioned along its course from its origin in the lumbosacral spine, its exit from the pelvis between the ischial tuberosity and the greater trochanter, along the posterior thigh, the posterolateral leg, and the lateral ankle and foot. The advancement of one leg a step forward in the standing position will traction the ipsilateral sciatic nerve and, if inflamed, will provoke pain over its distribution. The pain will exacerbate if the patient bends at the waist. Flexion of the hip with the patient supine is another way the sciatic nerve can be tractioned, especially if the knee is locked in extension during the process. Although the common denominator for both procedures is sciatic distraction, the first is commonly called advancement while the second is known as the Lasegue test.

A positive finding can then be confirmed by a variety of similar procedures including Lindner's sign, in which passive flexion of the patient's neck upon the chest tractions the dura and provokes pain in cases of sciatic root compression. Similar procedures have been developed to distract the femoral plexus in order to assess the possibility of root compression. Ely's test is a procedure in which the prone patient's knee is flexed until the heel approximates the ipsilateral buttock and tractions the femoral nerve as it passes along the anterior thigh. The motion is mechanically constrained in cases of articular damage of the hip or knee or significant inflammation of the iliopsoas muscle. A variation on this theme is conducted in the side-lying position with the patient's normal leg down. The affected leg is flexed at the knee and extended at the hip, again distracting the femoral plexus along the anterior thigh. Both procedures also distract the abdominal muscles and may help to identify an inflamed appendix.

Another example of distraction is the Halstead maneuver, designed to detect thoracic outlet syndrome, in which the examiner distracts the arm along its longitudinal axis while palpating the patient's radial pulse. Having depressed the clavicle through distraction, the patient is advised to extend and rotate the neck while the examiner feels for change in the amplitude of the radial pulse. A deficit in pulse amplitude is indicative of compression of the neurovascular bundle in the thoracic outlet.

Compression

The second common principle of motion testing is compression, wherein two adjacent structures are gently brought into apposition. Perhaps the most common example of compression is the articular end-range assessment so essential to the practice of chiropractic. The freedom of motion exhibited by a diarthrodial articulation necessitates some structural mechanism through which that motion can be checked when it reaches its normal limit. That mechanism is commonly ligamentous. When an articulation reaches the end of its range of motion in any direction, ligamentous structures that hold its articular components together undergo progressive changes in tension. Those that contain and support the articulation on the side to which it is being bent undergo compression while those on the opposite side are distracted. The limit of articular motion is eventually reached and the articulation moves no more.

Change detected by the patient's articular proprioceptors facilitates position sense—the ability to detect the slightest change in the position of a joint and to assess the rate at which that change occurs. Since the examiner cannot directly address the patient's position sense, he must develop the ability to discern fine gradations of articular tension during the passive assessment of an articulation's range of motion. A knowledge of the usual range of an articulation is helpful in judging its normalcy although variation may occur, especially after trauma. Motion is virtually unrestricted during the midrange of a normal diarthrosis. As movement encroaches into the last five degrees of end range it becomes progressively restricted due to the compressive mechanisms described above. When movement through the end range is exhausted, all play has been removed, the articular components are in complete apposition, and the articulation is said to be "taken to tension."

The abrupt restriction of passive motion without reaching end range is a strong indication that the disorder is intra-articular or inside the capsule, whereas an expanded end range and a prolonged and gradual restriction of motion are evidence that the disorder is extra-articular or outside the joint capsule. A clinician's inability to perceive this progressive restriction of motion accounts for the painful adjustive thrusts sometimes delivered into soft tissue before the articular surfaces are brought into full approximation.

Another example of the principle of compression is the iliac compression test, which involves the forced apposition of articular surfaces to detect inflammation of the sacroiliac articulation. The exertion of downward pressure on the iliac crest of a side-lying patient will cause the sacrum to move forward and exacerbate the pain of an inflamed, subluxed, or sprained joint. A variation on compressive sacroiliac assessment is the sacral apex test, a procedure in which a shear force is indirectly applied to the sacroiliac articulations of a prone patient by pressing down on the sacral apex. The procedure will exacerbate the pain of an inflamed articulation while pressure is applied.

Rotation

The third common principle is rotation, in which a structure is twisted around its longitudinal axis. Kemp's test, in which the patient's trunk undergoes active circumduction through the full range of motion, is an example. This screening procedure facilitates location of the vertebral level at which a problem exists but provides little indication as to its nature. Although the procedure may be conducted in either the standing or seated position, the former variation is commonly held to offer the greater range of assessment. The principle of the procedure is often mimicked by patients who circumduct their own spines by actively twisting their shoulders back and forth to determine whether the "catch" has been removed.

Rotation is also the mechanism underlying the Abbot-Saunders test, in which the fully extended arm is abducted and externally rotated to laterally stress the bicipital tendon. The externally rotated arm is then brought into complete adduction while the shoulder is palpated. Shoulder pain that is exacerbated by the rotatory component, or an audible or palpable click during the procedure, is presumptive evidence of a bicipital groove problem.

A third example is the Fabere-Patrick test, in which the thigh of a supine patient is sequentially flexed, abducted, and externally rotated before being brought into full extension at the completion of the test. This procedure is designed to move the ipsilateral acetabulum through its full range of motion in order to facilitate detection of inflammatory or degenerative arthritis of the hip. A certain level of discomfort during the procedure may be expected, but pain or restricted motion during abduction or external rotation is strongly indicative of abnormality and the need for diagnostic imaging.

Integrating Physical Examination into Responsible Patient Management

Just as physical examination procedures are selected and performed in order to confirm, modify, or discard the several clinical hypotheses that are generated during the acquisition of subjective data in the patient history, laboratory studies (radiologic, electrophysiologic, hematologic, or urinary) are selected, ordered, or conducted to further refine those clinical hypotheses that survive the initial scrutiny of subjective and objective evaluation.

A maxim commonly advanced in legal circles addresses the wisdom of a courtroom attorney who asks a question of a witness, the answer to which is not known by the attorney asking the question. Such "fishing expeditions" often net a catch that the attorney would rather the jury had not witnessed. While fishing in a diagnostic laboratory rarely produces the embarrassing results that can attend fishing in a court of law, other unwelcome consequences may ensue—there are those who contend that the indiscriminate selection of studies has driven the healing professions into managed care. Others contend that such practices reflect a defensive posture adopted in reaction to malpractice actions.

Without enjoining the argument, suffice it to say that the actions of an experienced clinician reflect alignment; the questions asked in the history, the procedures performed during the examination, and the laboratory studies that are ordered all reflect a reasoned and cogent attempt to solve the patient's problem in a clinically expedient manner. It is important to ask the questions that must be asked, to do the things that must be done, to order the studies that must be ordered, and most importantly, to integrate the subjective and objective data that is generated in order to arrive at a clear concept of the patient's problem and effect its appropriate resolution. As a practitioner of the healing arts, one can be expected to do no more and no less.

Terminology

apposition	caveat
auscultation	calor
bifurcate	clinical hypothesis
blepharoptosis	consanguinity
bruit	consolidation

crepitus
diplopia
direct inquiry
dolor
dysmetria
fremitus
functio laesa
hyperlipidemia
interphalangeal
inspection
labial
laminar
lingual
motion
mnemonic
nociception
oculomotion

objective
open-ended inquiry
palpation
parenchyma
pathophysiology
percussion
phoria
pleximeter
plexor
psychogenic
rarefaction
rhonchus
rubor
subjective
thrill
tumor
ulnar

Review Questions

1. Using general terms, construct a single paragraph in which you explain the clinical reasoning process you might use to assess your new patient's complaint and discover its cause.

2. Compare the method of open-ended inquiry to that of direct inquiry. Discuss the benefit of each, and describe a circumstance in which you would choose one over the other.

3. Compare the characteristics of visceral nociception to those of somatic nociception. What are three questions you might use to assess the pain your patient describes, and explain how the ability to elicit this distinction would be of value to your chiropractic practice.

4. List the six elements of patient inquiry with which the patient's complaint may be subjectively assessed. Describe each of the six elements in detail, and explain how the application of each element would be of value to your chiropractic practice.

5. List the five fundamental examination procedures with which the patient's complaint may be objectively assessed. Describe each procedure in

detail, and explain how mastery of each procedure would be of value to your chiropractic practice.

6. Describe the assessment of station and gait. Discuss the systems that are necessary to maintain normal station and gait, and explain the value of such assessments.

7. On abdominal palpation, you discover that the liver of your jaundiced patient presents below the right costal margin. What might account for this finding, and how would you ascertain what was actually responsible for this presentation. Other than palpation, which procedures would you select to support each hypothesis, and why?

8. Compare the mechanisms of rarefaction and consolidation of the pulmonary parenchyma, and discuss how each of these pathophysiologic mechanisms would affect inspection, palpation, percussion, and auscultation of the chest. How might these opposing pathophysiologic mechanisms affect the chest radiograph?

9. Describe the pathway through which oxygen reaches the brain. Explain how that pathway might be assessed, and explain why such assessment would prove to be of value to your chiropractic practice.

10. Why do those who are concerned with cost-benefit ratios frown on "fishing" in a diagnostic laboratory?

Concept Questions

1. Identify the systems that might be screened in the normal course of greeting a new patient seated in your reception area, as you engage in the civility of introduction and accompany the patient to your office.

2. Your patient presents with pain. How might you differentiate the pain generated by a neuromusculoskeletal source from that generated by a visceral or vascular source?

3. Discuss the separate concepts of risk-benefit and cost-benefit. Describe how the appreciation of these concepts will prove beneficial to your chiropractic practice.

6
Diagnostic Imaging
Christopher Kent

HISTORY

On the evening of November 8, 1895, less than 2 months after the discovery of chiropractic, Wilhelm Conrad Roentgen was working alone in his laboratory. As he passed a high voltage through an evacuated glass Crookes tube, a fluorescent screen nearby began to glow. Roentgen placed various objects between the tube and the screen, and found that only lead and platinum effectively stopped the glow. Upon placing his hand between the tube and the screen, Roentgen was astonished to see the shadow of the bones in his fingers. Roentgen called the newly discovered energy *x-rays*, as *x* classically represents the unknown in mathematics. He was awarded the first Nobel Prize in Physics in 1901.[1]

News of Roentgen's discovery spread quickly, and clinical applications were soon developed in medicine. It was 15 years later (although some historians suggest 13 years) that roentgenographic (now known as radiographic) procedures were introduced to the chiropractic profession. Bartlett Joshua Palmer had followed the progress of the fledgling science of diagnostic imaging, and in 1910 purchased a Scheidel-Western x-ray machine for the Palmer School of Chiropractic. Palmer coined the term *spinography* to define the use of spinal x-rays for chiropractic analysis.[2]

B.J. Palmer's original goals were to "verify or deny palpation findings and to verify or deny proof of the existence of vertebral subluxations."[3] He later found that x-rays could also provide information concerning developmental variants and spinal pathologies that could affect the chiropractic care of an individual. Despite resistance from some faculty members and practitioners, radiography soon became part of the regular curriculum at the Palmer School of Chiropractic (Fig. 6-1).

The evolution of x-ray techniques for chiropractic assessment progressed quickly. The Universal Chiropractic College in 1924 announced protocols for x-raying patients in the upright, standing position, rather than lying down. This procedure was said to permit imaging the spine under "all of the stresses to which it is normally subjected." Particularly noteworthy was the development of full spine radiography, which resulted in the entire spine being visible on one film. In 1931, Ray Richardson described the use of 8-inch × 36-inch film to visualize the full spine. The more popular 14-inch × 36-inch single-exposure full spine technique was developed by Warren Sausser in 1933.[4] Clarence Gonstead and Hugh B. Logan developed methods for spinal biomechanical assessment using upright 14-inch × 36-inch radiographs.

Fluoroscopic equipment permitted the examination of moving body parts, and the Palmer School of Chiropractic was equipped with fluoroscopic apparatus. Imaging the spine in motion became practical with the introduction of electronic image intensification. Fred Illi and Earl Rich were pioneers in the field of cineroentgenography, or x-ray motion pictures.[4] Modern equipment permits chiropractors to study the spine in motion with very low levels of radiation. The images may be recorded on videotape.

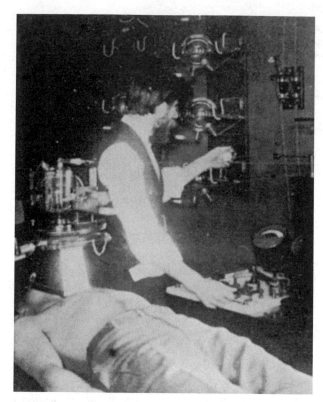

Figure 6-1. Early x-ray facility at the Palmer School of Chiropractic. (From Palmer College of Chiropractic, with permission)

Today, the chiropractic profession continues its commitment to excellence in the field of imaging. Chiropractic applications for advanced imaging techniques, including videofluoroscopy, computed tomography (CT), magnetic resonance imaging (MRI), and sonography are being explored. Specialized chiropractic radiographic techniques continue to be developed.

RADIOGRAPHY

Physical Principles

Radiography refers to any process used to produce photographic images by passing x-rays through the body. X-rays are a form of electromagnetic radiation with sufficient energy to penetrate the body. X-rays are produced in an evacuated glass tube when rapidly accelerated electrons collide with a dense target. The impact deceleration or "braking" of the electrons results in the production of x-ray photons.

The production of diagnostic x-rays is dependent upon the following four conditions:

1. *A source of free electrons.* A tungsten filament, similar to the filament in an incandescent lamp, produces a supply of free electrons. The filament is part of the negative electrode assembly, or cathode.
2. *Acceleration of the electrons.* The electrons are accelerated by a high voltage, typically 20,000 to 150,000 volts (20 to 150 kV). The high voltage is produced by a step-up transformer. A rectifier converts the alternating current from the transformer to direct current before it is applied to the tube.
3. *Impact deceleration of the electrons.* The electrons strike a dense tungsten target, resulting in the production of x-ray photons. In modern x-ray machines, the target is a portion of a positively charged disk known as a rotating anode.
4. *Quality and quantity control.* The quality of the x-ray beam is controlled by the kilovoltage (kV). The greater the kilovoltage, the greater the penetration. The quantity of x-ray photons is determined by the tube current (measured in milliamperes) and the exposure time.[5]

The x-ray tube is enclosed in an oil filled assembly called the tube housing. X-rays are emitted through an opening in the tube housing. A metal filter, usually aluminum, is placed over this opening to absorb weak x-rays, which lack the penetrating capability to contribute to the imaging process. The area of the x-ray beam is limited by a collimator. The collimator has moveable lead shutters which permit the operator to adjust the size of the beam[6] (Fig. 6-2).

The patient is placed between the X-ray tube and the image receptor. In radiography, the image receptor is a cassette that houses a sheet of photographic film and a pair of intensifying screens. Intensifying screens reduce the amount of radiation required by giving off visible light when exposed to x-rays. Modern intensifying screens are composed of rare earth phosphors.

The cassette is often placed in a grid cabinet or bucky diaphragm. The purpose of this assembly is to minimize the amount of secondary radiation reaching the film. Secondary radiation degrades the radiographic image. Thick, dense body parts produce a significant amount of secondary radiation. There-

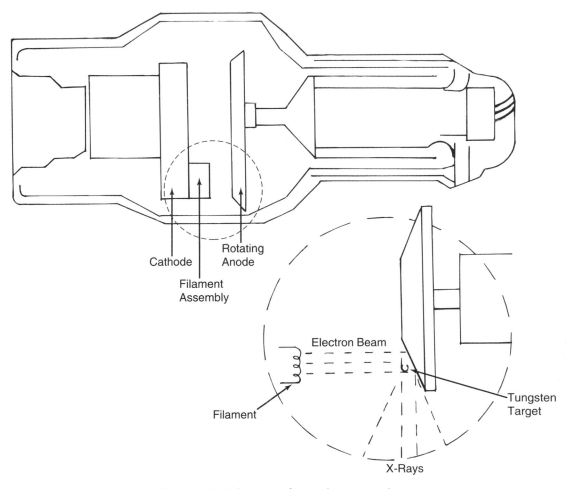

Figure 6-2. Schematic of a modern x-ray tube.

fore, grids or bucky diaphragms are frequently used in spinal radiography[7] (Fig. 6–3).

Radiographic Densities

The finished radiographs are a record of the shadows produced by the overlapping structures of the body. Structures which absorb most of the x-rays are termed radiopaque. Those which permit x-rays to pass through are radiolucent. Radiopaque structures appear light, while radiolucent objects appear dark. The interpretation of radiographs entails four basic radiographic densities:

1. *Bone:* Bone appears white on a radiograph. Some pathologies produce an ivory appearance due to increased bone density.

2. *Water:* Muscles, blood vessels, and most organs are water-density structures that appear gray on radiographs.
3. *Fat:* Fat offers less resistance to the x-ray beam than bone or water. Therefore, fat-density structures appear dark gray.
4. *Gas:* Gas offers little resistance to the x-ray beam. Therefore, structures containing gas (e.g., bowel gas) appear dark.[8]

Interpretation of radiographs depends upon an understanding of these densities and radiographic anatomy. There are three categories of deviations from normal:

1. *Altered density:* Pathology may cause an increase or decrease in the density of a structure. Thus, a

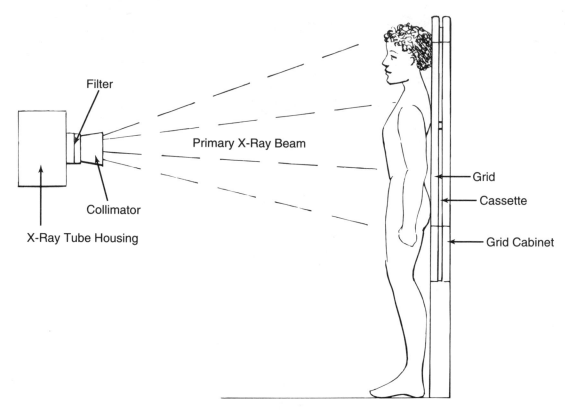

Figure 6-3. Components of an upright spinal x-ray system.

structure that appears too light or too dark may be abnormal.

2. *Edge sharpness:* Pathologies may produce a change in edge sharpness. For example, in many malignant processes, the "zone of transition" between healthy and malignant tissue may present an indistinct, permeative appearance.

3. *Anatomic relations:* A loss of normal anatomical relationships may indicate developmental variation, subluxation, dislocation, fracture, or pathology.

Indications for Radiographic Examination

I propose the following indications for radiographic examination:

1. History of trauma with clinical signs suggestive of fracture or dislocation

2. Clinical suspicion of infection or neoplasm

3. Clinical evidence of a congenital or developmental anomaly that could alter the nature of the chiropractic care rendered or that itself may require treatment

4. When clinical findings are equivocal, and the suspected condition can be detected or ruled out by plain-film radiography

5. When other examination procedures fail to disclose the nature of the condition and the patient is not responding favorably to care

6. To characterize the biomechanical component of the vertebral subluxation complex when such characterization is necessary to render chiropractic care, and less hazardous alternative examinations are not available

7. To evaluate patient response to chiropractic care when such evaluation may alter the nature of the care being rendered, and less hazardous alternative examinations are not available

Diagnostic Yield

As a primary health care provider, the doctor of chiropractic is responsible for determining the safety and appropriateness of chiropractic care. This responsibility includes the detection and characterization of vertebral subluxations, as well as examination for conditions for which certain chiropractic techniques are contraindicated or referral to another health care provider is indicated. Radiographic examinations should be conducted only after a benefits-versus-risks determination has been made, and it has been determined that the information to be provided by the examination justifies the exposure to ionizing radiation.

A detailed description of developmental variants and of the pathologies of interest to the doctor of chiropractic is beyond the scope of this text. The role of abnormal findings, however, can be defined. Patients may be classified according to how radiologic findings affect clinical management (Fig. 6-4):

Category 1: These patients have no skeletal or soft tissue abnormalities that make traditional adjusting techniques hazardous. They have good bone integrity, and thrust adjustments are not contraindicated.

Category 2: Congenital or developmental variants require the chiropractor to modify traditional adjusting procedures. However, appropriate thrust adjusting may be employed.

Category 3: Patients in this category have conditions that weaken or soften bone but that do not indicate dangerous conditions requiring consultation or referral. Adjusting procedures for such patients must be carefully selected. High-velocity adjustments to osteopenic bone should be avoided. Gentle, judiciously applied adjustments may be employed instead.

Category 4: These patients have dangerous conditions that contraindicate thrust adjustment of the affected area and may need medical attention. Examples include fractures, infections, and malignancies. It should be emphasized that I am not advocating that these patients be denied the benefits of chiropractic adjustments. Concurrent chiropractic care, skillfully and appropriately applied, should be considered.

Radiography and Vertebral Subluxation

The traditional chiropractic definition of the vertebral subluxation uses four criteria:

1. Loss of juxtaposition of a vertebra with the one above or the one below, or both
2. Occlusion of an opening
3. Nerve impingement
4. Interference with the transmission of mental impulses[9]

Contemporary definitions have proposed the concept of a "vertebral subluxation complex," which consists of five components. These components incorporate the structural, neurologic, and biochemical aspects associated with vertebral subluxation:

1. Spinal kinesiopathology
2. Neuropathology
3. Myopathology
4. Histopathology
5. End-tissue pathology and biochemical changes[10]

Subluxation degeneration is a process that may involve one or more pathophysiologic mechanisms. The common denominator in these processes appears to be altered biomechanics, which results in local tissue reactions. These local changes may compromise neurologic structures, causing abnormalities in peripheral structures.[11–21]

Biomechanical Analysis

Chiropractors have developed techniques to evaluate the biomechanical aspects of the vertebral subluxation complex. These systems vary in reliability and are generally applied to a single, specific technique. However, some methods of mensuration are well accepted by the healing arts community.

Evans[22] describes *anterior subluxation of the cervical spine* as a condition caused by flexion-rotational trauma and notes that the instability resulting from anterior cervical subluxation may result in neurologic sequelae and increasing displacement. Scher[23] defines *subluxation* as "anterior displacement of a vertebra in relation to the vertebra below, when the two apophyseal joints remain in contact." Dislocation is said to occur when the articular facets of the

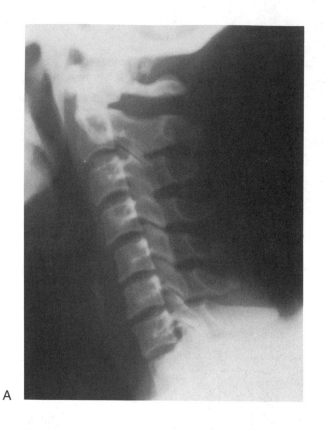

A

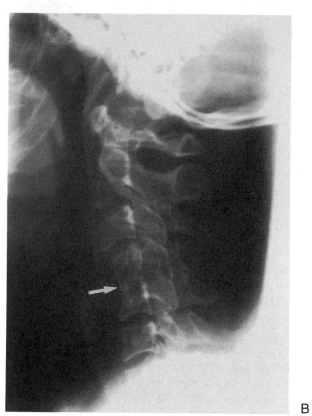

B

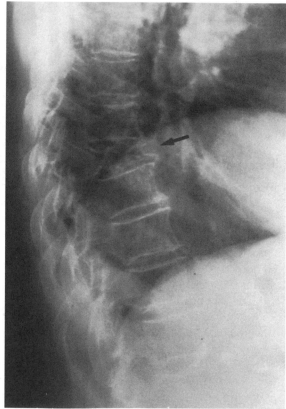

C

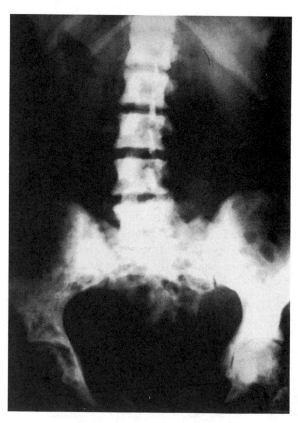

D

Figure 6-4. (A) Lateral cervical radiograph of a Category 1 patient. There is a loss of the cervical curve, although there is good bone integrity. **(B)** Lateral cervical radiograph of a Category 2 patient. Note congenital nonsegmentation at C4-C5. **(C)** Lateral radiograph of the thoracolumbar spine in a Category 3 patient. The patient has osteoporosis with an old compression fracture *(arrow)* **(D)** AP radiograph of the lumbar spine in a Category 4 patient. The "ivory vertebra" appearance is due to metastatic carcinoma.

apophyseal joints are no longer in contact. Green et al.[24] state that anterior displacement of 1 to 3 mm indicates subluxation, while displacement in excess of 3.5 mm indicates frank dislocation or fracture. Green and colleagues list six specific radiographic manifestations of anterior cervical subluxation:

1. Kyphous deformity at the level of subluxation.
2. Anterior rotation and/or displacement of the subluxed vertebra.
3. Anterior narrowing and posterior widening of the involved disc space.
4. Localized increase in distance between the subluxed vertebra and subjacent articular masses.
5. Alteration of configuration of interfacetal joints.
6. Abnormal widening of interspinous space.

Green et al.[24] noted that such manifestations are accentuated in flexion and are minimized or eliminated in extension. Thus, there is movement beyond the normal physiologic range. Dvorak et al.[25] reported statistically significant differences in measurements made on lateral cervical flexion/extension radiographs of soft tissue injury patients versus controls. Norris and Watt[26] found abnormal curves in the cervical spine to be more common in patients who had poor outcomes following rear-end vehicle collisions. Nagasawa et al.[27] found most patients with tension-type headaches have a straightened cervical spine. In assessing response to chiropractic care, favorable results were reported by two investigations. Leach[28] investigated the effect of chiropractic care on hypolordosis of the cervical spine. A significant improvement in the cervical curve was noted in patients receiving chiropractic care. Harrison et al.[29] reported that patients receiving adjustments and extension-compression traction demonstrated an improvement in the cervical lordosis compared to controls.

In an effort to standardize the reporting of vertebral malpositions demonstrated radiographically,

the following system was developed by a panel of chiropractic specialists in 1973 (Table 6-1).

Reliability of Spinographic Analysis

Jackson et al.[30] reported the results of a study designed to assess the reliability of geometric line drawings used on the lateral cervical radiograph in Chiropractic Biophysics Technique. Three examiners evaluated 65 radiographs. Parameters measured included anterior head translation, Jackson's cervical stress lines, and five relative rotation angles. In all measurements, the intra- and interexaminer reliabili-

Table 6-1. Radiographic Manifestations of Vertebral Subluxation

Static intersegmental subluxations
    Flexion malposition
    Extension malposition
    Lateral flexion malposition
    Rotational malposition
    Anterolisthesis
    Retrolisthesis
    Lateral listhesis
    Altered interosseous spacing
    Foraminal encroachment
Kinetic intersegmental subluxations
    Hypomobility
    Hypermobility
    Aberrant motion
Sectional subluxations
    Scoliosis or alteration of curves secondary to muscular imbalance
    Scoliosis or alteration of curves secondary to structural asymmetry
    Decompensation of adaptational curvatures
    Abnormal motion of a section
Paravertebral subluxations
    Costovertebral and costotranserve disrelationships
    Sacroiliac subluxations

ties were greater than 0.70, ranging from 0.72 to 0.99.[30]

Other studies have yielded results supporting the reliability of cervical spinographic techniques. Grostic and DeBoer[31] did a retrospective study of 523 patients evaluating radiographic measurements of atlas laterality and rotation pre- and post-adjustment. Statistically significant changes in the postulated direction of atlas positioning were reported. This establishes construct validity. Jackson et al.[32] studied the inter- and intraexaminer reliability of upper cervical radiographic marking. Six practitioners evaluated 30 radiographs. The study revealed very good intra- and interexaminer reliability for the procedure employed.[32] Rochester reported on a study in which four Orthospinology (Grostic) practitioners analyzed 10 sets of upper cervical radiographs. There was 100 percent agreement on the side of atlas laterality. Reliability of rotation measurement was less than the reliability of atlas laterality. However, acceptable reliability of atlas rotation was reported.[33]

Other systems of analysis have been developed for full spine assessment of intersegmental and postural changes associated with vertebral subluxation. Plaugher and Hendricks[34] evaluated the interexaminer reliability of the Gonstead pelvic marking system. Concordance on exact numeric values was poor. However, from a clinical standpoint, agreement for categorizing listings was impressive. Interexaminer concordance for listings of the ilia, sacrum, symphysis pubis, and femur head height was evaluated by calculating the κ-values for each. The resulting κ-values ranged from 0.4849 (moderate) to 0.8161 (excellent).[34]

In addition to Gonstead pelvic analysis, proponents of 14-inch × 36-inch full spine radiography also use the procedure to evaluate vertebral body rotation and lateral flexion malposition. Zengel and Davis[35] investigated how projectional distortion affects such determinations. They concluded, "as long as a given osseous segment is compared to its adjacent segment (as in analysis for subluxation), the apparent vertebral rotation may be regarded as a sufficiently accurate representation of the actual rotation of the vertebra." In reference to vertebral endplate lines used to assess lateral flexion malpositions, these investigators stated, "In every instance, off centering produced no measurable effect on the

position of the constructed Gonstead lines. We therefore conclude that these lines may be confidently used ... No correction for projectional distortion seems necessary."[36]

The judicious use of spinographic techniques can be valuable in characterizing the biomechanical component of the vertebral subluxation complex. The use of post-adjustment radiographs can assist the chiropractor in determining that the subluxation has been reduced when other examination techniques cannot reveal the desired information. Objective outcome assessments for chiropractic care are essential if chiropractic is to realize its potential in the health care delivery system.

VIDEOFLUOROSCOPY

Basic Principles

Videofluoroscopy is a technique used to produce x-ray motion pictures on videotape. A videofluoroscopic system consists of an x-ray generator capable of operating at low (0.25 to 5) milliamperage settings, an x-ray tube assembly, an image intensifier tube, a television camera, a videocassette recorder (VCR), and a monitor. The heart of the system is the image intensifier tube. This tube permits imaging at very low radiation levels. It is used instead of intensifying screens and film as an image receptor. When the fluoroscopic image is recorded on motion picture film, the term *cineradiography* is applied.

Clinical Applications

The role of videofluoroscopy in the evaluation of abnormalities of spinal motion has been discussed in textbooks, medical journals, and chiropractic publications. Observational and case studies have appeared in the literature comparing the diagnostic yield of fluoroscopic studies versus plain films. In addition, studies have been published reporting abnormalities detected by fluoroscopy that could not be assessed using plain films. Schaff[37] described cases in which instability of the upper cervical spine was appreciated on videofluoroscopic studies. It was observed that not all cases of upper cervical instability are revealed by static flexion-extension studies.

Wood and Wagner[38] reviewed the use of radiographic methods for the analysis of cervical sagittal motion. They reported that videofluoroscopic studies may reveal kinematic irregularities not detectable by examining the extremes of range of motion alone. Wallace et al.[39] studied the reliability of certain methods of fluoroscopic measurements, reporting that independent examiners could replicate the measurements reliably. Van Mameren et al.[40] used fluoroscopy to determine the variability of instantaneous centers of rotation in the cervical spine. These investigators concluded that their procedure "shows variability of such low extent that it seems feasible to use it to diagnose abnormal mobility or in assessing therapy in the neck region."

Bland[41] states, "Clearly, cineradiography is the best method for the study of biomechanics and dynamics of motion in the cervical spine ... The determination of normal motion, sites of greatest and least motion, contribution by joints, discs, ligaments, tendons, and muscles to motion (and their limitations), and the biomechanics of normal motion of the occiput-atlas-axis complex all have been studied very successfully through cineradiography."

Buonocare et al.[42] examined the cervical spines of 107 patients using cineradiography, including 57 who sustained flexion-extension injuries. They concluded, "The ability to demonstrate localized abnormal motion in the cervical spine allows one to predict soft-tissue injuries and the quality of spinal fusions, spinal stability, and early subluxation of the cervical spine—conditions that may not be identified on static roentgenograms nor at physical examination."

Chiropractors Foreman and Croft[43] in their textbook *Whiplash Injuries*, state, "This motion study of the spine may be quite useful in detecting abnormal biomechanics secondary to ligamentous damage that may be unappreciated with plain film radiography. ... Cineradiography or fluorovideo radiography plays an important role in the diagnosis of aberrant spinal biomechanics that may be secondary to chronic muscle contracture, scar tissue formation, or ligamentous instability."

Antos and coworkers[44] presented the results of an interexaminer reliability study of cinefluoroscopic detection of fixation in the mid-cervical spine. Two examiners reviewed 50 videotapes of fluoroscopic examinations of the cervical spine. The examiners achieved 84 percent agreement for the presence of fixation, 96 percent agreement for the absence of fixation, and 93 percent total agreement. The κ-value was 0.80 ($P < 0.0001$). Only the C4-C5 level was examined. The authors concluded, "The current data indicate that VF determination of fixation in the cervical spine is a reliable procedure."

Videofluoroscopy is an evolving technology in clinical chiropractic. Most current applications are related to evaluation of the post traumatic cervical spine. Nonclinical issues, such as availability and cost-effectiveness, will undoubtedly influence its future role in chiropractic practice.

COMPUTED TOMOGRAPHY

Basic Principles

Computed tomography (also referred to as CT or CAT scanning) is an imaging technique that produces axial (cross-sectional) images of body structures using x-rays. The procedure was developed in Great Britain by Godfrey Hounsfield in 1972.[1] In most CT scanners, a moving x-ray tube produces a fan-shaped beam of radiation. Sensitive electronic detectors record the amount of radiation passing through the body part under examination. The information from the detector array is processed by a computer. An image is displayed on a cathode-ray tube, which may be recorded on photographic film[45] (Fig. 6-5).

Although CT data are collected in the axial plane, computer reformatting permits the production of sagittal and coronal images. However, reformatting may produce artifacts. Furthermore, the reformatted images lack the high resolution of the axial images.[46]

An advantage of CT over conventional radiography is the ability to create "windows." Although the computer image consists of 2,000 or more levels of density, the ability of the human eye is the ultimate limiting factor in any diagnostic imaging procedure. The human eye can only perceive 16 to 20 shades of gray. To enable the viewer to see subtle differences between structures of similar densities, a "window" may be displayed.[47] The width and level of the window may be adjusted by the operator. In spine imaging, it is customary to provide two sets of images. One set displays a bone window, which optimizes visualization of osseous structures. The second set presents a soft tissue window, which permits effective

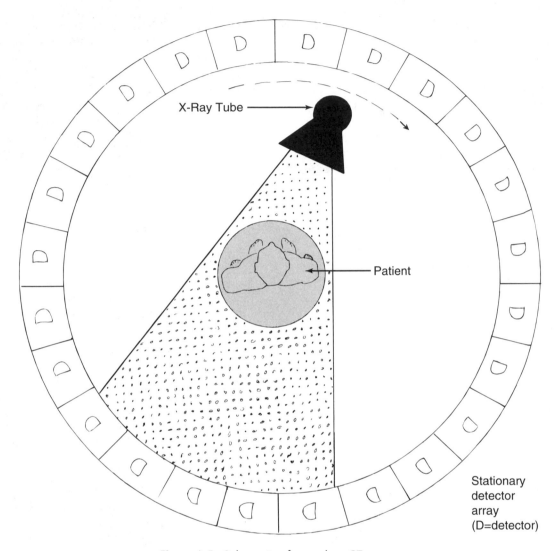

Figure 6-5. Schematic of a modern CT scanner.

visualization of the intervertebral disc, ligamentous structures, and neural tissues.

Manifestations of subluxation degeneration that may be demonstrated by CT scanning include disc lesions, spinal canal stenosis due to infolding of the ligamentum flava, osteophytosis, and bony sclerosis. CT applications for chiropractic analysis have been reported by Ebrall and Molyneux,[48] Richards et al.[49] Walker,[50] and Koentges.[51] In addition, CT may be used to evaluate developmental variants and pathologies that could affect the chiropractic man-

agement of a case. An important advantage of CT imaging is the ability to visualize the thecal sac, nerve roots, and intervertebral disc[52] (Figs. 6-6 and 6-7).

Disadvantages of CT scanning include a relatively high radiation burden and higher cost than are incurred with conventional radiography. When CT contrast media is used, there is the potential danger of an adverse reaction. Despite these shortcomings, CT has a place among the diagnostic options available to the chiropractor.

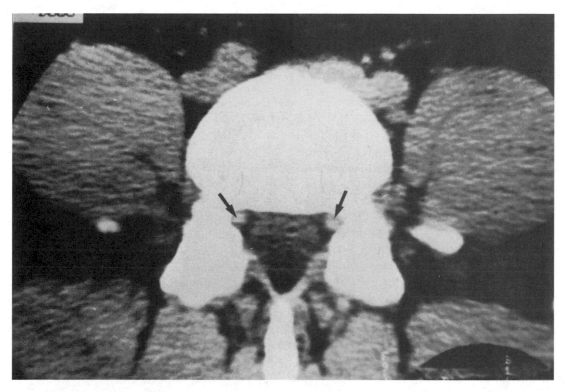

Figure 6-6. Normal axial CT scan. Note the symmetry of the nerve roots (*arrows*).

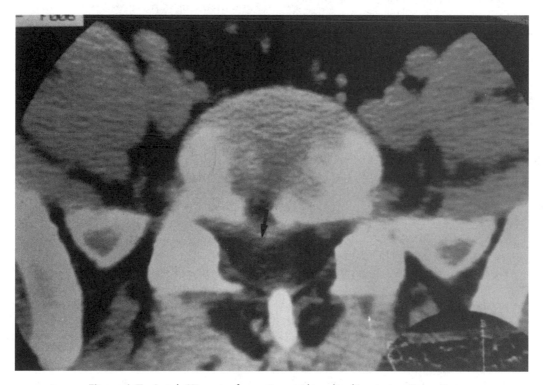

Figure 6-7. Axial CT scan of a patient with a disc herniation (*arrow*).

MAGNETIC RESONANCE IMAGING

Basic Principles

MRI provides high-resolution images of the body without exposure to ionizing radiation. In chiropractic practice, MRI may be useful in the detection and evaluation of vertebral subluxations, disc lesions, neoplasms, brain, cord, and nerve lesions.

The body part under examination is placed within a powerful magnetic field. The magnetic field may be produced by permanent magnets or superconductive electromagnets cooled with liquid helium and liquid nitrogen. Two absolute contraindications to MRI are cardiac pacemakers and ferrous cerebral aneurysm clips. Claustrophobic and uncooperative patients are poor candidates for MRI. The effects of strong magnetic fields on biologic systems, particularly during pregnancy, have not been fully explored. Ferromagnetic foreign bodies, implanted electrical stimulator wires, and metal prosthetic heart valves are relative contraindications to MRI studies.[53,54]

Most clinical MRI employs hydrogen as the element of interest. Because much of the human body is composed of water and fat, hydrogen imaging permits exquisite visualization of soft tissue structures. Hydrogen protons can be represented as tiny spinning magnets with north and south poles. When placed in a steady, powerful magnetic field, they align in the direction of the magnetic poles and "wobble," or precess, at a specific frequency. The scanner then introduces a powerful radiowave timed to this frequency, called the *Larmor resonance frequency*. This frequency is determined by the strength of the magnetic field and the element being imaged. This pulse of radiofrequency (RF) energy temporarily knocks the protons out of alignment.

After the RF pulse is turned off, the protons snap back into position, emitting a weak radiowave. This signal is received by a coil and processed by a computer. Images of the body part being examined are displayed on a cathode ray tube. Most MRI systems can produce axial, sagittal, and coronal images. Some equipment is capable of producing oblique images.[8] (Fig. 6-8).

Tightly bound hydrogen, such as the hydroxyapatite found in calcific structures, produces little or no signal. However, the hydrogen in water and fat will produce high signal intensity if appropriate parameters are employed. Depending on the parameters selected, the MRI will emphasize either structures with high concentrations of fat or structures with high concentrations of water. In clinical practice, two sets of images will normally be provided:

T₁-Weighted Images

T_1-weighted images are sometimes called "fat images." Structures containing fat appear bright. In the spine, the vertebral bodies contain marrow fat. In the absence of abnormality, vertebral bodies will appear relatively bright on T_1-weighted images. In conditions in which the marrow fat is replaced, the signal will be increased or decreased, and the vertebral bodies will appear lighter or darker. T_1-weighted images employ relatively short pulses and do not take as long to produce as T_2-weighted images.

T₂-Weighted Images

T_2-weighted images are often termed "water images." Water-rich structures, such as the nucleus pulposus and cerebrospinal fluid (CSF) appear light. Fat-containing structures appear dark. T_2-weighted images require longer imaging times than do T_1-weighted images. T_2-weighted images are useful in evaluating disc desiccation. These sequences also help identify edematous lesions and provide dramatic differentiation of disc, CSF, and cord.[11]

How Abnormalities Affect the MRI

Edema

Edema may occur secondary to infection, infarction, tumor, trauma, or demyelinization. On T_1-weighted images, edema appears dark. On T_2-weighted images, edema has an intense signal and appears white.[55,56]

Tumors

Tumors involving fluid-filled cysts behave similar to edematous tissues, while tumors involving calcification may be difficult to detect using present MRI techniques. Calcified tumors are better imaged using CT techniques. It is difficult to differentiate benign from malignant tumors reliably with current MRI techniques. Metastatic bone disease results in decreased signal on T_1-weighted images. This is due

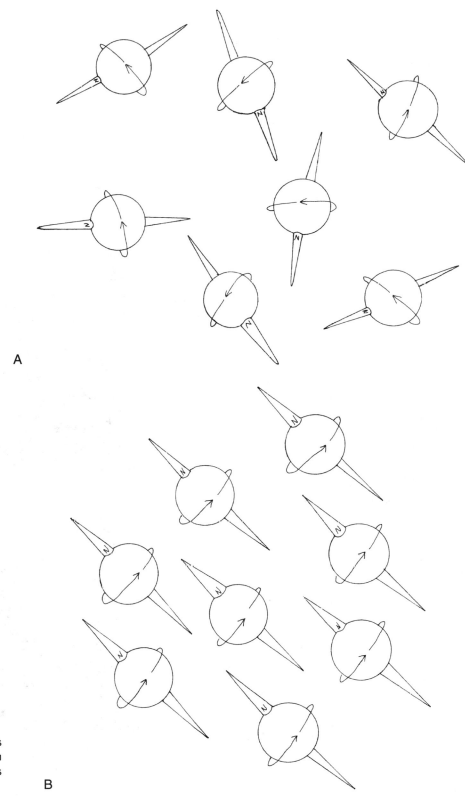

Figure 6-8. (A & B) Protons behave as tiny magnets. In a magnetic field, they align as shown in B.

A

B

to replacement of the marrow with tumor cells. T_2-weighted images may demonstrate increased signal intensity.[56–59]

Blood

Blood flowing rapidly appears dark because of turbulence and high velocity. Slow-flowing blood often appears bright.[60]

Inflammatory Diseases

Inflammatory diseases of the spinal cord, such as multiple sclerosis and transverse myelitis will demonstrate intense (bright) signals on T_2-weighted images when acute. Multiple sclerosis more frequently produces subtle changes in cord intensity. T_1-weighted images of the spinal cord demonstrate changes in cord contour, while T_2-weighted images demonstrate increased signal (brightness), where water content is high, such as CSF. Discitis and osteomyelitis may be evaluated using a combination of T_1- and T_2-weighted images.[61]

Intervertebral disc disease demonstrates low signal intensity (brightness) due to desiccation and degeneration. Herniations may also cause changes in cord contour, nerve root compression, and edema[62] (Figs. 6-9 and 6-10).

MRI Disc Degeneration and Spondylosis

Modic et al.[63] stated that MRI may be the appropriate first test for the evaluation of the cervical spine in degenerative conditions. The authors noted that disc herniation, canal stenosis, subluxation, and malalignment could be appreciated using MRI. They concluded, "MRI can certainly replace plain film myelography for the overwhelming majority of situations. … While the cost at first may seem prohibitive, the information that MRI is capable of providing in a noninvasive outpatient setting more than compensates for the expense."

Glenn et al.[64] and Modic et al.[63] proposed schemes for staging spinal degenerative disease. In the Modic scheme, signal intensity changes in vertebral body marrow adjacent to the endplates of degenerated discs are classified as follows:

- *Type I:*
Decreased signal on T_1-weighted images
Increased signal on T_2-weighted images

These changes are thought to represent acute disc degeneration.

- *Type II:*
Increased signal on T_1-weighted images
Iso- or hyperintense signal on T_2-weighted images
Histologic studies demonstrate yellow marrow replacement in the involved vertebral bodies and may represent a progression from type I changes.

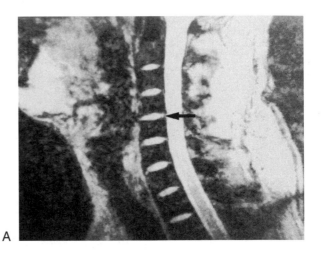

A

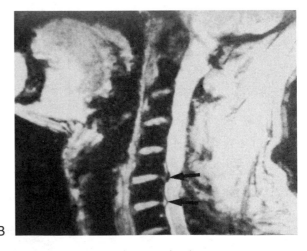

B

Figure 6-9. (A) Sagittal T_2-weighted magnetic resonance image demonstrating mild, early degenerative changes at C4-C5. **(B)** Sagittal T_2-weighted magnetic resonance image showing two subligamentous herniations at C5-C6 and C6-C7 (*arrows*).

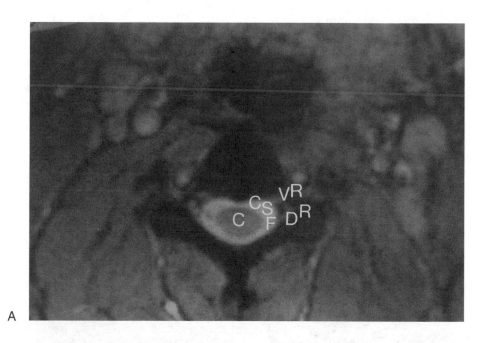

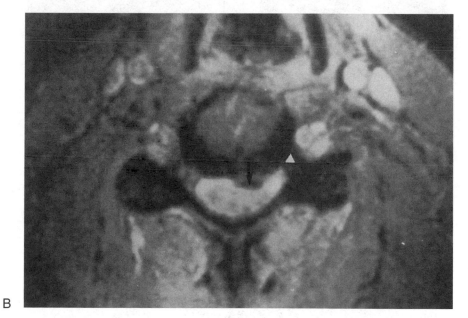

Figure 6-10. (A) Normal axial T$_2$-weighted magnetic resonance image through the lower cervical spine. Note spinal cord (C), cerebrospinal fluid (CSF), ventral root (VR), and dorsal root (DR). **(B)** Axial T$_2$-weighted magnetic resonance image through the lower cervical spine. Note disc herniation (*arrow*) causing impression on the spinal cord and osteophyte (*arrowhead*) causing foraminal encroachment.

- *Type III:*

Decreased signal on T_1-weighted images

Decreased signal on T_2-weighted images

Type III changes result from absence of marrow in areas of advanced bony sclerosis.

The Glenn scheme is based on the degree of foraminal and disc involvement, and has five stages as shown in Figure 6-11.

Karnaze et al.[65] compared CT and MRI findings in a retrospective study of 38 patients with suspected lesions of the cervical and thoracic spinal cord and canal. Nine of these patients demonstrated spondylosis. It was concluded that MRI was equal or superior to CT myelography in depicting

cases of cord enlargement, cord compression, and cord atrophy. Koyanagi et al.[66] reported that MRI studies in three patients with spondylosis were able to show directly compression of the spinal cord. These investigators noted that difficulty in detecting the abnormality at the thoracolumbar junction of plain radiographs often resulted in a delay in diagnosis.

Takahashi et al.[67] described the MRI changes evident in 128 patients with compressive lesions of the cervical spinal canal. They found that high-intensity lesions on T_2-weighted images were generally observed in patients with constriction or narrowing of the spinal cord. This abnormality is thought to be due to myelomalacia or cord gliosis secondary to long-standing cord compression.

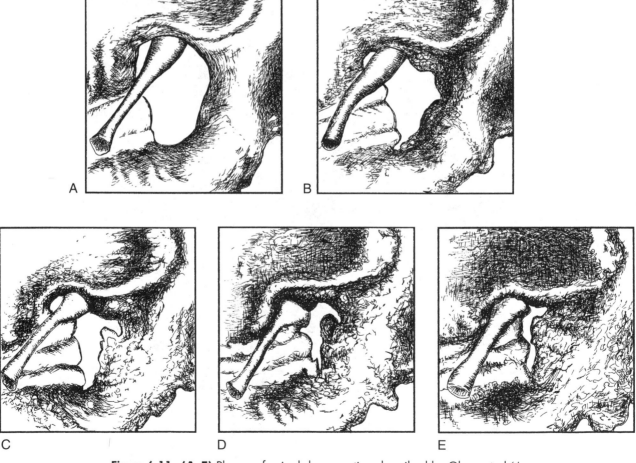

Figure 6-11. (A–E) Phases of spinal degeneration described by Glenn et al.[64]

Grenier et al.[68] did a retrospective study of 13 healthy subjects and 30 patients with degeneration of posterior spinal structures. These workers reported that sagittal MRI were useful in demonstrating hypertrophy of the ligamentum flava, facet degeneration, the degree of foraminal stenosis and measurement of the sagittal diameter of the spinal cord. Axial images facilitated the analysis of the facet joints, and permitted more accurate measurement of the thickness of the ligamentum flava and spinal cord diameter.

Batzdorf and Batzdorf[69] conducted an analysis of cervical spine curvature in 28 patients with cervical spondylosis. Plain films were used to evaluate spinal curves, and MRI was used to observe migration of the spinal cord. Although there was no clear correlation between severity of myelopathy and altered curvature, it was observed that neck pain was most severe in patients with a reversal of the cervical curve.

The CSF hypothesis of vertebral subluxation proposes that altered CSF dynamics result from alterations of sacral, vertebral, and cranial mobility. Klose et al.[70] employed MRI to evaluate CSF oscillation. These workers reported that oscillation of the CSF within the cardiac cycle is superimposed by a directed movement. The authors stated the movement was cranial directed in the lateral cervical subarachnoid spaces, and caudal in the ventral subarachnoid spaces. The use of this technology to evaluate the effects of subluxation on CSF circulation holds promise.

Support can be found in the literature[71–73] for the use of MRI for the detection and characterization of the following manifestations of subluxation degeneration (Fig. 6-12):

1. Subluxation and malalignment
2. Intervertebral disc desiccation and degeneration
3. Osteophytosis
4. Corrugation/hypertrophy of the ligamentum flava
5. Spinal canal stenosis
6. Foraminal stenosis
7. Disc herniation
8. Facet asymmetry
9. Facet degeneration
10. Altered CSF dynamics
11. Cord compression

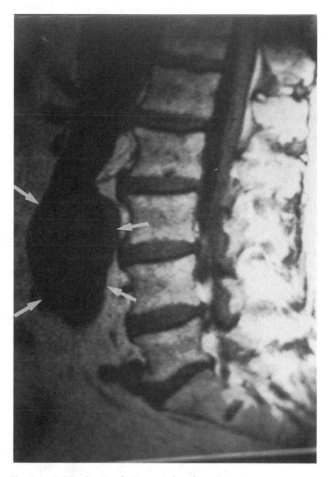

Figure 6-12. Sagittal T$_1$-weighted magnetic resonance image of a patient with an abdominal aortic aneurysm (*arrows*).

12. Gliosis and myelomalacia
13. Spinal cord atrophy

SONOGRAPHIC IMAGING

Basic Principles

Sonographic imaging uses echoes from ultrasonic waves to produce an image on a cathode-ray tube. Ultrasonic waves are transmitted and received by piezoelectric crystals. When an electrical signal is fed to a piezoelectric crystal, it vibrates at a specific frequency. Conversely, when ultrasonic energy is reflected back to the crystal, an electrical signal is produced. The strength of this signal is determined by how much energy is absorbed or reflected by the tissue being examined. This, in turn, determines the brightness of the spot on the screen. The assembly containing the crystals is known as a transducer.[74]

Pasto and Goldberg[75] described the factors influencing the appearance of echoes when performing sonographic imaging. Solid tissues have homogeneous or slightly granular reflectivity. This is referred to as *echogenicity*. By contrast, fluid structures lack internal structure, and therefore exhibit minimal echo return to the transducer. In clinical practice, the transducer may be oriented vertically along the spine to produce a longitudinal image or horizontally to produce an axial (cross-sectional) image. A coupling gel is used between the transducer and the skin to permit propagation of the ultrasonic waves. The procedure uses no ionizing radiation. Diagnostic ultrasound machines emit only a tiny fraction (typically 1/100) of the energy used in therapeutic ultrasound. Modern ultrasound imaging equipment also permits the precise measurement of anatomic structures and pathologic lesions. Images may be recorded on a printer. Or, in the case of dynamic (real-time motion) studies, on videotape.

Clinical Applications

Ultrasonic imaging is generally employed to evaluate soft tissue lesions and for functional vascular assessments with Doppler methods. It is also used to examine the fetus. Spinal applications have generally focused on the infant and pediatric spine. Because ultrasound does not penetrate bone, its clinical utility in evaluating the adult spine is limited. However, several applications for adult spinal sonography have been described in the literature.

Porter et al.[76] used sonography to measure the lumbar spinal canal in more than 700 subjects. Included in the study were persons ranging in age from newborn to 65 years. These investigators found that the canal was relatively wide in children, reached maximum diameter in the late teens, and then reduced slightly in adulthood. In examining more than 700 patients with back pain, the size of the canal was found to be significant in patients with neurogenic claudication and disc symptoms.

Other investigators have explored the use of sonographic measurement of the lumbar canal. Anderson et al.[77] measured the oblique parasagittal diameter of the lumbar canal in 49 hospital employees. Individuals with a canal diameter of less than 14 mm represented the lowest tenth percentile of the population. Being in the narrowest tenth percentile was reported as a risk factor for time missed from work due to low back pain. It was noted that ultrasound imaging may be useful for preplacement screening in industry. Chovil et al.[78] reviewed reports of the use of ultrasound imaging to measure the lumbar spinal canal, and suggested that ultrasound imaging may be a useful screening tool to identify narrow lumbar spinal canals.

In addition to spinal canal measurement, ultrasound imaging has been used to determine focal stenosis and disc disease. Engel et al.[79] used ultrasound imaging to evaluate the lumbar spines of 67 symptomatic patients. Focal stenosis was seen either as an isolated finding or in conjunction with diffuse stenosis in 44 patients. These investigators compared the results disclosed by the ultrasound imaging with myelographic and surgical findings. They described a "triple-density" sign representing soft tissue protrusion between two bony landmarks. In 19 cases where the sign was present, the sensitivity of this sign for indicating disc herniation was 89 percent. The specificity was 100 percent. For focal stenosis confirmed by surgery in 19 patients, the sensitivity was 95 percent, and the specificity was 100 percent.

Suzuki et al.[80] used ultrasound to measure vertebral body rotation in patients with idiopathic scoliosis. This was done by outlining the spinous process and laminae. The authors reported a strong linear relationship between the Cobb angle and the rotation of the apical vertebra in untreated patients but found that this relationship was lost in patients who had brace treatment. It was concluded that vertebral rotation can easily be measured by ultrasound.

A small study by Moore[81] compared sonographic results in patients with back pain previously examined by MRI, x-ray, and standard orthopedic examination. Moore stated, "Our correlation with MRI, x-ray, orthopedic and neurologic examination is approximately 90 percent."

The low cost, availability, ease of application, and noninvasive nature of sonographic imaging make it an attractive addition to the chiropractor's armamentarium. Furthermore, it has the potential to image various components of the vertebral subluxation complex, including spinal kinesiopathology, neuropathology, myopathology, histopathology, and pathology. However, caution must be exercised in evaluating the claims of promotors of sonographic equipment, particularly those relating to the assessment of nerve root or facet joint disease. Further research toward the establishment of chiropractic protocols should be undertaken to explore the clinical value of spinal sonography in chiropractic practice.

CONCLUSION

The chiropractic profession has made contributions to the field of diagnostic imaging. Diagnostic imaging procedures enable the doctor of chiropractic to determine the appropriateness of chiropractic care. Biomechanical analysis using chiropractic spinography may be used as an outcome assessment for chiropractic care. Advanced imaging procedures, such as videofluoroscopy, CT, and MRI imaging have established roles in chiropractic practice. Ultrasound imaging is a promising technology. Further research will determine the role of sonography in chiropractic practice.

Terminology

cineradiography
collimator
computed tomography (CT or CAT scanning)
image intensifier
magnetic resonance imaging (MRI)
radiograph
radiography
radiolucent
radiopaque
Roentgen, William
sonography
ultrasonography
videofluoroscopy

Review Questions

1. When were x-rays discovered? When were x-ray techniques first used in chiropractic?

2. What are the four requirements for x-ray production?

3. What are the four radiographic densities?

4. List the indications that were proposed for chiropractic radiographic examinations.

5. List the four patient classifications based on radiographic findings.

6. Describe any four radiographic manifestations of vertebral subluxation.

7. Define videofluoroscopy.

8. Describe the basic process of CT.

9. Describe the difference between T_1- and T_2-weighted magnetic resonance images.

10. List three possible applications for MRI in chiropractic practice.

Concept Questions

1. Under what circumstances do you feel x-ray examination is justified?

2. Compare the clinical value of CT with MRI.

References

1. Eisenberg RL: Radiology: An Illustrated History. Mosby-Year Book, St. Louis, 1992

2. Canterbury R, Krakos G: Thirteen years after Roentgen: the origins of chiropractic radiology. Chiro Hist 6:25, 1986

3. Palmer BJ: The Bigness of the Fellow Within. Palmer School of Chiropractic, Davenport, IA, 1949

4. Canterbury R: Radiography and chiropractic spinography p. 289. In Peterson D, Wiese G (eds): Chiropractic: An Illustrated History. Mosby-Year Book, St. Louis, 1995

5. Curry TS, Dowdey JE, Murry RC: Christiansen's Introduction to the Physics of Diagnostic Radiology. Lea & Febiger, Philadelphia, 1990

6. Shearer DR, Hendee WR: Roentgenography. p. 22. In Putnam CE, Ravin CE (eds): Textbook of Diagnostic Imaging. WB Saunders, Philadelphia, 1994

7. Hendee WR, Ritenour ER: Medical Imaging Physics. Mosby-Year Book, Chicago, 1992

8. Grossman CB: Magnetic Resonance Imaging and Computed Tomography of the Head and Spine. Williams & Wilkins, Baltimore, 1990

9. Stephenson R: Chiropractic Textbook, The Palmer School of Chiropractic, Davenport, IA, 1927

10. Dishman RW: Review of the literature supporting a scientific basis for the chiropractic subluxation complex. J Manipul Physiol Ther 8:163, 1985

11. Kent C, Gentempo P: The Documentary Basis for Diagnostic Imaging Procedures in the Subluxation-Based Chiropractic Practice. International Chiropractors Association, Arlington, VA, 1992

12. Akeson WH, Woo SL, Taylor TK et al: Biomechanics and biochemistry of the intervertebral discs. Clin Orthop 122:133, 1977

13. White AA, Johnson RM, Panjabi MM, Southwick WO: Biomechanical analysis of clinical stability in the cervical spine. Clin Orthop 109:85, 1975

14. Vernon H: Static and dynamic roentgenography in the diagnosis of degenerative disc disease: a review and comparative assessment. J Manipul Physiol Ther 5:163, 1982

15. Ressel OJ: Disc regeneration: reversibility is possible in spinal osteoarthritis. ICA Rev 45:39, 1989

16. Posner I, White AA, Edwards WT, Hayes WC: A biomechanical analysis of the clinical stability of the lumbar and lumbosacral spine. Spine 7:374, 1982

17. Nachemson A: Towards a better understanding of low back pain; a review of the mechanics of the lumbar disc. Rheumatol Rehabil 14:129, 1975

18. Huelke DF, Nusholtz GS: Cervical spine biomechanics: a review of the literature. J Orthop Res 4:232, 1986

19. Leach RA: The Chiropractic Theories. Williams & Wilkins, Baltimore, 1986

20. Reiter L: Apophyseal joint functional anatomy and experimental findings—a literature review. Res Forum 1:49, 1985

21. Bullough OG, Boachie-Adjei O: Atlas of Spinal Diseases. JB Lippincott, Philadelphia, 1988

22. Evans DK: Anterior cervical subluxation. J Bone Joint Surg 8B:318, 1976

23. Scher AT: Anterior cervical subluxation: an unstable position. AJR 133:275, 1979

24. Green JD, Harle TS, Harris JH: Anterior subluxation of the cervical spine: hyperflexion sprain. AJNR 2:243, 1981

25. Dvorak J, Froelich D, Penning L et al: Functional radiographic diagnosis of the cervical spine: flexion/extension. Spine 13:748, 1988

26. Norris S, Watt I: The prognosis of neck injuries resulting from rear-end vehicle collisions. J Bone Joint Surg 65B:608, 1983

27. Nagasawa A, Sakakibara T, Takahashi A: Roentgenographic findings of the cervical spine in tension-type headache. Headache 33:90, 1993

28. Leach RA: An evaluation of the effect of chiropractic manipulative therapy on hypolordosis of the cervical spine. J Manipul Physiol Ther 6:17, 1983

29. Harrison DD, Jackson BL, Troyanovich S et al: The efficacy of cervical extension-compression traction combined with diversified manipulation and drop table adjustments in the rehabilitation of cervical lordosis: a pilot study. J Manipul Physiol Ther 17:454, 1994

30. Jackson BL, Harrison DD, Robertson GA, Barker WF: Chiropractic biophysics lateral cervical film analysis reliability. J Manipul Physiol Ther 16:384, 1993

31. Grostic JD, DeBoer KF: Roentgenographic measurement of atlas laterality and rotation: a retrospective pre- and post-manipulation study. J Manipul Physiol Ther 5:63, 1982

32. Jackson BL, Barker W, Bentz J, Gambale AG: Inter- and intraexaminer reliability of the upper cervical x-ray marking system: a second look. J Manipul Physiol Ther 10:157, 1987

33. Rochester RC: Inter- and intra-examiner reliability of the upper cervical x-ray marking system: a third and expanded look. Chiro Res J 3:23, 1994

34. Plaugher G, Hendricks AH: The interexaminer reliability of the Gonstead pelvic marking system. J Manipul Physiol Ther 14:503, 1991

35. Zengel F, Davis BP: Biomechanical analysis by chiropractic radiography. Part II. Effects of x-ray projectional distortion on apparent vertebral rotation. J Manipul Physiol Ther 11:380, 1988

36. Zengel F, Davis BP: Biomechanical analysis by chiropractic radiography. Part III. Lack of effect of projectional distortion on Gonstead vertebral endplate lines. J Manipul Physiol Ther 11:469, 1988

37. Shaff AM: Videofluoroscopy as a method of detecting occipitoatlantal instability in Down's syndrome for Special Olympics. Chiro Sports Med 8:144, 1994

38. Wood J, Wagner N: A review of methods for radiographic analysis of cervical sagittal motion. Chiro Tech 4:83, 1992

39. Wallace H, Wagnon R, Pierce W: Inter-examiner reliability using videofluoroscope to measure cervical spine kinematics: a sagittal plane (lateral view). In Proceedings of the International Conference on Spinal Manipulation, Arlington, VA, May 1992

40. Van Mameren H, Sanches H, Beursgens J, Drukker J: Cervical spine motion in the sagittal plane II. Spine 17:467, 1992

41. Bland JH: Disorders of the Cervical Spine. WB Saunders, Philadelphia, 1987

42. Buonocare E, Hartman JT, Nelson CL: Cineradiograms of cervical spine in diagnosis of soft-tissue injuries. JAMA 198:143, 1966

43. Foreman SM, Croft AC: Whiplash Injuries: The Cervical Acceleration/Deceleration Syndrome. Williams & Wilkins, Baltimore, 1988

44. Antos J, Robinson GK, Keating JC, Jacobs GE: Interexaminer reliability of cinefluoroscopic detection of fixation in the mid-cervical spine. In Proceedings of the Scientific Symposium on Spinal Bimechanics, International Chiropractors Association, 1989

45. Kricun R, Kricun ME: Computed tomography. p. 376. In Kricun ME (ed): Imaging Modalities in Spinal Disorders. WB Saunders, Philadelphia, 1988

46. Grossman AD, Katz DS, Santelli ED et al: Cost-Effective Diagnostic Imaging: The Clinician's Guide. CV Mosby, St. Louis, 1995

47. Fullerton GD, Potter JL: Computed tomography. p. 43. In Putnam CE, Ravin CE (eds): Textbook of Diagnostic Imaging. WB Saunders, Philadelphia, 1994

48. Ebrall P, Molyneux T: Rotary subluxation of the atlas: an exploration of the diagnostic potential of the CT scan. Chiro J Aust 23:42, 1993

49. Richards G, Thompson J, Osterbauer P, Fuhr A: Use of pre- and post-CT scans and clinical findings to monitor low force chiropractic care of patients with sciatic neuropathy and lumbar disc herniation: a review. J Manipul Physiol Ther 13:58, 1990

50. Walker B: The use of computer-assisted tomography of the lumbar spine in a chiropractic practice. J Aust Chiro Assoc 15:86, 1985

51. Koentges A: Computerized axial tomography of the spine in the differential diagnosis of vertebral subluxations. Ann Swiss Chiro Assoc 8:25, 1985

52. Kent C: Contemporary technologies for imaging the vertebral subluxation complex. ICA Rev 45:45, 1989

53. Elster A: Magnetic Resonance Imaging: A Reference Guide and Atlas. JB Lippincott, Philadelphia, 1986

54. Zimmer W, Berqist T, McLeod R et al: Bone tumors: magnetic resonance imaging vs. computed tomography. Radiology 155:709, 1985

55. Moon K, Genant H, Helms C et al: Nuclear magnetic resonance imaging in orthopedics: principles and applications. J Orthop Res 1:104, 1983

56. Beltran J, Noto A, Herman L et al: Joint effusions: MR imaging. Radiology 158:133, 1986

57. Moon K Jr, Genant H, Helms C: Musculoskeletal applications of nuclear magnetic resonance. Radiology 147:161, 1983

58. Brady T, Gebhardt M, Pykett I et al: NMR imaging of forearms in healthy volunteers and patients with giant cell tumor of bone. Radiology 144:549, 1982

59. Aisen A, Martel W, Braunstein E et al: MRI and CT evaluation of primary bone and soft-tissue tumors. AJR 146:749, 1986

60. Wong W: Practical MRI: A Case Study Approach. Aspen, Rockville, MD, 1987

61. Modic M, Weinstein M, Pavlicek W et al: Nuclear magnetic resonance imaging of the spine. Radiology 148:757, 1983

62. Modic M, Steinberg P, Ross J et al: Degenerative disk disease: assessment of changes in vertebral body marrow with MR imaging. Radiology 166:193, 1988

63. Modic MT, Ross JS, Masaryk TJ: Imaging of degenerative disease of the cervical spine. Clin Orthop 239:109, 1989

64. Glenn WV, Burnett K, Rauschning W: Magnetic Resonance Imaging of the Lumbar Spine: Nerve Root Canals, Disc Abnormalities, Anatomic Correlations, and Case Examples. General Electric Company, Milwaukee, 1986

65. Karnaze MG, Gado MH, Sartor KJ, Hodges FJ III: Comparison of MR and CT myelography in imaging the cervical and thoracic spine. AJR 150:397, 1988

66. Koyanagi I, Isu T, Iwasaki Y et al: Radiological diagnosis of chronic spinal cord compressive lesion at thoraco-lumbar junction. No Shinkei Geka 16:1227, 1988

67. Takahashi M, Sakamoto Y, Miyawaki M, Bussaka H: Increased MR signal intensity secondary to chronic cervical cord compression. Neuroradiology 29:550, 1987

68. Grenier N, Kressel HY, Scheibler ML et al: Normal and degenerative posterior spinal structures: MR Imaging. Radiology 165:517, 1987

69. Batzdorf U, Batzdorf A: Analysis of cervical spine curvature in patients with cervical spondylosis. Neurosurgery 22:827, 1988

70. Klose U, Requardt H, Schroth G, Deimling M: MR tomographic demonstration of liquor pulsation. ROFO Fortsher Geb Rontgenstr Nuklearmed 147:313, 1987

71. Kent C, Gentempo P: MR imaging of subluxation degeneration. Chiro Res J 1:39, 1991

72. Kent C, Holt FJ, Gentempo P: Subluxation degeneration in the lumbar spine: plain film and MR imaging considerations. Int Rev Chiro 47:55, 1991

73. Kent C, Gentempo P: Subluxation degeneration in the cervical spine: plain film and MRI findings. Int Rev Chiro 47:47, 1991

74. Aldrete JA: Diagnostic ultrasound in pain management: an overview. Am J Pain Management 4:160, 1994

75. Pasto ME, Goldberg BB: Sonography. p. 598. In Kricun ME (ed): Imaging Modalities in Spinal Disorders. WB Saunders, Philadelphia, 1988

76. Porter RW, Hilbert C, Wellman P: Backache and the lumbar spinal canal. Spine 5:99, 1980

77. Anderson DJ, Adcock DF, Chovil AC, Farrell JJ: Ultrasound lumbar canal measurement in hospital employees with back pain. Br J Ind Med 45:552, 1988

78. Chovil AC, Anderson DJ, Adcock DF: Ultrasonic measurement of lumbar canal diameter: a screening tool for low back disorders? South Med J 82:977, 1989

79. Engel JM, Engel GM, Gunn DR: Ultrasound of the spine in focal stenosis and disc disease. Spine 10:928, 1985

80. Suzuki S, Yamamuro T, Shikata J et al: Ultrasound measurement of vertebral rotation in idiopathic scoliosis. J Bone Joint Surg 71B:252, 1989

81. Moore RE: Blind study: comparison of sonographic results in patients with back pain previously diagnosed by MRI, x-ray and standard orthopedic exam. Am J Clin Chiro 5:34, 1995

7

The Art of Manual Palpation and Adjustment

John G. Scaringe
David Sikorski

Palpation and chiropractic adjustive procedures are an art, not an exact science. Some individuals are gifted with the talents of manual therapy, while others have to practice hard to acquire the skill. A thorough understanding of basic and applied clinical sciences along with many hours of practice and concentration are necessary for the student and practitioner to master this art. Manual palpation and adjustment are the chiropractor's primary evaluative and therapeutic interventions and are used in combination with other diagnostic and treatment methods of chiropractic case management.

IDENTIFYING THE ADJUSTIVE LESION

Chiropractic has brought to the health sciences a special interest in the neuromusculoskeletal system that emphasizes the relations between alterations in structure and function. Clinical approaches that omit static and dynamic evaluation of the physical structure are incomplete. The chiropractic physician considering adjustive procedures must identify whether conditions exist that support manual ther-

apy. Haldeman[1] has referred to this process as the "identification of the manipulable lesion." This lesion, also described as the adjustive lesion, subluxation, joint fixation, or blockage (Table 7-1), is a complex clinical entity whose evaluation should not rely on a single evaluative tool. The following components will provide a system that uses various clinical indicators to identify the adjustive lesion.

Components of the Adjustive Lesion

The physician must always determine whether there is a clinical basis for treatment. Despite wide variation in the theorized mechanism of action of the adjustment, there is a reasonable amount of agreement on the clinical nature of the adjustive lesion. As with other aspects of patient evaluation, the chiropractor uses observation, palpation, percussion, and auscultation when identifying the adjustive lesion. Using the modified acronym *PARTS* used by Bourdillon and Day,[2] Bergmann[3,4] describes five diagnostic criteria (**P**ain/tenderness; **A**symmetry; **R**ange-of-motion abnormality; **T**issue tone, texture, and temperature abnormality; and **S**pecial tests) for the identification of joint subluxation/dysfunction.

Table 7-1. Definition of Terms Describing Functional or Structural Disorders of the Synovial Joints

Orthopedic subluxation
   A partial or incomplete dislocation
Chiropractic subluxation
   An aberrant relationship between two adjacent structures that may have functional or pathologic sequelae
Joint dysfunction
   Joint mechanics showing functional disturbances without structural changes
Somatic dysfunction
   Impaired or altered function or related components of the body framework (somatic system)
Osteopathic lesion
   A disturbance of musculoskeletal structure and/or function as well as accompanying disturbances of other biologic mechanisms
Joint fixation (restriction)
   The temporary immobilization of a joint in a position that it may normally occupy during any phase of normal movement

(Adapted from Bergmann et al.,[4] with permission.)

Pain and Tenderness

Pain is the localized sensation of discomfort, distress, or agony reported by an individual.[5] By contrast, tenderness is defined as abnormal sensitivity to touch or pressure.[5] Most patients with musculoskeletal disorders report pain as part of the clinical presentation. The location, quality, and intensity of pain or tenderness may help the clinician identify the origin of the patient's complaint. Pain of mechanical origin is characteristically aggravated by movement and often decreased or relieved by rest or inactivity. The location, quality, and intensity of tenderness produced by palpation of various structures (osseous and soft tissues) should also be noted. Pain and tenderness can be identified by taking a thorough history and evaluating the results of observation, percussion, and palpation. The chiropractor can use various reliable valid tools to measure and quantify pain. These include pain and functional capacity questionnaires, algometers, pain scales, diagrams, and drawings.

Asymmetry

Antalgic and asymmetric postures are common in acute presentations but are often within normal limits in mildly symptomatic patients. Asymmetric qualities can be noted on a sectional or segmental level. Alterations in segmental alignment may be noted by comparing adjacent osseous structures (e.g., spinous process, transverse process). These malalignments of the spine and extremity joints are of limited diagnostic value in the absence of other abnormal physical findings (e.g., normal variations and anomalies). Asymmetry is identified through observation (posture and gait analysis), static palpation, and static radiography.

Range of Motion

Changes in active, passive, and accessory joint motions should be noted. As with antalgic postures, global movements are characteristically guarded and restricted in acute presentations but often within normal limits in mildly symptomatic patients. Segmental motion palpation usually elicits local pain[6–8] or abnormal motion, or both. These abnormal motion changes may be either an increase or decrease of segmental range of motion, joint play, or end play. Range of motion abnormalities are identified through motion palpation procedures and stress radiography.

Tone, Texture, and Temperature

Changes in the characteristics of contiguous and associated soft tissues, including skin, fascia, muscle, and ligaments, should be noted. Reactive changes in these related soft tissues often lead to local muscle spasm. Long-standing joint dysfunction may be associated with areas of induration (abnormally hard spots), which palpate as deep sites of nodular or rope-like consistency. Tissue tone, texture, and/or temperature changes are identified through observation, palpation, instrumentation, muscle length, and strength testing.

Special Tests

Special tests include additional physical examination or laboratory procedures, or both, that aid in the differential diagnosis of joint dysfunction. Examples include orthopedic and neurologic tests, radiographic and imaging procedures, blood and urine testing, and electrodiagnosis. Testing procedures specific to a technique system such as leg-length assessment, specific radiographic marking techniques, and particular muscle testing procedures, should also be considered.

Palpation Procedures

Inspection, auscultation, and palpation are the three basic diagnostic methods used in clinical medicine.[9] In an age of rapidly growing technology with sophisticated diagnostic and laboratory equipment, palpation is underused in conventional medicine. Palpation is recognized as an essential skill by chiropractors, osteopaths, and physical and manual therapists and is one of the most important tools used by chiropractic physicians to identify the adjustive (manipulable) lesion. It should be noted that, after a well-executed history, palpation provides the first direct physical contact with the patient.[10] The quality of this contact may strengthen existing trust or destroy positive rapport between clinician and patient.

The foundations of palpatory literacy are knowledge of anatomy (cognitive) and the acute ability to touch and feel (psychomotor)[10] (Table 7-2). Although anatomic knowledge is primarily cognitive in nature, the development of psychomotor skill is a complex phenomenon that must be obtained by experience and practice. Thus, developing good palpation skills requires many hours of practice and concentration. The skillful palpator who develops both tactile and kinesthetic sensation will also find the art of adjusting and manipulation easier to master.

Table 7-2. Static Palpation Tips

1. Use the least pressure possible (touch receptors are designed to respond only when not pressed on too firmly).
2. Concentrate on the area and/or structure you want to palpate.
3. Try not to cause pain if possible (pain may induce protective muscle splinting and make palpation more difficult).
4. Carefully penetrate to deeper structures (brisk progress may induce reflexive muscle spasm).
5. Try not to lose skin contact before you are done with the palpation of the area.
6. Use broad contacts whenever possible.
7. Close your eyes to increase your palpatory perception.

(Adapted from Bergmann et al.,[4] with permission.)

Palpation procedures are commonly divided into static and dynamic assessments (Table 7-3). Static palpation is usually performed with the patient in a stationary position, and includes bony (joint structures) and soft tissue assessment. Dynamic, or motion, palpation is commonly performed to assess abnormal vertebral or extremity joint movements, as well as to evaluate accessory joint motion and is performed with the patient in a variety of positions.[3,4,8,11–16]

Static Palpation

Static palpation of bony landmarks of the spine and pelvis includes assessment of spinous, transverse, and mammillary processes of the vertebrae, and the posterior superior iliac spine (PSIS), ischial tuberosities, and iliac crest contours of the innominate bones. Bony landmarks such as femoral condyles, olecranon processes, and greater trochanters are examples of bony landmarks commonly palpated around extremity joints. The evaluator should note any asymmetries or anomalies, while keeping in mind that positional faults are unreliable and should be confirmed with additional evaluation procedures.

Palpatory tenderness has been shown to be a reliable method for identifying the adjustive lesion.[6–8] However, there is a difference between palpation of pain and tenderness and tactile palpation. Tactile palpation provides thermal and mechanical information that aids in structural assessment and may correlate with previous examination and historical findings. Tenderness palpation, on the other hand, may help distinguish healthy from unhealthy tissues.[10] Healthy tissues can usually tolerate greater pressure than can injured or diseased tissues. In the

Table 7-3. Types of Palpation

Static palpation
    Bony
    Soft tissue
Dynamic (motion) palpation
    Active
    Passive
        Joint play
        End play (end feel)
        Accessory

absence of a destructive lesion, these tissue changes are important indicators of joint subluxations/dysfunctions which may respond to manual treatment procedures.

Layer palpation is a systematic method of assessing the mobility and condition of myofascial and other soft tissue structures.[17] Palpation begins with the most superficial structures and proceeds to deeper tissues. Light palpation with the pads of the fingers is used to assess superficial tissues (Fig. 7-1). Deeper structures require increased pressure, and should be performed in a firm but gentle manner. Anatomic structure and tissue characteristics that can be palpated are listed in Tables 7-4 and 7-5.

On palpating the paraspinal tissues and myofascial structures of the extremities, areas of focal irritation with discrete palpable thickening or muscle contraction are commonly felt. These taut and tender fibers, or *trigger points*, can be found in the long paraspinal muscles, shoulder girdle muscles (infraspinatus, supraspinatus, trapezius, rhomboid, levator scapulae), the pelvis (iliopsoas, piriformis, quadratus, gluteal, tensor fascia lata), and extremity muscles (extensor carpi radialis, vastus medialis, soleus).[18–20]

Table 7-4. Structures Commonly Palpated

Blood vessels
Bones and bony processes
Fascia
    Subcutaneous
    Deep
Joint spaces
Ligaments
Muscle
    Bellies
    Sheaths
Musculotendinous junctions
Peripheral nerves
Skin
Tendons

Myofascial trigger points can be identified by flat or pincer palpation.[18] During flat palpation, the palpator's fingertips move the patient's subcutaneous tissue and skin across the taut muscle fibers. Pincer palpation is performed by grasping the muscle belly

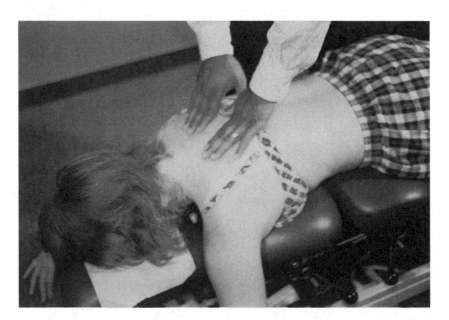

Figure 7-1. Static palpation over the transverse processes, bilaterally, of the thoracic spine.

Table 7-5. Tissue Characteristics

Contour
Crepitus
Elasticity
Mobility
Moisture
Pulses
Shape
Symmetry
Temperature
Tenderness
Texture
Thickness
Tone

between the thumb and fingers while gently squeezing the tissues with a back and forth motion to locate taut bands. Figure 7-2 demonstrates pincer palpation of the common wrist extensor muscle group.

Dynamic (Motion) Palpation

A widely held view on the primary effect of the adjustment is that it increases the range of motion of a joint.[4,11,14,21] The location and characteristics of the altered or restricted joint movement (fixation) must therefore be determined before an adjust-

ment/manipulation can be performed. The primary technique for this evaluation is the dynamic (motion) assessment of the various joints of the spine, pelvis, and extremities. Specific techniques for palpating motion in joints can be divided into active, passive, and accessory movements (Table 7-3).

Normally a joint will move through a certain range of *active motion*. Active movements are performed by the patient while the examiner guides the patient through a particular motion. The patient's voluntary muscle contraction causes the joint to move and the associated periarticular soft tissues are evaluated by the clinician for tension and resiliency. At the end of active motion, the clinician can passively push the bony lever (e.g., spinous process), thereby further assessing the quality of resistance called *end play* or *end feel*. Springing of the joint and the determination of end play are an integral part of the premanipulation examination (Fig. 7-3).

Joint play assessment "is the qualitative evaluation of the joint's resistance to movement when it is in a neutral position."[4] Joint play exists because the artic-

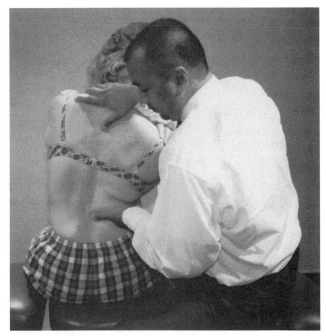

Figure 7-3. A motion (dynamic) palpation assessment for right lateral flexion of the L2 vertebra (L2-L3 motor unit) in the seated position.

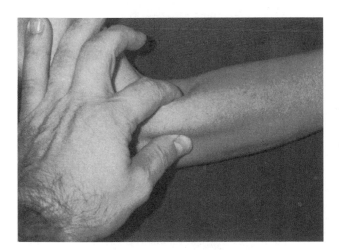

Figure 7-2. Pincer palpation of the patient's common wrist extensor muscle group.

ular surfaces do not perfectly fit. The incongruent articular surfaces also prevent a fixed axis of rotation from occurring during joint motion. The joint capsules and ligaments remain somewhat laxed to allow for rolling and gliding of the articular surfaces to accommodate for the changing axis of rotation around these irregular surfaces. The joint demonstrates "joint play" in the neutral position, or open-packed position, when it is under the least amount of stress, with the joint capsule and ligaments in the position of greatest laxity (Fig. 7-4). This joint play near the neutral position is followed by an active range of motion produced by voluntary muscle contraction. The end point of the active range of motion is called the *physiologic barrier*[22] (Fig. 7-4).

If active range of motion is under the control of the musculature, *passive movements* are involuntary. Passive range of motion is defined as "movements carried through by the operator (clinician) without the conscious assistance or resistance of the patient."[4] The passive range of joint motion is greater than the range of active joint movement (Fig. 7-4). During active joint movements, the muscles move the joint to the physiologic barrier. Further movement past this barrier, into the *end play zone*, is produced by additional overpressure per-formed by the examiner (Figs. 7-3 and 7-4). This end play zone, or increase in passive resistance, is thought to result from the elastic properties of the joint capsule and periarticular soft tissues. If the examiner releases the pressure while stressing the tissues in the end play zone, the joint springs back to its physiologic barrier. Movement beyond the end play zone is typically associated with a "cracking" noise followed by a slight increase in the range of motion and has been referred to by Sandoz[23] as the *paraphysiologic space*. Movement into the paraphysiologic space is within the normal boundaries of a joint and does not cause joint injury. At this point, another barrier is encountered called the *anatomic barrier*. Further movement beyond this point will damage anatomical structures associated with the joint (Fig. 7-4).

To illustrate this point, actively flex your right index finger at the metacarpophalangeal (MCP) joint as far as possible (active movement to the physiologic barrier). With a finger from your left hand, apply additional pressure to flex the right MCP joint further (passive movement into the end play zone) (Fig. 7-5). It is the quality of this resistance (increased, decreased, or normal) in the "end play" zone that the examiner evaluates during end play

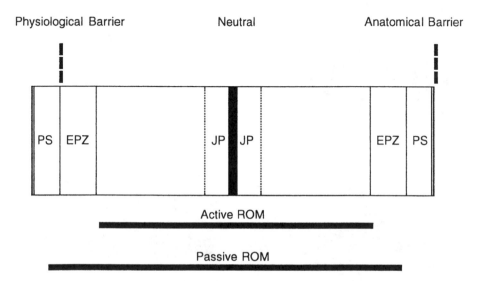

Figure 7-4. Active and passive components of joint motion. PS, paraphysiologic space; EPZ, end play zone; JP, joint play. Metacarpophalangeal joint end range palpation.

palpation. Now release the overpressure caused by your left finger and notice your right finger spring back toward the physiologic barrier (elastic properties of the capsule and periarticular soft tissues).

Accessory joint movements are small specific movements independent of voluntary muscle action.[4,8,16,21,24] Normal voluntary muscle action depends upon their character. If integrity of accessory movement is lacking, the active range of joint motion is decreased. Accessory movements are evaluated when performing joint play and end play procedures. As previously stated, joint play involves the qualitative assessment of resistance from the neutral joint position, while end play is resistance near the end of passive motion at the "end play zone."[4] The goals of accessory motion testing are to evaluate:

- Aspects of tissue compliance
- Amount of available range of motion
- Change in resistance relative to the range of motion
- Degree of resistance to motion.[16]

Information gained from accessory motion testing should be used with historical and other physical examination findings to establish a working diagnosis and treatment plan. As a diagnostic tool, however, accessory motion is primarily performed to determine relative joint resistance or stiffness (normal, hypermobility, or hypomobility). In the abnormal joint there is an increased resistance ("restriction") of movement in one or more directions forming a *pathologic (dysfunctional) barrier*. This resistance can vary in severity: it may be minor so that the range of movement is only slightly less than normal, or it may be major so that only a small range of joint movement remains.

An analogy or practical model to illustrate the qualitative assessment of joint play and end play would be to separate your thumb and index finger while having them wrapped with a rubber band (Fig. 7-6). The resistance felt with a single rubber band represents the normal tension and resiliency of a joint. Placing additional rubber bands around your fingers would represent the increased resistance felt with joint dysfunctions or restrictions.

CHIROPRACTIC ADJUSTIVE AND MANIPULATIVE PROCEDURES

Chiropractic adjustive and manipulative techniques fall within the broad classification of therapies known as manual procedures. As the term indicates, it encompasses all therapeutic procedures performed or administered by hand.[4] Although this form of treatment has been traced to numerous

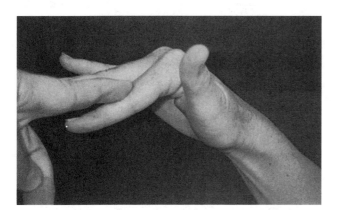

Figure 7-5. Passive movement into the end play zone of the metacarpophalangeal joint.

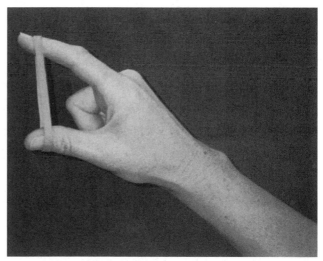

Figure 7-6. A practical model illustrating the qualitative assessment of joint end play using a rubberband wrapped around an index finger and thumb.

ancient civilizations throughout the world,[1,25,26] only within the last century has this method of treatment gained significance in the realm of mainstream health care, primarily via the growth and development of the chiropractic profession.[19,27,28]

Manual procedures may be divided into two general categories:

Joint manipulation, which includes the subcategories of the chiropractic adjustment, mobilization procedures, and traction-distraction procedures

Soft tissue manipulation, which encompasses point pressure techniques, massage, therapeutic muscle stretching, and visceral techniques[4] (Table 7-6)

A detailed study of all techniques and procedures in these categories is well beyond the scope of this chapter. This section offers the reader an overview of the more commonly used methods employed in the practice of chiropractic (Table 7-6).

Joint Manipulation Procedures

Joint manipulation procedures are techniques designed to introduce motion into a joint. They may involve the application of a dynamic thrust, as in adjustive procedures, or may be of a nonthrusting nature, as in mobilization and traction-distraction procedures.[4,19,29] In either case, the procedure is specifically intended to affect some element of the neuromusculoskeletal system, and in doing so, to produce therapeutically beneficial results for the recipient via the action on the tissues involved. Although the precise mechanism of the therapeutic

Table 7-6. Classification of Manual Therapies

Joint manipulation procedures
    Adjustments/Manipulation
    Mobilization
    Manual Traction/Distraction
Soft tissue manipulation procedures
    Point pressure techniques
    Massage
    Therapeutic muscle stretching/relaxation
    Visceral techniques

(Adapted from Bergmann et al.,[4] with permission)

action is not fully understood, it is believed by various authors to be the result of improved intra-articular relationship (alignment), restoration of proper joint range of motion, and reduction in tissue irritation and dysfunction.[4,19,30]

The terms *chiropractic adjustment* or *chiropractic manipulation* include a wide variety of manual and mechanical procedures applied with the intent of correcting a clinically identified adjustive lesion (e.g., subluxation, muscle dysfunction, motion dysfunction).[19] The adjustment is characterized by the application of a dynamic thrust to a joint of the axial or extremity skeleton, after the involved joint has been tensioned to the end of its physiologic limits. The speed, amplitude, and direction of the thrust must be precisely controlled by the clinician[4] in order to ensure the effectiveness of the procedure and minimize patient discomfort.

The adjustive or manipulative procedure forms the foundation of chiropractic treatment and constitutes the most common therapeutic procedure associated with the practice of chiropractic.[4] Simply stated, it is characteristic of the profession and represents application of the chiropractic art. As such, it is essential that the student as well as the practitioner of chiropractic devote significant time and energy to developing and maintaining the necessary cognitive and psychomotor skills.

Short Lever and Long Lever Adjustments

Adjustive procedures may be further classified according to the type of lever system employed in delivery of the dynamic thrust and the specificity associated with it. The two types commonly used are the *specific short lever adjustment* (Fig. 7-7) and the *nonspecific long lever adjustment* (Fig. 7-8). Although both involve administration of a controlled high-velocity, low-amplitude thrust, they vary in the method of doctor–patient contact relative to the target joint or joints, and consequently, in the specificity of the target area.

The *specific short lever* (Figs. 7-7 and 7-9) method incorporates a doctor contact directly on or over some part of the osseous structures directly associated with the manipulable lesion. Stabilization of the patient can be achieved with contacts in the immediate vicinity or at some distance away from the lesion.[4,19] Once contact and stabilization are

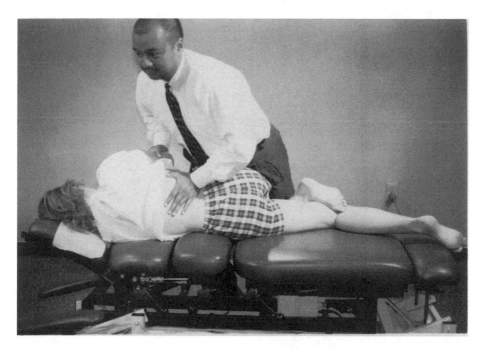

Figure 7-7. A short lever adjustment of the third lumbar vertebra using a soft pisiform contact over the right lateral aspect of the L3 spinous process.

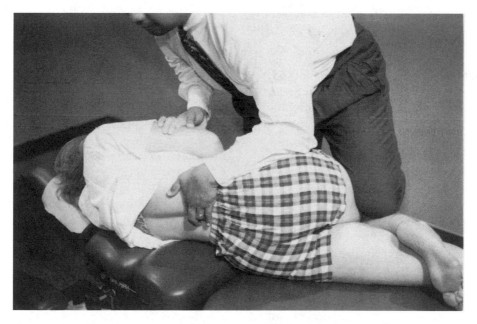

Figure 7-8. A long lever rotational adjustment of the lumbar spine using a digital contact on the patient's L3 spinous process. Note the use of the patient's right thigh as a lever to impart force to the patient's lumbar spine from the doctor's left leg.

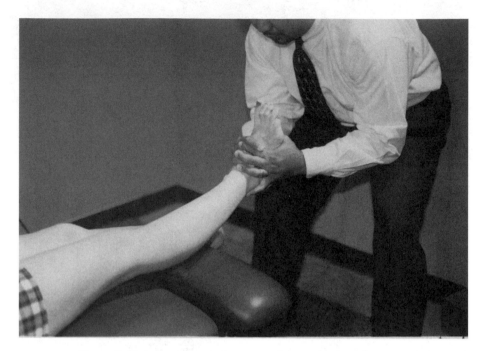

Figure 7-9. A distraction adjustment of the right tibiotalar joint.

established, the clinician tensions the joint to the end of its normal physiologic range ("locks" the joint) and delivers a controlled thrust, taking the joint into its paraphysiologic range. This movement into the paraphysiologic joint space is believed to initiate production of the audible "pop" or "click" associated with the adjustment. However, absence of this sound does not indicate that an effective adjustment was not achieved.[29] The short lever method is the most specific adjustive procedure available, allowing the experienced practitioner to affect individual target joints when skillfully applied.

By contrast, the *nonspecific long lever* (Fig. 7-8) method involves a doctor contact that may lie some distance from the targeted lesion or lesions. Although stabilization may be very similar to that employed in short lever methods, structures not directly associated with the manipulable lesion are positioned between the target area and the doctor contact.[4,19,29] Similarly, once contact and stabilization are established, the doctor delivers a controlled dynamic thrust, initiating the adjustment. This method of manipulation tends to be considerably less specific than the short lever technique, and is generally better suited for targeting an area or

region of the body rather than a specific joint. The skill, experience, and proficiency of the doctor, coupled with the clinical presentation of the patient, should be the major determining factors dictating the procedure of preference in any given situation.[31] With either method, the development and maintenance of the essential cognitive and psychomotor skills necessary to perform these procedures effectively with minimal risk to patient and doctor are crucial. It is the obligation of each practitioner to maintain the level of skill required for safe and effective practice.

Mechanical Devices to Aid Adjustment

Since the founding of the chiropractic profession and with the evolution of approximately one hundred technique systems[32] (Table 7-7), a number of mechanical devices and aids have been developed to assist in the effective delivery of the chiropractic adjustment. These range from a number of sophisticated adjusting tables, incorporating features such as spring or hydraulically operated drop pieces, to much simpler devices such as pelvic wedges, blocks, and anteriority boards (Fig. 7-10). All are designed to enhance the positioning of the patient or the doc-

Table 7-7. Named Chiropractic Techniques

Access seminars	Master energy dynamics
Activator technique	Mawhinney scoliosis technique
Alternative chiropractic adjustments	McTimody technique
Applied chiropractic distortion analysis	Mears technique
Applied spinal biomechanical engineering	Meric technique system
Applied kinesiology	Micromanipulation
Aquarian age health	Motion palpation
Arnholz muscle adjusting	Muscle palpation
Atlas orthogonality technique	Muscle response testing
Atlas specific	Musculoskeletal synchronization and stabilization technique
Bandy seminars	Nerve signal interference
Bio kinesiology	Network chiropractic
BioEnergetic synchronization technique (BEST)	Neuroemotional technique (NET)
Bioenergetics	Neuro-organizational technique
Biomagnetic technique	Neurolymphactic reflex technique
Blair upper cervical technique	Neurovascular reflex technique
Bloodless surgery	Olesky 21st century technique
Body integration	Ortman technique
Buxton technical course of painless chiropractic	Pettibon spinal biomechanical technique
Chiroenergetics	Pierce-Stillwagon technique
Chiro plus kinesiology	Posture imbalance patterns
Chirometry	Perianal postural reflex technique
Chiropractic concept	Polarity technique
Chiropractic spinal biophysics	Pure chiropractic technique
Chiropractic manipulative reflex technique (CMRT)	Reaver's 5th cervical key
Chiropractic neurobiomechanical analysis	Receptor tonus technique
CHOK-E system	Riddler reflex technique
Clinical kinesiology	Sacro-occipital technique (SOT)
Collins method of painless adjusting	Soft tissue orthopedics
Concept therapy	Somatosynthesis
Cranial technique	Spears painless system
Craniopathy	Specific majors
Diversified technique	Spinal stress (stressology)
Directional nonforce technique (DNFT)	Spinal touch technique
Distraction technique	Spondylotherapy
Endonasal technique	Thompson terminal point technique
Extremity technique	Tiezen technique
Focalizer spinal recoil stimulus reflex effector technique	Toftness technique
Freeman chiropractic procedure	Upper cervical technique (HIO)
Fundamental chiropractic	Top notch visceral techniques
Global energetic matrix	Tortipelvis/torticollis
Gonstead technique	Touch for health
Herring cervical technique	Total body modification
Holographic diagnosis and treatment	Truscott technique
Howard system	Ungerank specific low force chiropractic technique
Keck method of analysis	Variable force technique
King tetrahedron concept	Van Fox combination technique
Lemond brain stem technique	Zindler reflex technique
Logan basic technique	

(Adapted from Bergmann,[32] with permission.)

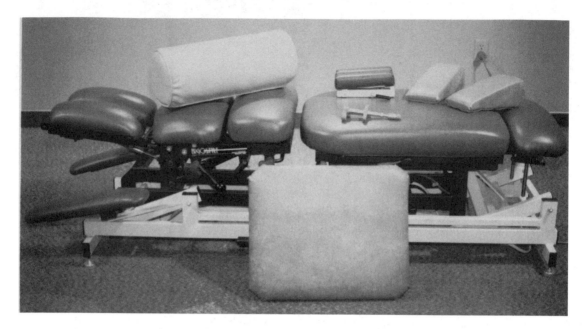

Figure 7-10. A Chattanooga hydraulic chiropractic table with adjustable cervical, thoracic, lumbar, and pelvic drop sections. On the table, from left to right, a Dutchman's (thoracic) roll, a portable toggle-recoil board (rear), an activator instrument (front), and a set of pelvic wedges. Resting on the floor, a thoracic anteriority board.

tor (Figs. 7-11 to 7-13) or to afford the doctor some mechanically assisted advantage in delivery of the dynamic thrust.

Tables that incorporate such features as cervical, thoracic, lumbar, or pelvic drop pieces, amplify the effect of the thrust and thereby allow less exertion or force by the adjustor. Devices such as cervical chairs, knee-chest benches (Fig. 7-14), and wedges, to mention a few, are designed to effectively position the patient so as to afford the doctor a biomechanical advantage in delivering a particular adjustment. The activator instrument, a spring-loaded percussion device (Fig. 7-10), is unique in that it is a precision device specifically designed to administer an impulse of a very controlled and uniform speed and amplitude. The activator instrument, with vectoring directed by the doctor, imparts the forces necessary for administration of the adjustment.

As is true in the effective application of all chiropractic manual adjustive procedures, safe and effective use of any equipment is dependent on the knowledge and skill of the user and the appropriateness of application in clinical situations.

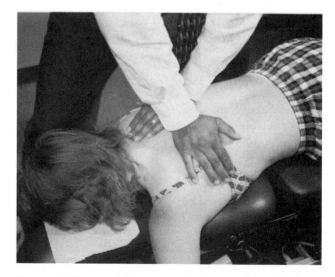

Figure 7-11. An adjustment of the mid-thoracic spine using a bilateral pisiform contact over the transverse processes of the patient.

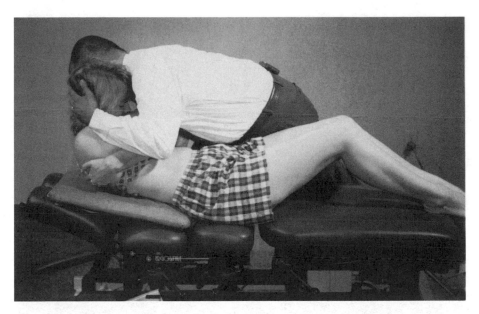

Figure 7-12. An anteriority adjustment of the thoracic spine using an anteriority board to assist the procedure.

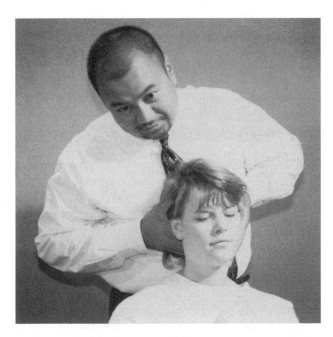

Figure 7-13. An adjustment of the cervical spine with the patient in the seated position.

Mobilization Procedures

Mobilization is a form of joint manipulation involving the passive movement of a joint within its physiologic passive range of motion.[4,19,29] Important to note is the absence of the dynamic thrust which is characteristic of the adjustive procedures. The target joint thus never enters its paraphysiologic range. As with the adjustive procedures, mobilization may involve a specific articulation, or a broader region of the body. In either situation, the primary goal of the procedure is to increase the range and quality of motion of the target joints.[4,19,29] As with other manipulative procedures, the effectiveness and safe application of mobilization procedures depend on the development of the necessary psychomotor and cognitive abilities. Application of mobilization techniques is only effective when performed with the level of skill that can produce positive therapeutic results, while minimizing risk of further injury to the patient.

Mobilization procedures may be an effective form of patient therapy in and of themselves, or used as a prelude to the administration of adjustive procedures. In fact, a large number of commonly used mobilization techniques both for the axial and

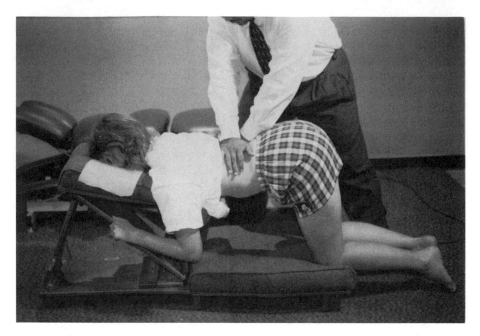

Figure 7-14. An adjustment of the thoraco-lumbar junction with the patient positioned on a knee-chest table.

for the extremity skeletal structures are identical in positioning and set up to adjustive procedures for the same joint, lacking only the dynamic thrust component characteristic of the adjustment process. As always, the practitioner must judge the type and extent of treatment required in each clinical situation.

Traction-distraction Procedures

Traction-distraction procedures, which include flexion-distraction and extension-distraction methods, are manual procedures designed to produce a pulling or distractive force at the target tissues and joints.[4] As with other manual procedures, they range from the very specific, targeting one joint, to the very general, targeting a region of the body. In either situation, the primary reason for applying the distractive force is to reduce joint compression, stretch tight painful tissues, and reduce intracapsular and intradiscal pressure as clinically indicated.[4,33] Traction-distraction techniques include purely manual procedures, and others that incorporate highly sophisticated mechanical tables specifically designed

to assist in precisely administering the appropriate force at a very specific target joint or area. Again, this method may be very effective as a primary or sole therapy or may be enhanced by the inclusion of adjustive and other procedures.

SOFT TISSUE MANIPULATION PROCEDURES

Soft tissue manipulation procedures (for further details, see Ch. 8) are manual therapies that apply forces to the non-osseous tissues of the body in order to improve function, reduce pain, or improve health. These procedures generally involve the application of a pressure, stretching, or distractive force to the involved tissues, with the desired effect of increasing circulation, reducing inflammation and edema, and reducing muscle spasm.[4] As with the previously mentioned manipulative procedures, soft tissue techniques may be therapeutically beneficial as a singular method of treatment, or used in combination with other manual procedures. It is not uncommon in the chiropractic practice for soft tissue procedures to be applied in preparation for a dynamic adjustment. Soft tissue procedures are believed to both facilitate and enhance the effects of the adjustment. Included under this heading are point pressure techniques, massage techniques, therapeutic muscle stretching techniques, and visceral procedures.[4,29]

Point Pressure Techniques

Point pressure techniques of soft tissue care, as the term suggests, involve the application of digital pressure to specific target tissues or areas. The applied pressure may be of a steady, sustained nature, or may be increased progressively, depending on the judgment of the practitioner and the response of the patient. In addition, the practitioner may apply vibratory and/or movement patterns to enhance the stimulation, and therefore, the therapeutic effect of the treatment.[4,29] This form of manipulation is commonly associated with such techniques as acupressure and reflexology, and various other techniques that employ primarily soft tissue methods.[4,29]

Massage Techniques

Massage techniques involve the manual application of forces to the body in order to stimulate the soft tissues.[4,19] The intended goal, as with most soft tissue procedures, is to increase blood flow, reduce inflammation and edema, and relax taut musculature. Included under this heading are procedures such as cross-friction massage (Fig. 7-15) and muscle stripping methods, which are particularly helpful in minimizing and reducing adhesions in myofascial and tendinous tissues.

Although there are numerous individual massage methods, many of them incorporate combinations or variations of basic massage techniques. The following list,[34] although not comprehensive, offers an overview of some of the methods not uncommon in chiropractic practice:

- *Cupping:* a quick tapping of the skin with palms cupped
- *Effleurage:* a light stroking procedure
- *Petrissage:* manipulation of large folds of skin and tissue
- *Pincement:* manipulation of small folds of skin

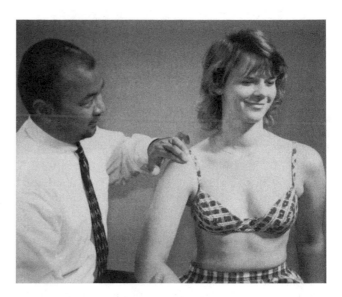

Figure 7-15. Cross-friction massage technique applied over the osteotendinous junction of the right supraspinatus muscle.

- *Pressure technique:* the application of full hand pressure, incorporating a simultaneous kneading component
- *Roulement:* the manipulation of large folds of skin with a progressive wave-like movement along the target tissue
- *Tapotement:* a quick tapping of the skin with the medial aspect of loosely held hands

The therapeutic effect of massage treatment, as with all other manual methods, is dependent on the skill of the practitioner, the clinical picture presented by the patient, and the individual patient response to the particular type of procedure.

Therapeutic Muscle Stretching/ Relaxation Techniques

Therapeutic muscle stretching and relaxation procedures include all techniques intended to produce the previously mentioned soft tissue effects through the stretching of muscles and their related fascia.[4] Commonly employed methods include the *post-contraction stretch* (*PCS*), *post-isometric relaxation* (*PIR*), and *reciprocal inhibition* (*RI*) techniques. As the name might suggest, post-contraction stretch (Fig. 7-16) involves the active contraction of the target muscles against resistance, followed by an aggressive passive stretch administered by the practitioner. This technique is especially useful in the treatment of chronic myofascial conditions.

Post-isometric relaxation methods incorporate a more gentle active muscle contraction or resistance, followed by a gentle stretch of the involved musculature. PIR can by more useful in the handling of some acute and subacute problems. Finally, reciprocal inhibition utilizes active contraction of antagonistic muscle groups in order to facilitate an inhibitory response in the targeted muscle or muscles, followed by a gentle stretch of the tissues. This method can be of significance in the treatment of acute and painful injuries.[35] The type, duration, and frequency of treatment using the noted procedures must be determined based on the clinical picture presented and on the skill and confidence of the practitioner.

Visceral Techniques

Visceral manipulation refers to all manual methods designed to improve or foster the mobility and/or motility of the internal organs of the body.[4] This effect is achieved by the application of very specific and very gentle forces or pressures over key areas of the body. The forces are intended either to manipulate the tissues in a particular direction or to stimulate the organ tissue or those tissues that may have a direct effect on the organ.[4]

ROLE OF DIFFERENT MANUAL METHODS

Although the adjustment, with its characteristic dynamic thrust, remains the backbone of the profession, the art of chiropractic is not limited to this singular method of treatment. The therapeutic procedures and equipment available to the contemporary chiropractor provide a wide array of treatment choices used in a variety of neuromusculoskeletal conditions. Each treatment method constitutes a legitimate therapeutic procedure that can be of substantial value to the needy patient in and of itself. In combination, they provide a repertoire well suited to the patient who desires an alternative or a complement to allopathic health care. The responsibility of the chiropractic student and practitioner lies in their willingness and ability to develop and maintain

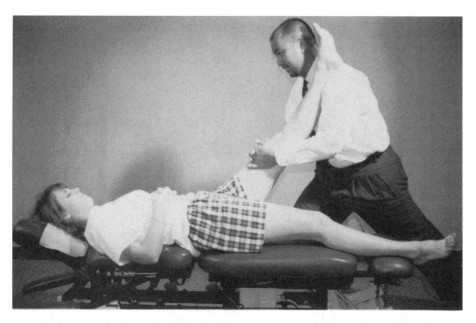

Figure 7-16. Post-contraction stretch (PCS) technique (also called post-facilitation stretch) applied to the left hamstring muscle group.

the necessary cognitive and psychomotor skills to successfully practice the art of chiropractic assessment and treatment.

Terminology

end play
adjustive lesion
accessory motion
somatic dysfunction
osteopathic lesion
joint play
physiologic barrier
anatomic barrier

Review Questions

1. Identify the four methods of examination employed by chiropractors to identify the adjustive lesion.

2. Using the acronym PARTS, describe the diagnostic criteria used for identification of joint dysfunction.

3. Name the cognitive and psychomotor foundations of palpatory literacy.

4. Briefly describe the difference between static and motion palpation.

5. Describe the difference between an anatomic barrier and a pathologic barrier with regard to joint movement.

6. What are the two basic categories of manual procedures?

7. Briefly contrast the short lever and long lever methods of delivering the chiropractic adjustment.

8. List some of the mechanical devices that can be employed to assist in the effective delivery of the chiropractic adjustment.

9. Define the term *mobilization procedures*.

10. List and briefly describe some of the soft tissue manipulation procedures discussed in this chapter.

Concept Questions

1. Is it possible at this time to reach an evidence-based conclusion as to which chiropractic techniques are more effective than others, and for which conditions? What sort of evidence would be needed to determine this accurately?

2. How should a chiropractor determine which technique or techniques to use in a particular case?

References

1. Haldeman S: Spinal manipulative therapy: a status report. Clin Orthop 179:62, 1983

2. Bourdillon JF, Day EA: Spinal Manipulation. 4th Ed. Lange Medical Publications, New Haven, CT, 1987

3. Bergmann TF: The chiropractic spinal examination. p. 97. In Ferezy JS (ed): The Chiropractic Neurological Examination. Aspen, Gaithersburg, MD, 1992

4. Bergmann TF, Peterson DH, Lawrence DJ: Chiropractic Technique. Churchill Livingstone, New York, 1993

5. Dorland's Illustrated Medical Dictionary. 26th Ed. WB Saunders, Philadelphia, 1981

6. Hubka MJ: Palpation for spinal tenderness: a reliable and accurate method for identifying the target of spinal manipulation. J Chiro Tech 6:5, 1994

7. Hubka MJ, Phelan SP: Interexaminer reliability of palpation for cervical spine tenderness. J Manipul Physiol Ther 17:591, 1994

8. Maher C, Adams R: Reliability of pain and stiffness assessments in clinical manual lumbar spine examination. Phys Ther 74:10, 1994

9. Lewit K, Liebenson C: Palpation: problems and implications. J Manipul Physiol Ther 16:586, 1993

10. Eder M, Tilscher H: Chiropractic Therapy: Diagnosis and Treatment. Aspen, Gaithersburg, MD, 1990

11. Schafer RC, Faye LJ: Motion Palpation and Chiropractic Technique: Principles of Dynamic Chiropractic. The Motion Palpation Institute, Huntington Beach, CA, 1989

12. Kaltenborn FM: Manual Mobilization of the Extremity Joints: Basic Examination and Treatment Techniques. 4th Ed. Orthopedic Physical Therapy Products, Minneapolis, MN, 1989

13. Kaltenborn FM: The Spine: Basic Evaluation and Mobilization Techniques. 2nd Ed. Orthopedic Physical Therapy Products, Minneapolis, 1993

14. Maitland GD: Vertebral Manipulation. 4th Ed. Butterworth–Heinemann, Boston, 1986

15. Maitland GD: Peripheral Manipulation. 3rd Ed. Butterworth–Heinemann, Boston, 1991

16. Binkley J, Stratford PW, Gill C: Interrater reliability of lumbar accessory motion mobility testing. Phys Ther 75:10, 1995

17. Cantu RI, Grodin AJ: Myofascial Manipulation: Theory and Clinical Application. Aspen, Gaithersburg, MD, 1992

18. Travell JG, Simons DG: Myofascial Pain and Dysfunction: The Trigger Point Manual. Williams & Wilkins, Baltimore, 1983

19. Haldeman S, Hooper PD, Phillips RB et al: Spinal manipulative therapy. In Frymore JW (ed): The Adult Spine: Principles and Practice. 2nd Ed. Lippincott–Raven, Philadelphia (in press)

20. Hammer WI: Functional Soft Tissue Examination and Treatment by Manual Methods: The Extremities. Aspen, Gaithersburg, MD, 1991

21. Mennell J McM: The Musculoskeletal System: Differential Diagnosis from Symptoms and Physical Signs. Aspen, Gaithersburg, MD, 1992

22. Greenman PE: Principles of Manual Medicine. Williams & Wilkins, Baltimore, 1989

23. Sandoz R: Some physical mechanisms and affects of spinal adjustive adjustments. Ann Swiss Chiro Assoc 6:91, 1976

24. Gonnella C, Paris SV, Kurtner M: Reliability in evaluating passive intervertebral motion. Phys Ther 62:436, 1982

25. Moritz U: Evolution of manipulation and other manual therapy. Scand J Rehabil Med 11:173, 1979

26. Gibbons RW: The evolution of chiropractic: medical and social protest in America. In Haldeman S (ed): Modern Developments in the Principles and Practice of Chiropractic. Appleton & Lange, Norwalk, CT, 1980

27. Halder NM, Curtis P, Gillings DB, Stinnett S: A benefit of spinal manipulation as adjunctive therapy for acute low back pain: a stratified controlled trial. Spine 12: 702, 1987

28. Cherkin DC, MacCornack FA: Patient evaluations of low back pain care from family physicians and chiropractors. West J Med 150:351, 1989

29. Haldeman S, Chapman-Smith D, Peterson DM Jr: Guidelines for chiropractic quality assurance and practice parameters. In Procedings of the Mercy Center Consensus Conference. Aspen, Gaithersburg, MD, 1993

30. Zusman M: Spinal manipulative therapy: review of some proposed mechanisms, and a new hypothesis. Aust J Physiother 32:89, 1986

31. Terrett A, Kleynhans AM: Complications from manipulation of the low back. Chiro J Aust 22:129, 1992

32. Bergmann TF: Various forms of chiropractic technique. Chiro Tech 5:53, 1993

33. Cox JM: Low Back Pain: Mechanism, Diagnosis, and Treatment. 5th Ed. Williams & Wilkins, Baltimore, 1990

34. States AZ: States Manual of Spinal, Pelvic and Extravertebral Technics. 2nd Ed. Kirk CR, Lawrence DJ, Valvo NL (eds): National College of Chiropractic, Lombard, 1985

35. Liebenson C: Rehabilitation of the Spine: A Practitioner's Manual. Williams & Wilkins, Philadelphia, 1996

8
Soft Tissue Therapies

Warren Hammer

A patient enters your office with a grade 2 traumatic cervical sprain due to a rear-end automobile accident. The patient's chief complaint is severe pain located at the anterior cervical area. How will you approach this case from a manual point of view? A professional piano player enters your office with pain and paresthesia in the first three and a half fingers of his right hand. Surgery for carpal tunnel syndrome failed to relieve his symptoms. What manual methods are appropriate in this case? Another patient enters your office with chronic lumbar pain; examination demonstrates a chronically shortened iliopsoas muscle. What is the manual approach for treating the shortened iliopsoas muscle? Still another patient has been to several orthopedists and chiropractors due to chronic mid-scapular pain. He has a forward head and forward shoulder posture. Adjustments have relieved the problem but have offered no sustained solution. What alternative manual approach could be the primary treatment for this condition?

All these conditions will benefit from spinal adjustments, but in each case soft tissue therapies can either completely cure the condition or (in the acute first case) provide symptomatic relief until an adjustment is feasible.

RATIONALE FOR SOFT TISSUE THERAPY

Differentiating Spinal from Peripheral Causes of Pain

As doctors of chiropractic dealing with the total locomotor system, our first responsibility is to find the source of the pain. The location of the source, along with its acuteness or chronicity, generally determines the type of treatment. In evaluating spinal subluxations related to musculoskeletal pain, the question that must always be asked is: what percentage of the pain is directly related to the subluxation? In many cases of peripheral soft tissue pain, the primary cause lies in the local soft tissue itself, not the spine. Thus, while the lumbar spine and sacroiliac joint may be indirectly related to an Achilles tendinitis or a trochanteric bursitis, in these cases the majority of the treatment must be directed to the involved soft tissue.

From a soft tissue point of view, the problem could be located in the muscle belly, musculotendinous portion, body of the tendon, insertion point of the tendon, bursa, ligament, or fascia. The tissue may be under tension due to a spinal source of pain; a postural, structural, or functional aberration; a viscerosomatic problem; or at the local soft tissue level.

Chiropractors pay particular attention to the subluxation, defined as a kinesiopathologic joint lesion (usually hypomobility) with many possible causes.[1] If the primary reason for a subluxation is degeneration in the muscular or connective tissue due to micro- or macrotraumatic injury, sedentary living, or altered motor patterns creating muscular imbalances, spinal adjustments alone will not fully correct the subluxation.

Spinal adjustments directly affect soft tissue. Facet movement externally elicted by an adjustment affects the joint capsules and surrounding periarticular connective tissue including muscles, ligaments, and fascia. A joint is a space built for motion and connective tissue structures surrounding that space are "soft tissues" affected by movement. The human spine, composed of vertebral bodies, discs, and supporting ligaments, lacks the ability to move on its own and depends on the dynamic muscular system as its prime mover. While spinal adjustments affect surrounding muscles, ligaments, and fascia, treatment of these soft tissue structures likewise affects the spine. It is important that chiropractors not limit their focus to only one side of this equation.

Evaluating and Treating the Whole System

Those seeking to develop expertise in treating functional conditions of the musculoskeletal system must evaluate and treat the whole system. The brain is a sensory and motor organ which delivers orders based on the sensory information it receives. Any persistent or chronic peripheral dysfunction (e.g., shortened muscle or fascia, trigger points, hyperpronation) will elicit from the central nervous system a compensatory response that may result in an altered movement pattern. A typical example of such an alteration is abnormal hip extension due to a weak gluteus maximus. The weakened gluteus maximus could be caused by its antagonist, a shortened iliopsoas, based on Sherrington's law of reciprocal innervation, or by a sacroiliac fixation. This could create a change in gait (weakened hip extension) resulting in compensatory lumbar lordosis and hypermobility at the L4 and L5 vertebral segments.

Many altered patterns of movement remain in place even after the original painful lesion has disappeared[2,3] and are a significant factor in subluxations that fail to respond to chiropractic adjustments or

refixate after being adjusted. Treatment of peripheral lesions not related to the spine, and treatment and prevention of spinal lesions (subluxations) require evaluation and treatment of soft tissue.

VARIETIES OF SOFT TISSUE TECHNIQUES

Literally hundreds of soft tissue techniques exist, among them friction massage, active release, postisometric relaxation, postfacilitation stretch, counterstrain, myofascial release, and muscle energy. This chapter surveys a variety of methods in common use. It will not make you an expert in these techniques, but it will provide a clear rationale for soft tissue work, and a basis for further education in these methods. All soft tissue techniques require hands-on supervision and practice.

Soft tissue techniques require the use of the hands as a sensor to evaluate the status of soft tissue. The practitioner learns to feel for end ranges, for barriers, for looseness, and for types of tissue organization described as "lumpy," "leathery," "stringy," "doughy," "boggy," "nodular," "mobile," "taut," and "springy." Manual palpation discerns changes in the tension of tissues, which helps determine the type of soft tissue treatment needed and monitor progress in the area under treatment. You can literally feel the pain. No technologic modality is capable of such sensitivity.

Some of these techniques are most effective in acute conditions, while others are effective in both acute and chronic conditions. The larger the number of effective techniques in your repertoire, the better the overall quality of care. If your toolbox contains only a hammer, you will look only for nails.

Mechanical load on soft tissues such as compression and tensile loading has been evaluated experimentally. Research has demonstrated that the form and function of musculoskeletal soft tissues are influenced by mechanical loading.[4] Loading methods such as transverse friction massage, myofascial release, and active release can presently be explained on a cellular level.

Kolega[4] found that stretching mobile clusters of epithelial fibroblasts caused the microfilaments within the cells to align along the long axis of that tension, thus offering a structural mechanism for fibroblast realignment with stress. Many studies[4] have shown that "cells in muscle, tendon, ligament, skin, and cartilage generally respond to windows of increased loading by increasing matrix synthesis, increasing metabolic activity, and increasing replication rates, and modifying their production of matrix components."

Transverse Friction Massage

Transverse friction massage (TFM) is a localized pressure that is usually administered on a ligament or muscle (belly, musculotendinous portion, body of the tendon and insertion), and recently described for use on chronically involved bursae.[5] This technique is extremely valuable in the treatment of tendinitis, ligamentous sprains, muscular lesions, and chronic bursitis. It is useful in both acute and chronic conditions depending on the condition and area involved. Light friction may be used on a recent partial tear and in recent ligamentous sprains; however, caution is required, as cells are then in an immature state. Stronger friction, respecting the patient's tolerance, is useful in the chronic stage.

Cyriax,[6] a medical physician, feels that the pressure and movement created in a small local area by TFM can create much greater (therapeutic) movement than strenuous exercise or manipulation. He states that TFM creates traumatic hyperemia and movement that breaks down adhesions. Recent studies on the effect of loading on cells has shown increased matrix synthesis, increased metabolic activity, increased cell replication rates, and remodeling of matrix.[7] The stimulation of TFM on the local mechanoreceptors may also create temporary anesthesia, allowing for increased levels of pressure. If the massage is terminated while anesthesia is still present after 10 to 20 minutes of TFM, functional isometric muscle testing of the involved area demonstrates decreased pain, providing positive feedback to both doctor and patient.[7]

The exact placement of the practitioner's finger is crucial. Cyriax emphasizes a functional evaluation of the area stressing particular tissues, thus allowing the practitioner to friction the precisely correct location. He notes that the most painful area is not necessarily the source of the pain and that painful isometric muscle testing often reveals a pain source that is not the most tender area.

The practitioner's finger and the patient's skin should move as if they are attached. Otherwise, the skin will be frictioned and bruising will occur. Knowledge of surface anatomy is necessary to ascertain that the exact location is being treated. Recent cadaver studies have indicated changes in previously accepted areas of palpation for some rotator cuff muscle and tendon areas.[8]

Figure 8-1 shows the new optimal position for maximally exposing the supraspinatus insertion. The patient sits arm behind back, in maximal adduction, medial rotation, and up to 30 to 40 degrees of hyperextension depending on patient tolerance. The maximal exposure for palpating and treating the insertion of the teres minor and infraspinatus is depicted in Figure 8-2, with the patient sitting with her shoulder in flexion to 90 degrees, 10 degrees of shoulder adduction, and 20 degrees of shoulder lateral rotation.

Cyriax,[5] who used injectable steroids for many conditions, considered others to be curable only by "deep friction":

- Belly of the subclavius
- Musculotendinous junction of the supraspinatus
- Long head and lower musculotendinous junction of the biceps
- Belly of the brachialis
- Belly of the supinator
- Ligaments about the carpal lunate bone
- Adductors of the thumb
- Interosseous belly at the hand
- Interosseous tendon at the finger
- Intercostal muscles
- Oblique muscles of the abdomen
- Lower musculotendinous junction of the iliopsoas (Fig. 8-3)
- Quadriceps expansion at the patella
- Coronary ligament of the knee
- Lower musculotendinous junction of the biceps femoris
- Musculotendinous junction of the anterior and posterior tibial and peroneal
- Posterior tibiotalar ligament
- Anterior fascia of the ankle joint
- Interosseous belly at the foot

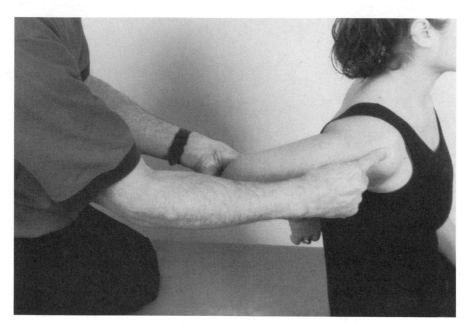

Figure 8-1. Optimal position for palpating and treating supraspinatus tendon insertion.

Active Release Techniques

Developed by chiropractor P. Michael Leahy, active release techniques are used for the examination, diagnosis, and treatment of cumulative injury disor-

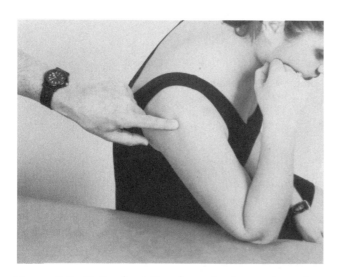

Figure 8-2. Optimal position for palpating and treating insertion of infraspinatus and teres minor (just below infraspinatus).

ders.[9–12] Leahy[9] states that acute injury or repetitive injury of a constant pressure/tension may lead to a cumulative injury cycle resulting in a state of adhesion-fibrosis. Unless tissue is free of adhesions, a "traction neurodesis"[9] may occur resulting in peripheral nerve entrapment. Peripheral nerves must be able to glide during movement. For example, the brachial plexus moves 15.3 mm during shoulder abduction/adduction and median nerve excursion proximal to the elbow is 7.3 mm during full elbow flexion and extension.[9] Any restriction to this motion will affect transmission of impulses through the peripheral nerve. Peripheral nerve entrapment is far more common than spinal nerve root entrapment.

As with all other soft tissue techniques, active release requires a hands-on learning process. The practitioner must evaluate tissue texture, tension, movement, and function. Leahy[9] states that it is possible to determine the duration of a condition through palpation. For example, in the inflammatory phase (24 to 72 hours post-injury) a movable, fluid-like swelling with the associated signs of inflammation may be palpated. After 2 days to 2 weeks, a "stringy, guitar string" feeling will be elicited. A

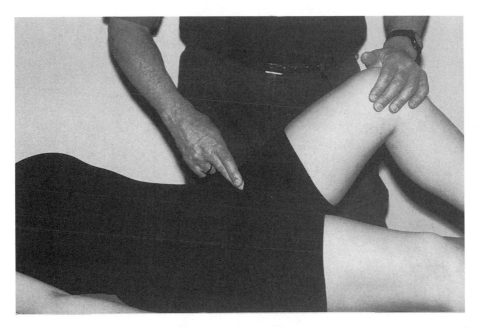

Figure 8-3. Position for friction massage of lower musculotendinous junction of iliopsoas.

lumpy feeling will be palpated after 2 weeks to 3 months have passed, and finally after 3 months a leathery feeling will be present.

In the active phase of the technique, the practitioner applies a specific contact on the muscle in its shortened position just below the site of the lesion. The patient actively lengthens the muscle to draw the lesion under the contact from the muscle's shortest to its longest length. The practitioner's contact passively strips the muscle in a longitudinal manner with the patient providing most of the motion. Usually three to five passes every other day are recommended. Significant improvement should occur in two to three visits. It is necessary to trace the nerve to a variety of locations along its pathway to be certain that the nerve is no longer entrapped.

Active release is an appropriate treatment for the failed carpal tunnel surgery mentioned at the beginning of this chapter. It is an excellent procedure for treatment of entrapment of the median nerve as it passes through or under the pronator teres muscle. Often percussion of the pronator teres at its midbelly elicits a positive Tinel sign, referring paresthesia to the median nerve distribution in the hand. Figure 8-4 depicts treatment of the pronator teres using

active release. The original entrapment in this condition may also originate at other locations of possible median nerve compression, such as beneath the subscapularis or the ligament of Struthers.

Postisometric Relaxation

Lewit[13] uses postisometric relaxation (PIR) to relax tense muscles, comparing this method to the Travell's spray and stretch technique. For muscle tension due to spinal fixation or viscerosomatic reflexes, this technique will not be effective. The acute whiplash patient with muscle spasm offers the classic case for appropriate use of PIR.

The technique is as follows (see Figures 8-5 and 8-6 for upper trapezius);

1. Lengthen the muscle until the slack (barrier) is taken up, at the point where slight resistance is encountered without creating pain.
2. Instruct the patient to contract the muscle isometrically with minimal force (this should cause little or no pain) and to inhale and look with the eyes to the side of contraction. Patient should contract the muscle for 10 seconds. Gaymans[14]

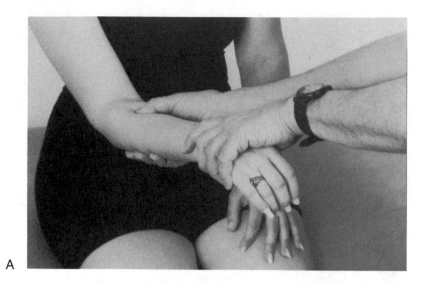

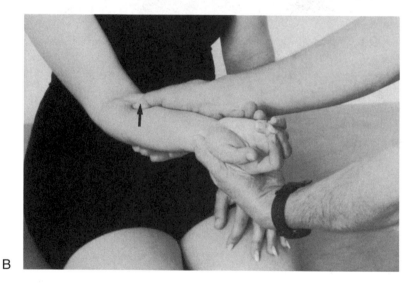

Figure 8-4. (A) Position of pressure on pronator teres in its shortened position just before the site of the lesion. **(B)** Patient actively supinates forearm while doctor maintains pressure with flat surface of thumb, allowing lesion to pass under thumb.

has shown that inhalation has a facilitating and exhalation an inhibiting effect on muscles, and that moving the eyes toward the side of muscle activity facilitates that muscle, while looking away from the side of contraction inhibits the contracting side.

3. Instruct the patient to "let go," to relax, exhale, and look in the opposite direction. The practitioner allows the muscle to lengthen by spontaneous decontraction. Relaxation can last 10 to 20 seconds, as long as the muscle lengthens, at which point a new barrier is reached. The procedure can be repeated three to five times. If the patient has difficulty relaxing, the isometric contraction phase can be increased up to 30 seconds.

Figure 8-7 demonstrates PIR technique for a patient in acute pain who is forward flexed due to

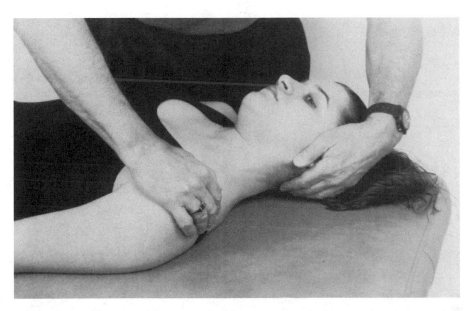

Figure 8-5. Postisometric relaxation of upper trapezius. Slack is gently taken up while patient inhales and looks to side of muscle contraction for 10 seconds.

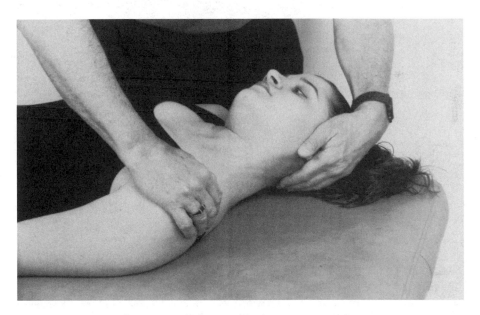

Figure 8-6. Patient "lets go," exhales, and looks in opposite direction as practitioner allows muscle to lengthen by spontaneous decontraction.

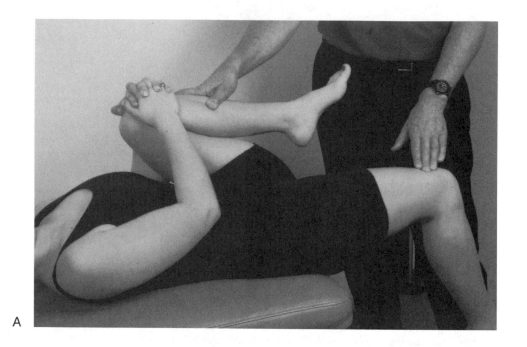

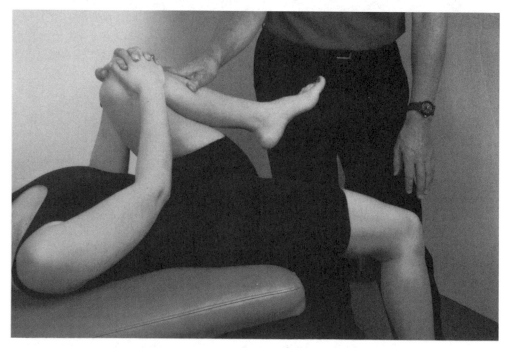

Figure 8-7. (A) PIR for iliopsoas. **(B)** Relaxation phase of PIR for iliopsoas.

iliopsoas spasm. The patient is in a modified Thomas position (see Fig. 8-8 in the section *Post-facilitation Stretch*) showing a flexed right hip due to spasm of the right iliopsoas. The patient performs the same procedure as for the upper trapezius, but in this case looking up with the eyes during inspiration. The doctor exerts minimal pressure on knee, feeling the psoas contract (Fig. 8-7). During inspiration phase, the patient may minimally contract isometrically, as long as pain is not elicited. Figure 8-7B shows the patient "letting go" with expiration and eyes downward for 10 to 20 seconds or until relaxation occurs.

Unlike the Travell spray and stretch method, in this case an attempt is made to avoid the stretch reflex. Lewit[13] feels that this method should eliminate trigger points and pain points where the tendon is attached to the periosteum. Methods that relax muscles usually improve joint range of motion.

Post-facilitation Stretch

Post-facilitation (PFS) stretch is used primarily to stretch chronically shortened muscles. This technique for restoring muscle balance was popularized by Janda, a medical physician. Certain muscles, principally postural slow twitch muscles, such as the iliopsoas, tensor fascia lata, piriformis, and erector spinae, tend to tighten while other phasic muscles including the serratus anterior, and gluteus maximus, medius, and minimus tend to become weak and inhibited.[15] By using PFS, often for as few as six treatments over 2 weeks, tight muscles normalize. Janda[3] describes typical "muscle imbalance patterns" that perpetuate many spinal problems. Often a tight muscle is the cause of a weak, inhibited antagonistic muscle and after using PFS the inhibited muscle spontaneously strengthens.

The iliopsoas, which can be evaluated with the modified Thomas test (Fig. 8-8A), is considered tight if the extended femur does not easily reach 5 to 15 degrees extension below the table. The PFS technique for the iliopsoas is as follows:

1. Place the shortened psoas in the mid-position. The patient isometrically resists for 7 seconds (Fig. 8-8B) and then "lets go" (Fig. 8-8C); doctor stretches the muscle for 12 seconds.

2. The patient may have to be taught to relax completely, as any tension exerted by the patient after they "let go" will inhibit the relaxation phase, which is necessary for this stretching procedure.

3. Wait 20 seconds before you attempt to restretch. Three to 5 passes may be applied. Do not continue if pain ensues. As range of motion increases, begin isometric contraction at the new range.

4. The patient should then perform active movement of the muscle in its new range of motion.

One reason that some low back problems never completely resolve is that a tight iliopsoas may be responsible for a weak gluteus maximus, creating an abnormal pattern of hip extension. Normal hip extension begins with contraction of the ipsilateral gluteus maximus and hamstrings, followed immediately by contraction of the contralateral lumbar muscles. This sequential muscular contraction creates a lever that crosses the lumbosacral area to stabilize the lower spine and pelvis during hip extension.

When the gluteus maximus is weak, the hamstrings work harder, creating abnormal sequences of motion. Contraction of the ipsilateral lumbar muscles, instead of the contralateral lumbar muscles, can occur, as can contraction of the ipsilateral thoracic muscles or even the trapezius muscles, as the body attempts to accomplish hip extension. Abnormal hip extension may result in an increased lumbar lordosis and hypermobility of the lower lumbar spinal segments.

Treatment of the tight iliopsoas by post facilitation stretch or active release technique could allow the inhibited weak gluteus maximus to spontaneously regain its strength.

Figure 8-9 demonstrates PFS for the left upper trapezius. Figure 8-9A shows the patient's neck in maximum flexion, contralateral side bending, and ipsilateral rotation. The patient isometrically pushes her left shoulder cephalad against the doctor's resistance for 7 seconds. In Figure 8-9B, the patient was told to "let go" and allow the doctor to push the shoulder caudal for 12 seconds. The position in Figure 8-9B is also used for screening to determine the end-feel for tightness. This end-feel is compared with the opposite side. The precise mechanism for proprioceptive neuromuscular facilitation techniques such as PFS is still under examination.[16,17]

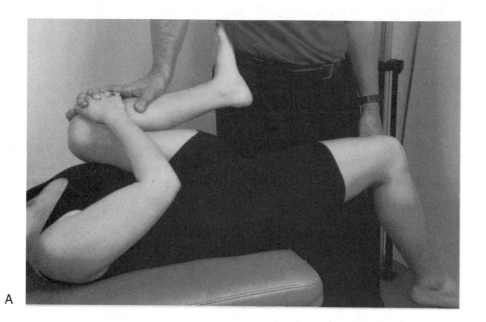

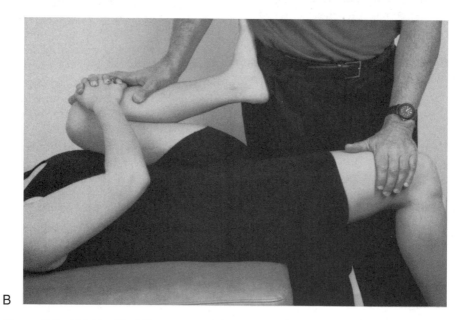

Figure 8-8. (A) Modified Thomas test indicating a tight iliopsoas. **(B)** Patient isometrically resists doctor's pressure for 7 seconds. *(Figure continues.)*

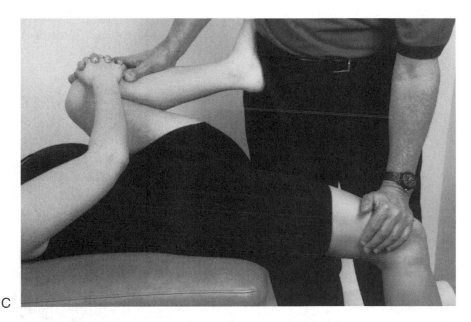

Figure 8-8. *(Continued)* **(C)** Patient "lets go" and doctor stretches iliopsoas for 12 seconds.

Strain and Counterstrain

In *Strain and Counterstrain*,[18] osteopath Lawrence H. Jones relates the discovery of this technique. A patient was unable to stand erect or sleep due to continuous pain and had failed to respond to 2 months of treatment by two chiropractors or to 2 more months of treatment by an osteopath, himself. Dr. Jones finally spent 20 minutes attempting different positions that relieved the patient until he "achieved a position of surprising amount of comfort." When the patient stood, he was "overjoyed." His posture was erect, and the pain substantially decreased. No manipulation was performed. In subsequent years, Jones found almost 200 "small zones of tense, tender, edematous muscle and fascial tissue about a centimeter in diameter" all over the body, along with specific associated positions that relieved the local tender points.

Counterstrain is a system of evaluation and treatment of joint pain based on the idea that joint pain results from a strain of the proprioceptive and neuromuscular reflexes that cause muscular imbalance and joint dysfunction. Uses for this technique have been described for supraspinatus tendinitis,[19] for-

ward and backward torsions of the sacrum,[20] acute ankle sprains,[21] and a variety of conditions in a hospital population.[22]

Irwin Korr's Theory of Proprioception

The work of physiologist Irwin Korr,[23] the premier osteopathic researcher of the 20th century, offers a model to explain counterstrain. A good illustration is a cervical trauma, wherein as the head extends posterior, the anterior cervical muscles are stretched while the posterior cervical muscles are maximally shortened. Spindle activity is reduced to almost zero in the passively shortened posterior muscles, reflecting lack of stimulation of primary afferent Ia fibers. Getting no feedback from the muscle spindle, the central nervous system (CNS) then activates the gamma system (high gamma gain), which reactivates the spindle. But the high gamma gain does not return to normal and continues to provide inaccurate information to the CNS regarding muscle length. The posterior muscle in its shortened position therefore reports that it is being stretched.

Korr[23] feels that the muscle resists returning to its resting length due to the increased spindle dis-

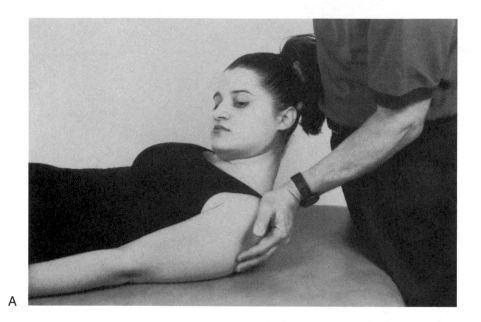

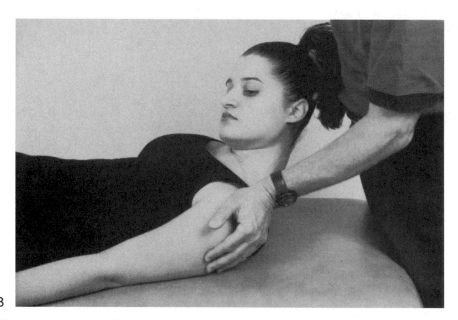

Figure 8-9. (A) Postfacilitation stretch for left upper trapezius. **(B)** Postfacilitation stretch for left upper trapezius. See text for explanation.

charge. The sustained contraction prevents the spinal segment from returning to its original resting position. Eventually segmental facilitation occurs, which can last for years. Counterstrain points may overlap with trigger points or acupuncture points but tend to be more segmental.[24]

General Counterstrain Technique

1. Find the tender point.
2. Move the muscle or joint into a position of comfort until a pain level estimated at "ten" is reduced to "two." This position shortens the muscle containing the dysfunctional proprioceptors and allows the primary endings to "shut off" the abnormal elevated activity. As the gamma system shuts off, the annulospiral endings reduce the output to the alphas and the muscle relaxes. You will feel the tender points shut off.
3. Hold the position of comfort for no less than 90 seconds. This is the minimum time required to allow the gamma system to return to normal.
4. Return very slowly to the neutral position in order not to reactivate the sensitive proprioceptors.

Counterstrain Technique for Cervical Muscles

As an example of counterstrain technique for anterior neck pain, let us consider a tender point at the anterior surface of the tip of the left transverse process of C5. Such tenderness may be due to involvement of the scalenus anticus and longus colli. In Figure 8-10 the patient's neck is flexed (position of comfort for this point) while the doctor presses the sensitive point with up to 2 lb of pressure. For this particular point the neck is brought into increasing flexion while the doctor palpates for diminution of the tender point. The point is then "fine-tuned" by contralateral rotation and possible lateral bending away from the pain until the patient feels no more than 25 percent of the original pain. The point is held for 90 seconds and the neck is then slowly returned to its neutral position.

In treating the anterior cervical points, treat the most painful point first. This technique is very beneficial in acute cervical problems in this case with anterior cervical pain on active or passive cervical extension. The painful point usually reduces in two visits, with a 50 percent reduction in pain typically noted after the first visit.

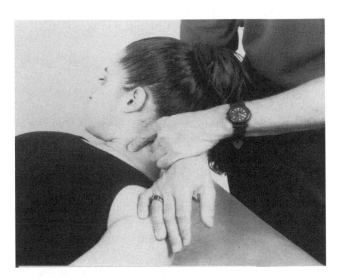

Figure 8-10. Counterstrain position for treatment of anterior cervical tender point.

Figure 8-11 depicts the position for counterstrain treatment of a painful psoas point. Follow the above procedure. The iliopsoas muscle is treated similarly to the anterior cervical muscles, since the points in both situations are on the anterior portion of the body and are therefore treated in flexion. There are rare occasions in which an anterior point is treated

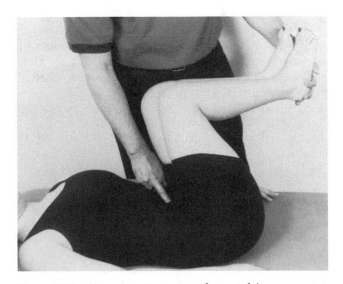

Figure 8-11. Counterstrain position for painful psoas point.

in extension or a posterior point is treated in a flexed position.

Myofascial Release Technique

Myofascial release technique is a method of evaluating and treating the fascia. Barnes[25] estimates that 90 percent of patients treated with musculoskeletal problems have myofascial dysfunction and asserts that this physiologic system has been widely ignored, resulting in poor or temporary results from many treatments.

The fascia is a three-dimensional web of connective tissue that spreads throughout the body without interruption. Fascial restriction can cause abnormal pressure on nerves, muscles, blood vessels, osseous structures, and visceral organs.[25] An obvious fascial restriction occurs in "compartment syndrome" in which an increase in lower extremity blood pressure prevents a runner from continuing. Blood vessels are supported and surrounded by fascia which upon shortening restricts the blood supply to the muscles. Pain due to ischemia and increased blood pressure prevents the runner from continuing. This condition is often treated by a surgical fasciotomy.

Barnes[25] finds that restrictions are most commonly caused by chronic poor posture, inflammation, or trauma. Pelvic torsion, forward head and shoulders, lumbar lordosis, and spinal fixations are among the structural aberrations directly related to restricted fascia. Fascia from low back patients evaluated by light and electron microscopy has been found to display "a primary ischemic pathoanatomy in the fascia that may be of relevance to back pain syndromes.[26]

Greenman[27] states that "there are a wide variety of myofascial release techniques in use by many practitioners." He describes a technique taught by Ward, an osteopath, in which the practitioner evaluates the fascia by applying compression and transverse shear in opposite directions, sensing for tension or laxity in both superficial and deep fascial levels. Contact is applied against the barrier, and the practitioner follows the "inherent tissue motion," during which time the patient performs enhancing motions using the eyes or breathing for physiologic summation.[3] Physiologic summation refers to the facilitative use of the eyes or breathing on the muscular system, as discussed under Postisometric Relaxation.[13]

Lewit[13] simply takes up the slack (engages the barrier) and with minimal change in pressure waits until release occurs, which generally takes between a few seconds and half a minute. He then follows the release.

Barnes[25] maintains that some myofascial techniques only affect the elastic and muscular components rather than the collagenous viscous portion of the ground substance embedded in the interstitial spaces of the fascial system. He states that the ground substance loses some of its fluid content and undergoes colloidal solidification, thereby restricting both local and distal areas. Manual intervention provides a mechanical, electromagnetic, and thermal force that can change the consistency of the colloid to a more liquid gelatinous arrangement.

Barnes Myofascial Release Technique

1. First palpate the skin for deeper restrictions and determine the direction of the barrier.
2. Make contact against the barrier with one hand, while the other hand provides a counter pressure.
3. Wait 1 to 2 minutes until the barrier releases; follow the direction of release.

Barnes emphasizes that waiting for the release is essential since early motion is due to the elastic rather than the viscous component of the fascia.

Figure 8-12 depicts a release on the side of an anterior ilium due to a restriction of fascia on the anterior thigh. Figure 8-13 depicts a position for fascial release in the area of the psoas. The thigh is shifted through its range of motion to palpate for fascial restrictions.

A cross-handed position on the pectoral areas of the chest is an excellent method of freeing fascia responsible for causing forward shoulders. Forward shoulders and head are often responsible for chronic upper thoracic pain due to pressure on the posterior upper thoracic spine. Releasing the anterior chest fascia will often allow the shoulders to shift posterior, taking the strain off the posterior thoracic spine.

Muscle Energy Technique

Developed by osteopath Fred L. Mitchell, muscle energy technique involves voluntary contraction of the patient's muscles in a precisely controlled direction, at varying levels of intensity, against a distinctly

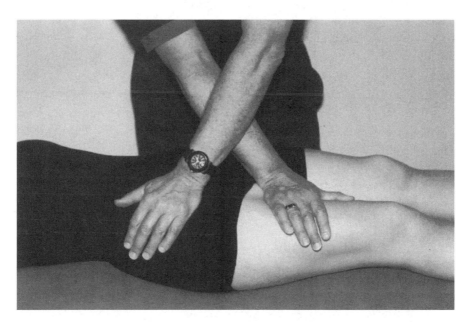

Figure 8-12. Fascial release of the anterior thigh fascia. Doctor's left hand is pressing cephalad against the anterior superior iliac spine (ASIS) while right hand is pressing against barrier.

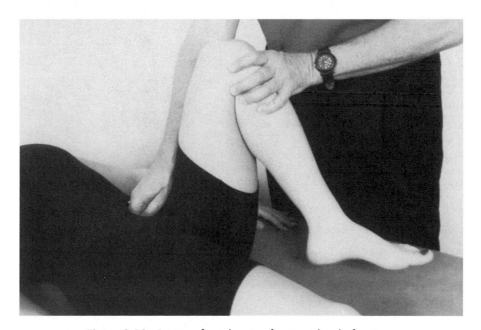

Figure 8-13. Position for releasing fascia at level of psoas.

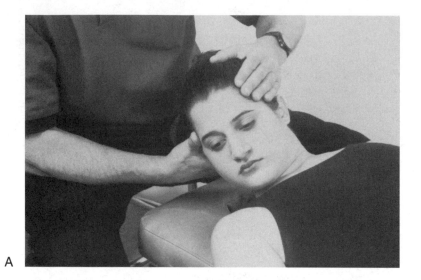

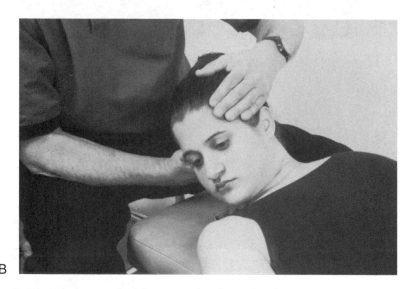

Figure 8-14. (A) Patient's head is rotated rightward to barrier. She is then asked to resist against rotation to her left. **(B)** Patient has increased range of rotation to a new barrier and again is resisting against rotation to her left.

executed counterforce applied by the practitioner.[27] According to Greenman,[27] this technique can be used to mobilize a restricted articulation. Other uses are lengthening shortened, contracted, or spastic muscles, strengthening physiologically weakened muscle groups, and reducing localized edema caused by congestion by using muscles to pump the lymphatic and venous systems.

Muscle Energy Technique for the Cervical Spine

The muscle energy method used for the cervical spine is based on the theory of reciprocal innervation. A short hypertonic muscle prevents normal motion in the opposite direction and also inhibits its antagonistic muscle. After isometrically contracting the hypertonic muscle, the hypertonic muscle can be stretched to a new resting length. At the same time, the weakened antagonist develops increased tone, thereby balancing the area. Muscle energy treatment takes into consideration coupled motions of the cervical spine in which for C1 to C7 side bending and rotation occur to the same side. Therefore, both side bending and rotation are treated. These coupled motions are evaluated in both flexion and extension. If the segment is fixed in flexion and/or extension, treatment would also include the additional coupled motion of flexion and/or extension.

For example, first palpate for restricted lateral motion in both flexion and extension. If lateral motion is restricted in the flexed position due to localized hypertonicity at C5 pushing from right to left, you can assume that C5 is restricted in flexion, right lateral bending, and right rotation (coupled motions).

1. Contact the articular pillar of C6 so that C5 can move upon it.
2. Flex the patient's head forward as far as the C5–C6 interspace.
3. Next, move the neck into the barrier of right rotation and right side bending. From this position the three coupled motions are treated with muscle energy.
4. Have the patient rotate isometrically left against resistance for 3 to 5 seconds, 3 to 5 times (Fig. 8-19A).
5. Then, have the patient move her head laterally left against resistance for 3 to 5 seconds, 3 to 5 times.
6. Finally have the patient resist isometrically into extension for 3 to 5 seconds, 3 to 5 times.

After each of these movements, the practitioner may observe enhanced mobility, with barriers becoming progressively less restrictive (Fig 8-14B).

If C5 were fixed in extension, right lateral bending, and right rotation, something would be preventing the right facet from closing. The same procedure would be used, except that isometric resistance by the patient towards flexion would be used because of the restriction found in cervical extension.

While chiropractic adjustments can in many cases accomplish all of the above, in certain circumstances high-velocity, low-amplitude thrusts are inadvisable. These include various acute pain situations, severe osteoporosis, and bony abnormalities. In such cases, muscle energy technique and other soft tissue methods offer a valuable addition to the chiropractor's repertoire.

Terminology

active release technique
counterstrain
muscle energy technique
myofascial release
soft tissue
Sherrington's Law of Reciprocal Innervation
periarticular
postisometric relaxation
post-facilitation stretch
transverse friction massage

Review Questions

1. Name two causes of a weakened gluteus maximus.

2. What is the effect of manual soft tissue techniques on connective tissue cells?

3. In what situations is light rather than strong friction massage appropriate?

4. What is the benefit of creating soft tissue anesthesia by manual methods?

5. Describe the ideal position for transverse friction of the supraspinatus muscle.

6. Why is it necessary for peripheral nerves to have freedom of motion?

7. In palpating soft tissue, how would you distinguish between a lesion of two weeks compared to a lesion of over 3 months?

8. How does Lewit's PIR technique differ from Travell's spray and stretch method regarding the muscle stretch?

9. Describe Irwin Korr's theory relating to counterstrain.

10. Why is the muscle put into a shortened position in the counterstrain technique?

Concept Questions

1. Based on your chiropractic philosophy, do you believe that the spinal component supersedes the soft tissue component sometimes, always, or never? Explain.

2. What percentage of patients requires a soft tissue evaluation? Explain.

References

1. Seaman D: Subluxation: causes and effects. Dynamic Chiro 14:22, 1996
2. Lewit K: Manipulative Therapy in Rehabilitation of the Locomotor System. 2nd Ed. Butterworth–Heinemann, Boston, 1991
3. Janda V: Muscles and motor control in low back pain: assessment and management. p. 253. In Twomey LT, Taylor J (eds): Physical Therapy of the Low Back. Churchill Livingstone, New York, 1987
4. Frank CB, Hart DA: Cellular response to loading. p. 555. In Leadbetter WB, Buckwalter JA, Gordon SL (eds): Sports-Induced Inflammation. American Academy of Orthopedic Surgery, Park Ridge, IL, 1989
5. Hammer WI: The use of transverse friction massage in the management of chronic bursitis of the hip or shoulder. J Manipul Physiol Ther 16:107, 1993
6. Cyriax J: Textbook of Orthopaedic Medicine. Vol. 2. 11th Ed. Baillière Tindall, London, 1984
7. Hammer WI: Friction massage. p. 236. In Hammer WI (ed): Functional Soft Tissue Examination and Treatment by Manual Methods: The Extremities. Aspen, Gaithersburg, MD, 1991
8. Mattingly GE, Mackarey PJ: Optimal methods for shoulder tendon palpation: a cadaver study. Phys Ther 76:236, 1996
9. Leahy PM: Active release techniques. In Hammer WI (ed): Functional Soft Tissue Examination and Treatment by Manual Methods, 2nd Ed. Aspen, Gaithersburg, MD, 1998
10. Leahy PM, Mock LE: Myofascial release technique and mechanical compromise of peripheral nerves of the upper extremity. Chiro Sports Med 6:139, 1992
11. Leahy PM, Mock LE: Altered biomechanics of the shoulder and the subscapularis. Chiro Sports Med 5:62, 1991
12. Leahy PM, Mock LE: Synoviochondrometaplasia of the shoulder: a case report. Chiro Sports Med 6:5, 1992
13. Lewit K: Manipulative Therapy in Rehabilitation of the Locomotor System. 2nd Ed. Butterworth, Boston, 1991
14. Gaymans F: Die Bedeutung der Atemtypen fur Mobilisation der Wirbelsaule. [Manuell Medizin 18:96, 1980.] p. 145. In Lewit K (ed): Manipulative Therapy in Rehabilitation of the Locomotor System. 2nd Ed. Butterworth–Heinemann, Boston, 1991
15. Jull GA, Janda V: Muscles and motor control in low back pain. p. 253. In Twomey LT, Taylor JR (eds): Physical Therapy of the Low Back. Churchill Livingstone, New York, 1987
16. Moore MA, Kukulka CG: Depression of Hoffmann reflexes following voluntary contraction and implications for proprioceptive neuromuscular facilitation therapy. Phys Ther 71:321, 1991
17. Guissard N, Duchateau J, Hainaut K: Muscle stretching and motoneuron excitability. Eur J Appl Physiol 58:47, 1988
18. Jones LH, Kusunose R, Goering E: Jones Strain-Counterstrain. Jones Strain-Counterstrain, Boise, 1995
19. Jacobson EC, Lockwood MD, Hoefner VC Jr et al: Shoulder pain and repetition strain injury to the supraspinatus muscle: etiology and manipulative treatment. J Am Osteopath Assoc 89:1037, 1989
20. Cislo S, Ramires MA, Schwartz HR: Low back pain: treatment of forward and backward torsions using counterstrain technique. J Am Osteopath Assoc 1(3): 255, 1909
21. Jones LH: Foot treatment without hand trauma. J Am Osteopath Assoc 72:481, 1973
22. Schwartz H: The use of counterstrain in an acutely ill in-hospital population. J Am Osteopath Assoc 86:433, 1986
23. Korr I: Proprioceptors and somatic dysfunction. J Am Osteopath Assoc 74:638, 1975
24. Kusunose RS: Strain and counterstrain. p. 323. In Basmajian JV, Nyberg R (eds): Rational Manual Therapies. Williams & Wilkins, Baltimore, 1993
25. Barnes JF: Myofascial release: A Comprehensive Evaluatory and Treatment Approach. MFR Seminars, Paoli, PA, 1990
26. Bednar DA, Orr FW, Simon GT: Observations on the pathomorphology of the thoracolumbar fascia in chronic mechanical back pain. Spine 20:1161, 1995
27. Greenman PE: Principles of Manual Medicine. 2nd Ed. Williams & Wilkins, Baltimore, 1996

9
Clinical Nutrition

Jerrold Simon
Juanee Surprise

*H*uman health is dependent on adequate intake and assimilation of essential nutrients. Emphasis on proper nutrition is an important part of chiropractic practice. For many years, chiropractic college curricula have included required courses in nutrition, in contrast to most allopathic training institutions. Some chiropractic colleges also offer a separate degree in nutrition.

Nutrition should be part of any complete treatment program. However, except for specific diseases (cardiovascular, celiac, diabetes), conventional physicians often omit or underemphasize nutrition in patient care. By contrast, chiropractors consider nutrition an integral part of disease processes. Chiropractic clinical nutrition encompasses recommendations for proper diet, and where permitted by state law also includes the use of vitamins, minerals, micronutrients, enzymes, herbs and botanicals, phytochemicals, "nutraceuticals," and homeopathic medicines. These are used in comprehensive programs to restore and maintain health and wellness.

The American Chiropractic Association Council on Nutrition offers an extensive and rigorous educational program. To attain diplomate status with the American Chiropractic Board of Nutrition, chiropractic physicians must (1) attend and pass a 300-hour course with a college holding status with the Council on Chiropractic Education or the United States Department of Education, (2) demonstrate a minimum of 3 years practice experience, teaching or performing research in

nutrition, and (3) pass written and practical diplomate examinations.

DIET AND LIFESTYLE CONSIDERATIONS

The typical diet of people in western industrialized nations is high in fat and low in fiber, and characterized by excessive intake of processed carbohydrates and fats, protein, soft drinks, alcohol, and milk products.[1,2] Insufficient intake of vitamins, minerals, trace elements, complex carbohydrates, and pure water is also common. The relationship between these dietary failings and the rising incidence of chronic degenerative diseases such as heart disease and cancer has been explored increasingly over the past few decades and is discussed later in this chapter, as is the responsibility of chiropractors to educate patients on the critical implications of the foods and beverages they consume. Discussion of the full range of nutritional interventions is beyond the scope of this chapter.

Some practitioners fail to investigate and address potential nutritional components of patient complaints adequately out of concern that the process will be too time-consuming. While it is true that the doctor must offer direct personal involvement on recommendations for supplements and lifestyle changes, much of the patient education process can be accomplished through use of handouts and audio- or videotapes. In addition, support staff such as chiropractic assistants or certified clinical nutritionists can handle follow-up where the doctor's direct intervention is not required.

Recording Dietary Intake

To assess a patient's nutritional status, begin with a record of dietary intake. Among the methods used are the dietary history, 24-hour recall diary, 7-day food diary, and food frequency questionnaire. Each method has strengths and weaknesses. The goal is to acquire an accurate record of food intake without burdening the patient with cumbersome procedures.

The 24-hour recall diary is probably the least demanding procedure. The patient is asked to write down everything he or she ate or drank the previous day while logging the time, place, type of food, and amount consumed. Patients usually find this easy to accomplish. Disadvantages include the possibility of inaccurate recall, as well as selective "forgetting" of items such as sweets and alcohol. In addition, food intake on one particular day may not be representative of the patient's typical diet.

More representative is the dietary history (Fig. 9-1), which is quantitatively and qualitatively more accurate than the 24-hour recall. Although more time-consuming, the information gathered from the dietary history takes into account significant data that may be missed in the 24-hour recall, including the impact of medications on food consumption and the patient's supplementation with vitamins, minerals, and herbs.

The food frequency questionnaire provides information on the frequency of consumption of various foods and is fairly easy to standardize. Patients can administer the questionnaire without the aid of nutritionist interviewers. This procedure is particularly useful in determining whether a single nutrient or food group is deficient or missing. A disadvantage is that it is not inclusive of all foods and therefore may provide an incomplete picture of the patient's total food intake.

The data on dietary intake elicited in the diary or questionnaire are then compared with standard criteria for an adequate diet. While there is no single pattern of diet that must be followed to ensure good nutrition,[3] there is general consensus on dietary guidelines. Individual dietary recommendations, however, should take into account factors such as the person's age, ethnic food preferences, socioeco-

nomic background, availability of foods, and ease of food preparation.

Food Groups

For the past several decades, the United States Department of Agriculture (USDA), has suggested dietary guidelines in the form of food groups.[4] Each food guide in its day served as a benchmark in standardizing the American diet.

In 1916, the USDA proposed food groups that consisted of:

- Milk, meat, fish, poultry, eggs, and meat substitutes
- Fruits and vegetables
- Breads and other cereal foods
- Butter and wholesome fats

The Basic Seven Guide in 1943 divided the fruit and vegetable category into three parts and established allowances for the number of daily servings in each category. In 1956, the USDA reduced the Basic Seven to the Basic Four food groups:

- Milk and milk products (two servings)
- Meat, fish, poultry, eggs (two servings)
- Fruits and vegetables (four servings)
- Bread, flour, cereal (four servings)

In 1979, the Hassle-Free Food Guide increased the serving size for milk and milk products (cheeses) from 2 to 2 to 4 and added a cautionary fifth category of fats, sweets, and alcohol. The Food Wheel in 1984 was significant in that the serving sizes were more variable than the Hassle-Free Food Guide and, more importantly, the recommended serving size of breads and cereals was increased from 4 servings to 6 to 11 servings. It was suggested that more than one serving of this food group should be eaten with each meal.

In 1992, the USDA endorsed the Food Guide Pyramid, which takes into account factors of proportion, moderation, and variety. At the top of the pyramid are foods to be eaten sparingly, including fats, oils, and sweets. Farther down the pyramid are foods to be eaten with greater frequency: milk and cheeses (2 to 3 servings); fruits (2 to 4 servings); vegetables

DIET HISTORY

Name _____ Date _____

Occupation _____ Sex _____ Age _____ Marital Status: _____

Highest level of education:
grade school _____ college _____
junior high _____ professional school _____
high school _____

Ethnicity (check one):
Caucasian _____ African American _____
Hispanic _____ Oriental _____
Indian _____ Other _____

Weight: _____ Height (inches) _____ Body Fat % if known: _____

Max. weight ever:(lbs) _____ Age at max. weight: _____ Desired weight:(lbs) _____

Food likes: _____ Food dislikes: _____ Food craving: _____
_____ _____ _____
_____ _____ _____

Food allergies (sensitivities): _____

Medications (check those you are currently taking):

Antacid _____ blood pressure _____ antidepressants _____
heart _____ antibiotics _____ oral contraceptives _____
ulcer _____ laxatives _____ hormone (i.e. estrogen) _____
thyroid _____ chemotherapy _____ muscle relaxants _____
diuretic _____ steroids _____ antiinflammatories _____

Number of meals eaten daily: _____ What % of weekly meals are eaten out: _____

What is the major source of your home food:
grocery store _____ bulk _____
garden _____ home preserved _____
other _____

What preparation methods do you use: (check all that apply)
oven _____ microwave _____
frying pan _____ wok _____
crock pot _____

What method is used for storing food:
refrigerator _____ freezer _____
food cellar _____ other _____

Figure 9-1. Dietary history. *(Figure continues.)*

What size is your average meal: small_____ medium_____ large _____ extra large _____

How much of the following (per glass, cup or can) do you consume daily?

coffee	_____	tea	_____
soda	_____	beer	_____
wine	_____	liquor	_____

Describe your average consumption of sweets per week (give examples): _____
_____

How many times per week to you consume the following?

milk	_____	salt	_____
fatty foods	_____	eggs	_____
fruits	_____	vegetables	_____
red meats	_____	water	_____

What diets have you been on in the past five years? (check all that apply):

low fat	_____	low sugar	_____
low salt	_____	low cholesterol	_____
bland	_____	hypoglycemic	_____
low purine	_____	liquid	_____
weight loss	_____	other	_____

Do you take vitamin/mineral/herbal supplements? (type, brand name and quantity) _____
_____
_____
_____
_____

Signature _____ date _____

Figure 9-1. *(Continued)* Dietary history.

(3 to 5 servings); and breads, cereals, and rice (6 to 11 servings) (Fig. 9-2).

In 1995, the USDA and the Department of Health and Human Services released the fourth edition of Dietary Guidelines for Americans. Without altering the Food Guide Pyramid, these new guidelines propose seven summary steps to healthy eating:

- Eat a variety of foods.
- Balance the food you eat with physical activity; maintain or improve your weight.
- Choose a diet with plenty of grain products, vegetables, and fruits.

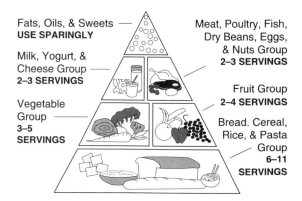

Figure 9-2. USDA Food Guide Pyramid.

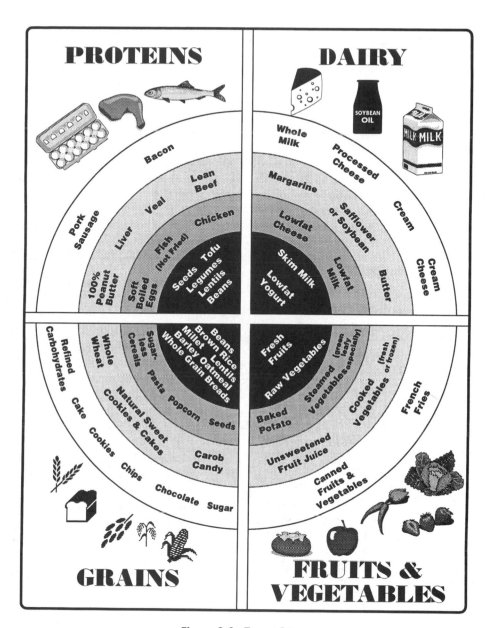

Figure 9-3. Target Diet.

- Choose a diet low in fat, saturated fat, and cholesterol.
- Choose a diet moderate in sugars.
- Choose a diet moderate in salt and sodium.
- If you drink alcoholic beverages, do so in moderation.

Nutritionally oriented chiropractic physicians may also provide an easy-to-follow dietary guide to the patients. Known as the Target Diet (Fig. 9-3), this guide keeps the patient focused on targeting food choices toward the center of the circle.

VITAMINS AND MINERALS

The term *vitamin* was coined by the Polish chemist Casimir Funk. Experimenting with the food supply of pigeons, he noted that certain nitrogenous compounds appeared to be essential for the growth and sustenance of the birds. These *amines* vital to the birds' health were thus dubbed "vitamines," and later "vitamins."

There are two broad categories of vitamins: fat soluble and water soluble. The fat-soluble vitamins A, D, E, and K tend to be stored in the body and are readily absorbed with dietary fats and hence unlikely to be excreted in the urine. The water soluble vitamins include the B vitamins (B_1, B_2, B_6, B_{12}), niacin, pantothenic acid, biotin, folic acid, inositol, and choline, and vitamin C. These are not stored in the body and are readily excreted in the urine.

Minerals are inorganic, solid substances widely distributed in the earth's crust. Although not as dynamic and complex as the vitamins, minerals are important contributors to human metabolism. Minerals are divided into two broad categories: major minerals and trace (rare earth) minerals.

Major minerals include calcium, phosphorus, magnesium, sodium, potassium, chlorine, and sulfur. Trace minerals are more numerous. Their functions are in many cases lesser known and more elusive than the major minerals. Trace minerals include, but are not limited to, aluminum, bismuth, boron, cadmium, chromium, cobalt, copper, europium, fluorine, gallium, iodine, iron, manganese, molybdenum, nickel, selenium, silicon, silver, tin, tungsten, vanadium, and zinc.

Deficiency of any of these minerals or vitamins may lead to various forms of nutritional deficiency disorder. Because of their ability to be stored in human tissues, vitamin toxicity (hypervitaminosis) although rare, is more common with fat-soluble rather than with water-soluble vitamins.

Recommended Daily Allowances

The US recommended daily allowance (RDA) is defined as the level of a nutrient necessary to meet the needs of practically all healthy persons.[5] RDAs are determined by the Food and Nutrition Board of the National Research Council, which is a composite group drawn from the Council of the Institute of Medicine, the National Academy of Sciences, and the National Academy of Engineering.

RDA must be understood within the context in which it was derived. In particular, it is crucial to differentiate RDA from the dietary needs of people with nutritionally related illnesses. RDA is not intended to suggest therapeutic dosages. Furthermore, it may not reveal optimal nutrient dosage for the average individual. The quantities of nutrients needed to prevent nutritional deficiency may be lower than the amounts necessary for optimal function of body systems.

CONSEQUENCES OF NUTRIENT DEFICIENCY

Malnutrition, defined as faulty nutrition resulting from malassimilation, poor diet, or overeating,[6] is common in the United States due to insufficient intake of necessary nutrients (vitamins, minerals, trace elements), complex carbohydrates, fiber, and pure water along with excessive intake of highly processed carbohydrates and fats, protein, soft drinks, alcohol, and milk products.[7–9] Malnutrition affects various functions of the body, increases risk of injury and disease, and decreases healing potential.

The standard American diet has been linked to the chronic degenerative diseases of our time. The concerned clinician should review patients' diet histories and offer counseling on better food and beverage choices, and lifestyle habits, such as smoking, alcohol consumption, and stress-control techniques. When indicated, a detoxification program[10] and/or basic nutritional supplementation should be instituted. The ACA Council on Nutrition recommends basic nutritional supplementation consisting of: a high quality, multiple vitamin/mineral and trace mineral supplement without iron unless need for iron is indicated; additional calcium from two or more sources to meet the RDA for age and sex; and additional vitamin C, preferably in ascorbate form. With continuing research into the advantages of additional antioxidant nutrients, some doctors are also including these in a basic nutrition program.

Approximately one-half the coursework of the diplomate program of the American Chiropractic Board of Nutrition is concerned directly or indirectly with nutritional deficiencies and excesses.

Nutrient deficiencies can lead to disorders in the endocrine, gastrointestinal, hematologic, genitourinary, immune, and nervous systems. In addition, certain nutrient deficiencies may systemically manifest in particular aspects of the life cycle, such as infancy, adolescence, or old age, or in women during pregnancy and lactation.

That the full range of these conditions cannot be covered in this chapter should not imply that they are of minor significance. With heart disease and cancer responsible for more than one-half of all deaths in the United States,[11] it behooves all health practitioners to understand the nutritional influences affecting these disorders.

Detecting Nutritional Deficiencies

Knowing how to detect vitamin D deficiency is essential for the chiropractor. Known as the "bone vitamin," vitamin D plays an important role in the growth, maturation, and sustenance of the skeletal system. The RDA is 400 international units (IU). Since the synthesis of vitamin D from 7-dehydrocholesterol to cholecalciferol is sunlight dependent, people living in warmer climates with more direct skin exposure to sunlight are less likely to become deficient in vitamin D.

In children, vitamin D deficiency can lead to rickets, characterized by misshapen bones (bowed legs, pigeon breast, and rachitic rosary ribs) and retarded growth.[12] Adult vitamin D deficiency is known as osteomalacia, which involves a softening of the skeletal framework, bone demineralization, and involuntary muscle spasms.

The RDA of vitamin A (retinol) is 5,000 IU for men and 4,000 IU for women. Deficiencies of this vitamin are best identified in the eye (retina, conjunctiva, and cornea), skin, and bone. Vitamin A is synthesized from β-carotene (provitamin A), which is naturally found in crystalline form in plant cells.[4]

This fat soluble vitamin can lead to devastating effects in both deficiency and toxicity states. Vitamin A deficiency can lead to corneal ulceration with or without xerosis, multiple areas of desquamated, keratinized cells in the conjunctiva known as Bitot's spots, or dry and roughened skin with spinous papules located at the hair follicles known as perifollicular hyperkeratosis. Toxicity is detected not only in the skin but also the skull, blood, nervous system, gastrointestinal tract, liver, and spleen.[13] Hypervitaminosis A, in some cases the result of uninformed self-supplementation, can yield bright red gingival discoloration, widening of the sagittal and coronal sutures, increased deoxyhemoglobin, irritability, loss of appetite, jaundice, and splenomegaly. In the skin, hypercarotenosis from ingesting excessive quantities of carrots or dark green leafy vegetables or carotene supplements can yield orange-yellow discoloration most noticable on the face, palms, and soles of the feet. It can be reversed by decreasing dietary intake of these vegetables or supplements to acceptable levels.

The average adult requirement for thiamin (vitamin B_1) is 1 mg/day. Deficiencies of this vitamin adversely affect the neuromusculoskeletal and cardiovascular systems. Vitamin B_1 deficiency is uncommon in developed nations and can be avoided by ingesting pork, beef, grains, or legumes. Deficiency can result in dry beriberi with subsequent wrist and foot drop, or wet (cardiac) beriberi with resultant biventricular heart failure and pulmonary congestion.[12] In addition, severe deficiencies can lead to Wernicke-Korsakoff syndrome, a state of mental dysfunction involving confusion, polyneuropathy, dysphonia, and even coma. Alcoholics are particularly at risk since alcohol inhibits assimilation of thiamin.

Deficiencies of other B vitamins also affect the nervous system. Deficiency of riboflavin, vitamin B_2 (RDA 1 mg/day), can also impair wound healing. Riboflavin deficiency is detected by the presence of magenta tongue or angular stomatitis (fissuring at the angles of the mouth).

Reddening or soreness of the tongue can also be seen in pyridoxine (vitamin B_6), cobalamin (vitamin B_{12}), folic acid, and niacin deficiencies.

The hallmark of niacin deficiency (RDA 20 mg/day) is pellagra, a discolorating dermatitis that largely affects the extremities bilaterally.[12] Niacin deficiency can also lead to mental confusion, neuritis, lassitude, generalized weakness, and psychosis.

Pyridoxine is essential to the function of the nervous system. It is involved in amino acid reactive mechanisms including transamination, decarboxylation, transsulfuration, and deamination. Its RDA of 2 mg/day can be found in corn, wheat, yeast, and organ meats. Deficiencies result not only from lack of this nutrient but also from pyridoxine antagonists such as desoxypyridoxine or isoniazid (a drug used to treat tuberculosis). Manifestations of pyridoxine deficiency include dermatitis, glossitis, and nervous disorders such as hyperirritability, abnormal brain patterns, and convulsions.

The RDA for cobalamin (vitamin B_{12}) is 3 μg. B_{12} deficiency is usually due to impairment of absorption rather than inadequate dietary intake. This is the case in pernicious anemia, where intrinsic factor is lacking. The result is megaloblastic anemia characterized by histamine fast achlorhydria, lemon-yellowish skin, and marked fatigue. Of particular relevance to the practicing chiropractor is the peripheral nervous system degeneration that often accompanies cobalamin deficiency.

NUTRITION AND MUSCULOSKELETAL CONDITIONS

Finding the Source of the Pain

Pain is associated with both acute and chronic problems, and the majority of patients seeking care from a chiropractic physician present with pain as part or all of their chief complaint.[14] It is imperative to know why pain is being produced in order to correctly address it nutritionally. For example, a patient with pain in the right, medial scapular region may have a local acute or chronic inflammatory response due to subluxation, trauma, bursitis, extension neuralgia from a cervical whiplash injury, or referred pain from an active trigger point or from the gallbladder. Moreover, there is always the possibility that more than one cause is present. In the example of scapular pain, the chiropractic physician must also rule out causes such as fracture, pneumonia, or cancer which necessitate medical referral. Even where referral is required, nutritional support can often be helpful and co-treatment may be in the patient's best interest.

Nutritional Approach for Inflammation

Whether caused by trauma, injury, joint fixation, or subluxation, chemical irritants such as lactic acid, histamine, bradykinin, prostaglandin E_2, leukotriene B_4, and others are released, producing irritation and inflammation. Appropriate nutrition can serve as a "biochemical adjustment"[15] to influence the healing process. A basic nutritional protocol for inflammation or pain should start with dietary suggestions, including elimination of red meat, dairy, highly processed and fried, high-fat foods, while adding whole grains, fresh fruit, and vegetables, especially green leafy vegetables. This will decrease proinflammatory arachidonic acid and increase the anti-inflammatory prostaglandins 1 and 3.

In addition to a high-quality multivitamin/mineral formula without iron, the following supplements have been found to be of benefit in inflammatory conditions. Iron is not given during inflammation because of its role in free radical formation. Once the inflammation is controlled, iron can be supplemented if symptoms and laboratory tests indicate need.[16]

Proteolytic Enzyme Formula

Proteases are known to decrease proinflammatory and increase anti-inflammatory eicosanoids; to reduce pain and the progression of inflammation by destroying or inactivating bradykinins; to increase transport to and from cells, decreasing edema and increasing cell metabolism; to prevent excess thrombin clot formation; and to aid in phagocyte functions to reduce edema and remove necrotic tissue. This can decrease healing time by as much as 50 percent.[16] Indications for use include acute, traumatic injuries such as sprains, strains, bruises, wounds, fractures, sciatica, acute low back pain, and acute exacerbation of chronic joint conditions.[17,18]

Proteolytic enzymes found in oral products are pancreatin, trypsin, chymotrypsin, bromelain, papain, and other plant origin proteases. Dosage will vary depending on the enzyme and the potency of the product. Typically, 2 to 10 tablets are taken 3 to 5 times per day for 7 to 14 days. When used for treatment of inflammation rather than aiding digestion, proteolytic enzymes should be taken between meals. They are contraindicated in patients with ulcers and gastritis. Bloating, abdominal cramps, and flatulence are common side effects corrected by reducing the dosage.

Vitamin C

Scurvy, which results from frank vitamin C deficiency, is rarely seen in industrialized nations but evidence of vitamin C insufficiency is common. Symptoms include skin, gum, and bone lesions, capillary fragility, joint pain and effusions, edema, anemia, muscle weakness, fatigue, bone pain, osteopenia, decreased resistance to infection, elevated plasma histamine and increased membrane lipid peroxidation.[19] Vitamin C is also critical to the formation of proteoglycan and collagen which play a major role in strengthening connective tissue, including the intervertebral disc, ligaments, and tendons. It is also important in glandular function, especially adrenal function, and for blood vessel integrity.[19] The RDA of 60 mg is adequate to prevent scurvy but below the amount needed for connective tissue and blood vessel integrity and hormone gland function.[20]

Rath and Pauling[21] concluded that 1,320 mg/day is necessary to prevent heart disease. Other investigators have found that traumatic or surgically induced wounds and ulcers heal faster and degenerative joint disease pain is lessened by ascorbate supplementation varying from 100 to 4,000 mg/day.[22–25] One way to determine individual ascorbate need is by having the patient perform a vitamin C flush using the ascorbate form of the vitamin.[26]

Evening Primrose, Borage, Marine, and Flaxseed Oils

These oils contain γ-linolenic acid (GLA), the precursor to prostaglandin 1, and eicosapentaenoic acid (EPA), the precursor to prostaglandin 3. Both have anti-inflammatory actions.[7]

Vitamins B₅ and B₆

Vitamins B_5 and B_6, along with vitamin C, are necessary for adrenal gland function. The adrenals produce cortisol, a natural anti-inflammatory steroid.

Bioflavonoids and Quercetin

Flavonoids inhibit many of the inflammatory pathways, and histamine release from basophils and mast cells and decrease lipid peroxidation, leukotriene release, and collagen breakdown by hyaluronidase.[27,28]

Glucosamine

Important in the synthesis of synovial fluid and cartilage matrix including collagen and proteoglycans, glucosamine has been shown to decrease pain and increase mobility and joint function in mild to moderate osteoarthritis.[29,30]

Turmeric, Ginger, and Curcumin

The action of the spices turmeric, ginger, and curcumin is thought to include an antihistamine effect, inhibition of neutrophil function, and stabilization of lysosomal membranes which release enzyme mediators of inflammation.[31–34]

Phenylalanine

Phenylalanine is an amino acid that increases production of endorphins and enkephalins, the body's natural pain killers. It also slows enzymatic destruction.[35]

Osteoporosis

Osteoporosis is a debilitating disease of bone that occurs mainly in females, aggravated by a diet high in protein and phosphorus, lack of exercise, smoking, and heavy antacid use, including calcium carbonate.[20] The use of calcium by itself, even in high doses, does not stop bone loss. Estrogen helps reduce bone loss by decreasing the rate of turnover; however, studies have not shown it to be consistent in reducing fracture rate.[19] Vitamins C and D, along with the trace minerals zinc, copper, manganese, boron, silicon, and chromium, all play important roles in bone formation and in the prevention and treatment of osteoporosis.[19,36,37]

The best way to prevent osteoporosis is to have good bone formation prior to age 35.[38] This can only be accomplished by a good diet from childhood, with supplemental nutrients added if the diet is insufficient. Parents should be educated about the importance of giving their children a good start on bone health. After age 25, starting or continuing a program designed to decrease bone loss is the best way to prevent osteoporosis in later years.[39]

NUTRITION AND CARDIOVASCULAR DISEASE

Heart disease is the leading cause of untimely death in the United States,[12] and is also the second most common debilitating chronic disorder plaguing the elderly, after arthritis.[40] As such, knowledge of cardiovascular nutrition is of paramount importance to chiropractors and all health care providers.

The incidence of cardiovascular mortality has declined during the past few decades,[41] apparently due to increased awareness of risk factors, advances in medical care, and earlier clinical intervention. Nonetheless, it remains a serious problem and more needs to be done to educate patients. Without patient awareness and self-care, atherosclerosis can go unchecked and progress to coronary heart disease.

Waiting until adulthood to begin the educational process is a costly error, as signs of cardiovascular disease can appear in adolescence. Cardiovascular disease in adults may be traced back to childhood obesity, lack of exercise, pediatric hypertension, and teenage smoking habits.[42] The pathologic process involves atherogenesis of the arterial intima originating with a "fatty streak." This streak usually develops in the aorta or other large diameter arteries and is the result of elevated serum lipids (especially cholesterol) combined with vascular wall injury. In time, the fatty streak becomes fibrous, forming a raised atherosclerotic plaque known as a thrombus that can subsequently block arterial flow. Thrombi are said to be precipitated by the platelet proaggregatory prostaglandin thromboxane A_2.

Risk factors for the development of CHD include[43]

- High low-density lipoprotein (LDL) cholesterol
- History of myocardial infarction
- History of angina pectoris
- Male sex
- Family history of coronary heart disease
- Cigarette smoking
- Hypertension
- Low high-density lipoprotein (HDL) cholesterol
- Diabetes mellitus
- History of other vascular disease
- Obesity

In addition, the Framingham heart study indicates that excessive alcohol consumption might also be a factor.[44]

Many studies have documented dietary interventions for CHD. In a 1985 study in the *Journal of the American Medical Association*, Sacks et al,[45] scrutinized the effects of a lactovegetarian diet on plasma lipoproteins. The parameters included plasma levels of total cholesterol, LDL, and HDL in 75 adult vegetarians for whom dairy products were the major source of fat and cholesterol. These results were then compared with levels recorded in vegans (vegetarians who eat no animal products). The study concluded that adding fatty dairy products to a vegetarian diet tends to raise plasma LDL levels approximately three times higher than HDL levels.

Ornish et al.[46] examined the effects of comprehensive lifestyle changes with respect to coronary atherosclerosis in a prospective, randomized, controlled study that compared 28 patients in an experimental group with 20 in a "usual care" control group. Lifestyle changes in the experimental group consisted of a very low-fat (10 percent) vegetarian diet, stopping smoking, training in stress management, and exercising moderately. Following the 12-month study, positron emission tomography (PET) scan results revealed a statistically significant reduction of the average percentage of arterial stenosis in the experimental group from 40.0 percent to 37.8 percent, while the control group showed an increase from 42.7 percent to 46.1 percent. Ornish and colleagues concluded that certain comprehensive lifestyle changes may have a significantly positive effect in bringing about regression of even severe coronary atherosclerosis.

It is within the purview of the chiropractor to counsel patients on the steps needed to reduce the risk of heart disease. Suggestions for lowering the risk of atherogenesis and its resultant cardiovascular complications come in three categories: lifestyle changes, dietary changes, and dietary supplementation.

Lifestyle changes include the following steps:

- Stop smoking
- Increase physical exercise (if sedentary)
- Lose weight (if overweight)

Dietary suggestions include the following approach:

- Decrease alcohol consumption (if excessive)
- Decrease salt intake, especially if hypertensive or sodium sensitive

- Decrease fat intake, especially saturated fats
- Decrease cholesterol intake
- Decrease whole milk dairy products
- Decrease refined carbohydrates
- Increase dietary fiber
- Increase fruits and vegetables
- Increase fish (especially deep-sea varieties)

There is evidence supporting the use of supplements in the prevention and treatment of coronary heart disease in humans. Among these are magnesium,[47] niacin,[48] folic acid,[49] vitamin B$_6$,[50] potassium,[51] vitamin E,[52] vitamin C,[53] chromium,[54] and coenzyme Q-10.[55]

NUTRITION AND CANCER

Cancer is a plague of modern civilization. It is the second most common cause of mortality in the United States, after heart disease.[12] Alarmingly, its incidence continues to increase, having more than tripled in the past century.[56] According to the American Cancer Society, there are an estimated 1.35 million new cases of cancer annually in the U.S.[57]

Ever since German physician Rudolph Virchow theorized in 1853 that new cells arise from preexisting cells in a process of division, pathologists have postulated that cancer can be understood as cell division gone awry. Cell division occurs in four distinct phases known as prophase, metaphase, anaphase, and telophase. At some point in the process, normal cells can be transformed into cancerous cells.

When this occurs, it is the role of the immune system to attack and destroy these potentially harmful cells with specific T-cells or B-cells. T-cells arising from the thymus gland activate an inflammatory process to wall off the foreign invader and initiate its destruction through phagocytosis. B-cells arising from gut lymphoid tissue are responsible for producing immunoglobulins that yield a type of memory imprint of the antigenic intruder.

Immune system function depends on high-quality nutrition. Nutritionally aware doctors can offer cancer patients information geared toward strengthening the body's efforts to deal with associated symptoms and related disorders attributed to the

cancer. Such nutritional intervention is particularly important in light of estimates by the National Academy of Sciences that 60 percent of women's cancers and 40 percent of men's cancers are related to nutritional factors.[58]

A preponderance of data suggest a strong, direct relationship between certain cancers and high-fat diets.[59] Moreover, there is significant evidence of an inverse relationship between cancer (especially of the colon and breast) and high-fiber diets. However, some research has disputed the therapeutic effects of fiber.[60]

As in the case of cardiovascular disease, suggestions for combating cancer also fall into the three categories of lifestyle changes, dietary changes, and dietary supplementation.

Suggestions for lifestyle changes include the following steps:

- Stop smoking
- Avoid excessive direct sunlight
- Avoid smokeless tobacco
- Minimize exposure to ionizing radiation
- Minimize exposure to industrial agents such as asbestos, nickel, vinyl chloride, iron particulate, and silicon
- Reduce other lifestyle stressors (neuroendocrine related)

Dietary suggestions include the following approach:

- Reduce dietary fat
- Avoid smoked, pickled, or salt-cured foods
- Avoid preservatives such as sodium nitrate, and sodium benzoate
- Avoid sugar
- Avoid partially hydrogenated oils
- Reduce intake of foods high in oleic acid (e.g., olive oil, beef tallow)
- Increase dietary fiber
- Increase intake of fruits and vegetables

There is evidence supporting the use of supplements in the prevention and treatment of certain cancers in humans. Among the nutrients for which there is such evidence are folic acid for cervical dysplasia in users of oral contraceptives,[61] calcium[62] for those at high risk of colon cancer, as well as alkylglycerols[63] for uterine and cervical cancer and γ-linoleic acid[64] for a wide range of malignancies.

Other Applications for Nutrition in Practice

Conservative nutritional approaches are appropriate in the management of many diseases.[65] While discretion is necessary in life-threatening illnesses, such as myocardial infarction, stroke, or fulminating infection, which require aggressive treatment and medical intervention, a concurrent nutritional approach may be of benefit to the patient. Certain gastrointestinal ailments, including those of associated organs such as the liver and gallbladder, are amenable to nutritional intervention,[66] as are disorders related to the menstrual cycle,[67,68] vaginal candidiasis,[69,70] urinary tract infections,[71] and prostate problems.[72] Nutritional research also shows promise for neurologic diseases, including multiple sclerosis,[73] Parkinson's disease,[74,75] and epilepsy[76] and psychological disorders such as depression.[77]

Terminology

dietary history
fat-soluble vitamins
food frequency questionnaire
Food Guide Pyramid
malnutrition
mineral
osteoporosis
proteolytic enzymes
RDA
7-day food diary
Target Diet
24-hour recall diary
USDA
vitamin
water-soluble vitamins

Review Questions

1. What are some common failings in the typical diets of people in industrialized nations?

2. Name and describe three methods for recording dietary intake.

3. According to the USDA Food Guide Pyramid, which categories of foods should constitute the majority of a healthy diet?

4. Does the recommended daily allowance indicate the nutrient needs for people with nutritionally related illnesses?

5. What are the possible consequences of vitamin D deficiency?

6. List four nutritional supplements with anti-inflammatory effects.

7. What is the best way to prevent osteoporosis?

8. What did the Ornish study demonstrate about treatment of heart disease? What dietary and nondietary interventions were utilized?

9. What are the first and second most common causes of mortality in the United States?

10. What are three nutritional recommendations for decreasing the likelihood of developing cancer?

Concept Questions

1. What is the chiropractor's role in offering nutritional advice to patients? Should this be part of chiropractic case management for all patients?

2. If a chiropractor does not include nutrition in patient care, what possible consequences may result from this?

References

1. Williams SR: Nutrition and Diet Therapy. 4th Ed. CV Mosby, St. Louis, 1981

2. Werbach M: Nutritional Influences on Illness. 2nd Ed. Third Line Press, Tarzana, CA, 1983

3. Shils ME, Young VR: Modern Nutrition in Health and Disease. 7th Ed. Lea & Febiger, Philadelphia, 1988

4. Madigan E: News Division, Office of Public Affairs. United States Department of Agriculture, Washington, DC, 1992

5. National Research Council Food and Nutrition Board: Recommended Daily Allowances. 8th Ed. National Academy of Sciences, Washington, DC, 1974

6. Steadman's Medical Dictionary. 22nd Ed. Williams & Wilkins, Baltimore, 1972

7. Williams SR: Nutrition and Diet Therapy. 6th Ed. CV Mosby, St. Louis, 1989

8. Kretchmer N: Nutrition is the keystone of prevention. Am J Clin Nutr 60:1, 1994

9. Pryor WA: The RDAs: past, present and future. Nutr Rep 12:33, 1994

10. Bland J, Barrager E, Reedy RG, Bland K: A medical food-supplemented detoxification program in the management of chronic health problems. Alternative Ther 1:62, 1995

11. Leaf A: The aging process: lessons from observations in man. Nutr Rev 46:40, 1988

12. Maclaren DS: A Colour Atlas of Nutritional Disorders. Wolfe, London, 1981

13. Whitney E, Hamilton M: Understanding Nutrition. West, St. Paul, MN, 1977

14. Job Analysis of Chiropractic: A Project Report, Survey Analysis and Summary of the Practice of Chiropractic Within the United States. National Board of Chiropractic Examiners, Greeley, CO, 1993

15. Seaman DR: Chiropractic and Pain Control. 3rd Ed. DRS Systems, Atlanta, GA, 1995

16. Biemond P, Swaak AJG, van Eijk JG, Koster JF: Superoxide dependent iron release from ferritin in inflammatory diseases. Free Radical Biol Med 4:85, 1988

17. Taussig SJ, Batkin S: Bromelain, the enzyme complex of pineapple (*Ananas comosus*) and its clinical application, an update. J Ethnopharmacol 22:191, 1988

18. Tassman G: Evaluation of a plant proteolytic enzyme for the control of inflammation and pain. J Dent Dis 19:73, 1994

19. Shils ME, Olson JA, Shike M: Modern Nutrition in Health and Disease. 8th Ed. Lea & Febiger, Philadelphia, 1994

20. Levine M, Conry-Cantilera C, Wang Y et al: Vitamin C pharmacokinetics in healthy volunteers: evidence for a recommended dietary allowance. Proc Natl Acad Sci USA 93:3704, 1996

21. Rath M, Pauling L: Solution to the puzzle of human cardiovascular disease: its primary cause is ascorbate deficiency, leading to the deposition of lipoprotein(a) and fibrinogen/fibrin in the vascular wall. J Orthomolec Med 6:125, 1991

22. Hunt C, Duncan LA: Hyperlipoproteinemia and atherosclerosis in rabbits fed low level cholesterol and lecithin. Br J Exp Pathol 66:35, 1988

23. Hunter T, Rajan DT: The role of ascorbic acid in the pathogenesis and treatment of pressure sores. Paraplegia 8:211, 1971

24. Greenwood J: Optimum vitamin C intake as a factor in the preservation of disc integrity. Med Ann DC 33:274, 1964

25. Schwartz ER: Metabolic response during early stages of surgically induced osteoarthritis in mature beagles. J Rheumatol 7:788, 1980

26. Lytle RL: Chronic dental pain: possible benefits of food restriction and sodium ascorbate. J Appl Nutr 40:95, 1988

27. Bauman J, Bruchnausen FW, Wurm G: Prostaglandins. Prostaglandins 20:627, 1980

28. Middleton E: The Flavonoids. Elsevier Science, Amsterdam, 1984

29. Crolle G, Este E: Glucosamine sulfate for the management of arthritis: a controlled clinical investigation. Curr Med Res Opin 7:104, 1980

30. Vaz AL: Double-blind clinical evaluation of the relative efficacy of ibuprofen and glucosamine sulfate in the management of osteoarthrosis of the knee in outpatients. Curr Med Res Opin 8:145, 1982

31. Middleton E, Drzewicki G: Naturally occurring flavonoids and human basophil histamine release. Arch Allergy Appl Immunol 77:155, 1985

32. Leibovitz V: Polyphenols and bioflavonoids, the medicines of tomorrow. Part 1. Townsend Letter for Doctors, April 1994

33. Srivastava KC, Mustafa T: Ginger (zingiber officinale) in rheumatism and musculoskeletal disorders. Med Hypotheses 39:342, 1992

34. Fewtrell C, Gomperts B: Effects of flavone inhibitors of transport ATPases on histamine secretion from rat mast cells. Nature 265:635, 1977

35. Budd H: Advances in Pain Research and Therapy. Raven Press, New York, 1983

36. Heaney RB: Calcium in the prevention and treatment of osteoporosis. J Intern Med 231:169, 1992

37. Kidd PM: An integrative lifestyle: nutritional strategy for lowering osteoporosis risk. p. 400. Townsend Letter for Doctors, May 1993

38. Cook A: Osteoporosis: review and commentary. JHMS 2:9, 1994

39. Kamen B: New Facts About Fiber. Nutrition Encounter, Novato, CA, 1992

40. Rudman D: Nutrition and fitness in elderly people. Am J Clin Nutr 49:1090, 1989

41. United States Department of Health and Human Services, National Center for Health Statistics. Monthly Vital Stat Rep 44: 1996.

42. Kannel WB: Pediatric aspects of lipid-induced atherogenesis. J Am Coll Nutr 3:139, 1984

43. Goodman DS: Report of the national cholesterol education program expert panel on detection, evaluation and treatment of high blood cholesterol in adults. Arch Intern Med 148:36, 1988

44. Castelli WP, Garrison RJ: Incidence of coronary heart disease and lipoprotein cholesterol levels: the Framingham study. JAMA 256:2835, 1986

45. Sacks FM, Ornish D, Rosner B et al: Plasma lipoprotein levels in vegetarians. JAMA 254:1337, 1985

46. Ornish D, Brown SE, Scherwitz LW et al: Can lifestyle changes reverse coronary heart disease? Lancet 336:129, 1990

47. Rasmussen HS, Aurys P, Hojberg S et al: Magnesium and acute myocardial infarction. Arch Intern Med 146:872, 1986

48. Hoeg JM, Gregg RE, Brew HB: An approach to the management of hyperlipoproteinemia. JAMA 255:512, 1986

49. Brattstrom LE, Hultberg BL, Hardebo JE: Folic acid responsive postmenopausal homocystenemia. Metabolism 34:1073, 1985

50. Serfontein WJ, Ubbink JB, De Villiers et al: Plasma pyridoxal-5-phosphate level as risk index for coronary heart disease. Atherosclerosis 55:357, 1985

51. Nordrehaug JE, Johannessen KA, von der Lippe G: Serum potassium concentration as a risk factor of ventricular arrhythmias early in acute myocardial infarction. Circulation 71:645, 1985

52. Steiner M, Anastasi J: Vitamin E: an inhibitor of the platelet release action. J Clin Invest 57:732, 1976

53. Bordia A, Verma SK: Effect of vitamin C on platelet adhesiveness and platelet aggregation in coronary artery disease patients. Clin Cardiol 8:552, 1985

54. Simonoff M: Low plasma chromium in patients with coronary artery and heart diseases. Biol Trace Elem Res 6:431, 1984

55. Kamikawa T, Kobayashi A, Yamashita T et al: Effects of coenzyme Q-10 on exercise tolerance in chronic stable angina pectoris. Am J Cardiol 56:247, 1985

56. Department of Health, Education and Welfare. Cancer Questions 77:1040, 1975

57. American Cancer Society: Cancer Facts and Figures. American Cancer Society, Atlanta, 1996

58. National Academy of Sciences: Nutrition, Diet and Cancer. National Academy of Sciences, Washington, DC, 1982

59. Miller AB, Howe GR: Food items and food groups as risk factors in a case control study of diet and colo-rectal cancer. Int J Cancer 32:155, 1983

60. Riley V: Cancer and stress: overview and critique. Cancer Detect Prev 2(2):163, 1979

61. Butterworth CE Jr, Hatch DK, Gore H et al: Improvement in cervical dysplasia associated with folic acid therapy in users of oral contraceptives. Am J Clin Nutr 35:73, 1982

62. Lipkin M, Newmark H: Effect of added dietary calcium on colonic epithelial-cell proliferation in subjects at high risk for familial colonic cancer. N Eng J Med 313:1381, 1985

63. Brohult A, Brohult J, Brohult S, Joelsson I: Reduced mortality in cancer patients after administration of alkoxylglycerols. Acta Obstet Gynecol Scand 65:779, 1986

64. Van der Merwe CF, Boovens J, Katzeff IE: Oral gamma-linoleic acid in 21 patients with untreatable malignancy. An ongoing open clinical trial. Br J Clin Pract 41:907, 1987

65. Gabel L, Fahey PJ, Gallagher-Alred et al: Dietary prevention and treatment of disease. AFP J 41S:415, 1992

66. Moerman CJ, Smeets FW, Kromhout D: Dietary risk factors for clinically diagnosed gallstones in middle-aged men: a 25-year follow-up study (Zutphen study). Ann Epidemiol 4:248, 1994

67. Cassidy A, Bingham S, Setchell KD: Biological effects of a diet of soy protein rich in isoflavones on the menstrual cycle of premenopausal women. Am J Clin Nutr 60:333, 1994

68. Posaci C: Plasma copper, zinc, and magnesium levels in patients with premenstrual tension syndrome. Acta Obstet Gynecol Scand 73:452, 1994

69. Fong IW: The rectal carriage of yeast in patients with vaginal candidiasis. Clin Invest Med 17:426, 1994

70. Mikhail MS, Palan PR, Basu J et al: Decreased beta-carotene levels in exfoliated vaginal epithelial cells in women with vaginal candidiasis. Am J Reprod Immunol 32:221, 1994

71. Avorn J, Monane M, Gurwitz JH et al: Reduction of bacteriuria and pyuria after ingestion of cranberry juice. JAMA 271:751, 1994

72. Adlercreutz H, Markkanen H, Watanabe S et al: Plasma concentrations of phyto-estrogens in Japanese men. Lancet 342:1209, 1993

73. Reynolds EH: Multiple sclerosis and vitamin B_{12} metabolism. J Neurol Neurosurg Psychiatry 55:339, 1992

74. Juncos JI: Diet and Related Variables in the Management of Parkinson's Disease Current Concepts in Parkinson's Disease Research. Hogrefe and Huber, London, 1993

75. Karsteadt PJ, Pincus JH: Protein redistribution diet remains effective in patients with fluctuating parkinsonism. Arch Neurol 49:149, 1992

76. Botez MI, Botez T, Ross-Chaumand A: Thiamine and folate treatment of chronic epileptic patients: a controlled study with the Wechsler IQ scale. Epilepsy Res 16:157, 1993

77. Creilin R, Bolligeliere T, Reynolds EF: Folate and psychiatric disorders: clinical potential. Drugs 45:623, 1993

10
Musculoskeletal Disorders Research

Anthony L. Rosner

*D*espite the fact that chiropractic has existed as a formal profession for over a century, most of the rigorous research that supports this modality of health care has emerged in just the past two decades. The year 1975 was a watershed, during which an assessment of the research status of spinal manipulation was conducted and published by Murray Goldstein of the National Institutes of Neurological Diseases and Stroke (NINDS)—with results that were not encouraging. Goldstein's report concluded that there was a paucity of rigorous outcomes research in support of chiropractic intervention for back pain and other musculoskeletal disorders.[1]

Besides lacking sufficient numbers of randomized controlled clinical trials published in established medical journals, early outcomes trials suffered from several design flaws:

- Often lacking an adequate description of manipulation, these trials commonly described mobilization rather than manipulation. Furthermore, the methods often lacked adequate descriptions to permit their replication.
- Qualifications of those administering treatment were not reported.
- There was ambiguity in the sample clinical characterizations.

- Physician–patient contact times were not uniform across compared groups.
- Blinding of participants and investigators was not always assured.
- Sample sizes were often too small to approach statistical significance.
- Experimental bias was often introduced into the trial and often implicit in the recruitment process.
- A failure to observe or control baseline characteristics was common.
- In a laboratory setting under tightly controlled conditions, the intervention tended to be very individualized and as such was difficult if not impossible to generalize to the clinical situation.

Twenty years later, dramatic changes are in evidence. Regarding back pain as assessed by a U.S. government agency, the Agency for Health Care Policy and Research (AHCPR), chiropractic appears to have vaulted from last place to first. According to the 1994 monograph *Acute Low Back Pain in Adults*, an AHCPR clinical practice guideline, the strength of the evidence found to support manipulation was rated sufficiently high to place this intervention among the *first* two options (together with the use of analgesics and nonsteroidal anti-inflammatory drugs [NSAIDs] to be considered from 22 different types of interventions reviewed.[2] This conclusion was based on 112 articles screened, 12 randomized clinical trials meeting the criteria for review[3–14] plus two meta-analyses[15,16] and a cost analysis.[17]

This chapter describes the progression of musculoskeletal disorders research with primary emphasis on back and neck pain, as well as headache. The focus is on research since the watershed NINDS conference during the mid-1970s, seeking as well to identify the key events influencing this dramatic reversal of fortune.

HISTORICAL PERSPECTIVE

Through the 1920s, the chiropractic profession remained largely unfamiliar with research methodology, relying primarily on testimonials from cured patients to document its effectiveness.[18] This was the era when allopathic medicine was just beginning to follow experimental research regimens as first proposed by Claude Bernard in 1865.[19] Chiropractic research was significantly hampered at this time and for decades to come by staunch opposition from the American Medical Association (AMA).[20]

In the early years of the profession, most chiropractic professional schools were proprietary and depended on tuition and clinical fees for survival. Under those conditions, little research was possible, except for some case studies, many of which provided valuable clinical insights. Many of these early investigations followed the interests of B.J. Palmer and the Palmer School of Chiropractic, beginning with the establishment of a "spinographic" laboratory in 1910, in which it was believed that radiographs would provide the opportunity for detecting spinal displacements.[21] After the introduction of this technology, it was asserted by some that patient recovery increased dramatically.[22] B.J. himself proposed that:

> Spinography does more than read subluxations, it proves the existence, location, and degree of exostosis, anyklosis, abnormal shapes and forms, all of which may prevent the early correction to normal position of the subluxation.[23] The growth of interest in radiography continued with the introduction of full spine radiography by Thompson,[23] later refined in 1931 by the use of a single film.[21]

H.E. Crowe's description of the term *whiplash* in 1928—used to describe soft tissue injuries in the vicinity of the cervical spine, often caused by automobile accidents[24]—introduced the importance of the soft tissue injury. Although now accepted as a medical term, the condition is often associated with litigation[25] and suffers from a scanty literature base.[26]

Largely through the efforts of Joseph Janse and Fred Illi, the sacroiliac joint became the next key focus in chiropractic research. Starting in 1943 at his laboratory at the Institute for the Studies of Statics and Dynamics of the Human Body in Geneva, Switzerland, Illi's ongoing work provided insight into the functioning of the sacroiliac joint as a synovial articulation required for fully upright bipedal locomotion.[27]

During World War II, European chiropractic researchers developed the practical spinal analysis called motion palpation as a collective work. A group of Belgian chiropractors including Marcel and Henri Gillet, Maurice Liekens, Fenande De Mey, Henri Poeck, and Paul de Borchgrave drew upon chiropractic pioneer O.G. Smith's theory that the vertebral joint has both a circumscribed field and center of motion, which are offset when a subluxation occurs.[28] Now, publications described the methods available to help the practitioner find and demonstrate the evident changes in mobilities of the vertebral and sacroiliac articulations before and after an adjustment.[29,30]

Then in 1975 the NINDS conference drew a line in the sand regarding chiropractic research. Responding to political pressure from chiropractors, the Senate Appropriations Labor-HEW Subcommittee recommended in its 1974 report to the Senate that, "This would be an opportune time for an 'independent, unbiased' study of the fundamentals of the chiropractic profession." Consequently, Congress authorized up to $2 million of the 1974 DHEW appropriation for that purpose.[18]

Organized and chaired by osteopath Murray Goldstein, Associate Director of NINDS, the conference topic was termed *spinal manipulation*, in order to emphasize the common ground shared by the multidisciplinary group leading clinicians and scientists who met for 3 days in Washington. Although the conference failed to deliver a consensus as to the indications, contraindications, and precise scientific basis for the results obtained by manual manipulation of the spine,[1] it did produce the following comments by its organizer which set the stage for the next 20 years of chiropractic research:

But perhaps of most far reaching importance, the Workshop documented that although there are a number of meaningful basic and clinical research questions about manipulative therapy and vertebral biomechanics that are amenable to investigation, there was relatively little quantitative data either in support or in opposition to the several clinical hypotheses. ... I suspect the NINCDS Workshop cleared the air by demonstrating that there are precise scientific issues relevant to manipulative therapy that deserve research attention.[31]

Over the past two decades, the chiropractic profession has heeded this call, producing an extensive body of research.

BACK PAIN RESEARCH

Methods of Measurement

As in other clinical outcomes research, chiropractic investigations require reproducible and verifiable measurements from multiple viewpoints involving both the patient and the clinician. Table 10-1 illustrates three such perspectives: (1) functional ability, (2) patient perception regarding pain and satisfaction, and (3) general health (global) perceptions on the part of the patient. All the indices noted have been verified in the literature; use of the measures represented on this list is indicated for any outcome study to achieve sufficient construct validity.

At the same time, outcomes research is bedeviled by what appears at first glance to be a conundrum.

Table 10-1. Outcome Instruments in Chiropractic Research

Functional outcome assessments
    Oswestry Back Disability Index
    Roland-Morris Low Back Pain Disability Questionnaire
    Neck Disability Index
    Range of Motion
Patient perception outcome assessments
    Pain
        Visual Analog Scale (VAS)
        Verbal Rating Scale (VRS)
        Behavioral Rating Scale (BRS)
    Patient satisfaction
General health outcome assessments
    SF-36
    COOP Charts

Table 10-2 lists outcome studies in order of decreasing rigor, from the most fastidious, demanding (and expensive) randomized clinical trial to anecdotes arising from everyday personal experiences. One would assume that the most controlled investigation, the clinical trial, would yield the most useful information; indeed, the clinical trial is often referred to as the "gold standard"[32] in clinical research. Paradoxically, because it is so controlled, the most rigorous member of the clinical research hierarchy presents its own difficulties in its generalizability. In using a presumably broad, cross-sectional patient base rather than the individual retellings from unique patients in the case report or anecdote, it does offer a means to offer a general predictive outcome pattern to patients outside the study. What is often overlooked, however, is the fact that the *intervening conditions* are restricted, screening out potentially important and perhaps undefined elements which occur in the natural setting of the patient's visit to the doctor's office. Thus, the experimental designs at the "low" end of the spectrum offer their own unique brand of generalizability, although of an uncontrolled and often confounded nature.

What is needed to support a particular type of intervention are research results from both ends of the spectrum to obtain both the rigor and different types of generalizability sought after in clinical documentation. It is, in fact, the material from the anecdotes and clinician's office that provides the impetus—the food for thought—to design and conduct a randomized clinical trial.

Clinical Trials on Back Pain

As of this writing, close to 40 clinical trials including spinal manipulation therapy have been reported; at least 25 controlled trials published in English were confirmed as of 1992.[16] Suffering from the design flaws mentioned above, the earlier trials tended to suggest only short-term benefits for spinal therapy, eliciting a widespread belief from the allopathic medical community that spinal manipulation therapy was beneficial in the alleviation of acute pain but that there existed no convincing documentation of its efficacy with severe problems or long-term complications.[33]

Fourteen of the leading clinical trials and prospective (cohort) studies addressing the role of spinal manipulation therapy in the treatment of

Table 10-2. Hierarchy of Clinical Research Designs, in Decreasing Rigor

Design Classification	Definition
1. Randomized clinical trial (RCT)	Defined treatment to one group, placebo, or sham to a second (control)
2. Prospective (cohort) study	Defined treatment to one group, no control blank or sham group
3. Retrospective (case control) study	Study done after treatment (many cases)
4. Cross-sectional study	Study of all subjects done at one point in time
5. Single-subject time series	Following of response of 1 case over time
6. Case series	Report on a group of cases
7. Case report	Report on 1 single case
8. Anecdotes	Recollections of case responses, lacking the details of case report

back pain are summarized in Table 10-3. From these results, many characteristics are evident:

1. Chronic and subacute complaints have now begun to be addressed.
2. More robust statistical analyses are now available due to the inclusion of both larger sample sizes (many in the hundreds) and more objective, reproducible outcome measures such as those proposed in Table 10-1.
3. The difference between manipulation and mobilization has been more clearly understood, especially evident from the inclusion of the latter intervention as an entirely discrete arm of the clinical trial, often called a "sham" or "mimic" procedure.
4. Practitioners have become more clearly identified as chiropractors with proper training in manipulation, having the liberty to treat as they would in actual clinical practice. In this manner, the research becomes more pragmatic and gains external validity, helping to solve the conundrum proposed in Table 10-2.[33,34–47]

Regarding the coming of age of chiropractic research on back pain, the 1985 Kirkaldy-Willis and Cassidy study is noteworthy in that it represents the first time a chiropractor (Cassidy) coauthored an article published in a medical journal.[36] A more recent trial by Koes et al.[39] shows that improvement in the main complaint produced by manual therapy was not only superior to standard medical treat-ment, but that the latter intervention even failed to keep pace with the placebo, in which no intervention took place (Table 10-3 and Fig. 10-1).

Probably one of the most important current trends is that, in contrast to some of the earlier trials in which the relief provided by chiropractic adjustments appeared to be short-lived (less than 2 weeks),[45–47] some of the more recent larger trials demonstrate that the beneficial effects of spinal manipulation therapy are uniquely long-lived, persisting for as much as 12 months[39] to 2 years.[37] In fact, Meade's recent follow-up to his previous study[37] indicates that, from the viewpoint of the Oswestry pain scale, spinal manipulation therapy is superior to an outpatient hospitalization regimen for up to 3 years following the treatment regimen.[38] One problem that has been raised regarding the Meade study, however, is that only 28 percent of its patients were randomized into the chiropractic branch of treatment.[37]

The RAND Appropriateness and Utilization Study

A second facet of musculoskeletal disorders research relating to back pain and chiropractic can be credited to the RAND Corporation, a nonprofit research and development company which first gained prominence with research for the U.S. military in World War II. RAND now conducts research in the health sciences as well as education, applied economics, sociology, defense, and civil justice.

Several years and millions of dollars in the making, the 1992 RAND Appropriateness and Utiliza-

Table 10-3. Summary of Leading Low Back Pain Clinical Trials/Cohort Studies Involving Chiropractic Intervention

Investigator	Design	Branches	No. of Subjects	Presenting Condition	Outcomes	Follow-up
Bronfort[35]	Prospective	SMT	298	LBP (acute, chronic)	Ability to work Bed rest Use of medication Subjective feeling	12 mo
Kirkaldy-Willis/ Cassidy[36]	Prospective	SMT	283	LBP (chronic)	Improved grade Patient impression of pain relief Loss of disability	1 mo 3 mo 6 mo 9 mo 12 mo
Meade[37]	RCT	SMT Hospitalization	741	LBP (acute, chronic)	Oswestry pain disability Straight leg raising Lumbar flexion	2 yr
Meade[38]	RCT	SMT Hospitalization	741	LBP (acute, chronic)	Oswestry pain disability Satisfaction	3 yr
Koes[39]	RCT	SMT Physiotherapy Gen pract Placebo	256	Nonspecific back, neck (subacute, chronic)	Severity of main complaint Global perceived effect Pain Functional states	3 wk 6 wk
Pope[40]	RCT	SMT Massage Corset TMS	164	LBP (subacute)	Pt confidence VAS Range of motion Maximum voluntary extension Straight leg raise Biering-Sorenson fatigue test	3 wk
Blomberg[41]	RCT	Medical Mechanical Mobilization Stretching Autotraction Cortisone SMT	101	LBP (acute, subacute)	Pain Sick leave	1 mo 6 mo
Triano[42]	RCT	SMT Mimic Back education	209	LBP (chronic)	Self-reported pain Activity tolerance	2 wk 4 wk
Waagen[43]	RCT	SMT full spine Sham/massage	19	LBP (acute)	Pain relief Spinal mobility	2 wk

(Continues)

Table 10-3. *(Continued)*

Investigator	Design	Branches	No. of Subjects	Presenting Condition	Outcomes	Follow-up
Farrell and Twomey[44]	RCT	Mobilization plus SMT PT (diathermy, exercises, ergonomic inst)	48	LBP (acute)	Pain symptoms	1st trtmt 3rd trtmt Last trtmt 3 wk
Halder[45]	RCT SMT	Sham mobiliz.	54	LBP (acute)	Pain	Day 1 post Every 3 days 3 wk
Hoehler[46]	RCT	SMT Massage	95	LBP	Pain	Variable Discharge 3 wk post
Glover[47]	RCT	SMT Placebo (detuned SWD)	84	LBP	Pain	15 min 3 days 7 days 1 mo
Berquist-Ullman, Larsson[3]	RCT	Back school Combined PT + SMT Placebo (detuned SWD)	197	LBP (acute, subacute)	Pain Sick leave	10 d 3 wk 6 wk 3 mo 6 mo 1 yr

Abbreviations: LBP, low back pain; PT, physical therapy; RCT, randomized clinical trial; SMT, spinal manipulation therapy; SWD, short wave diathermy; TMS, transcutaneous muscle stimulation; trtmt, treatment

tion Study sought to provide "a comprehensive set of indications for performing spinal manipulation with low back pain," with the guidelines based on a review of the literature, appropriateness ratings by both multidisciplinary and all-chiropractic panels of experts, and field studies abstracted from five North American cities: Portland, Oregon; Minneapolis, Minnesota; Miami, Florida; San Diego, California; and Toronto, Ontario.

The literature review of 67 articles and 9 books published between 1952 and 1991 established that chiropractors within the United States performed 94 percent of all the manipulative care for which reimbursement was sought, with osteopaths delivering 4 percent and general practitioners and orthopedic surgeons accounting for the remainder. Support was consistent for the use of spinal manipulation as a treatment for patients with acute low back

pain and an absence of other signs or symptoms of lower limb nerve root involvement. For low back pain with minor lower limb neurological findings or sciatica, the evidence was judged to be either insufficient or conflicting. There was no systematic report on the frequency of complications due to spinal manipulation therapy.[48]

The appropriateness of chiropractic spinal manipulation was assessed by two expert panels, one multidisciplinary and one all-chiropractic, each rating a comprehensive array of more than 1,500 clinical scenarios for appropriateness or inappropriateness of chiropractic intervention. These scenarios varied according to the duration of symptoms, clinical course of the pain, presence of comorbid diseases, history in response to previous treatments for back pain, findings upon physical examination, and findings on lumbosacral radiographs as well as com-

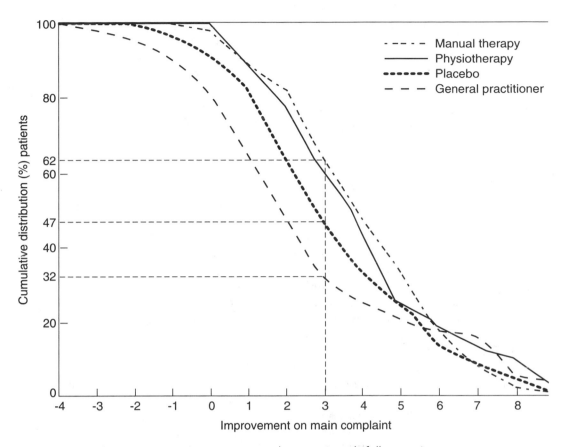

Figure 10-1. Improvement on main complaint at 6-week follow-up (intention-to-treat analysis). (From Koes et al.,[39] with permission.)

puted tomography (CT) or magnetic resonance imaging (MRI).

Among the conditions recognized by the multidisciplinary panel[49] as appropriate for chiropractic intervention were acute (under 3 weeks' duration) back pain with the absence of neurologic findings, and acute back pain with minor neurologic findings and uncomplicated lumbosacral neurologic radiographs. In the final ratings, panelists rated 7 percent of all conditions as appropriate for spinal manipulation therapy, although these conditions represent the majority of back pain patients. As might be anticipated, the all-chiropractic panel[50] rated a higher percentage (27 percent) of all conditions as appropriate. Inappropriate ratings by the multidisciplinary and all-chiropractic panels were 60 percent and 48 percent, respectively.

On the all-chiropractic panel, there was a higher level of intra-panel agreement than was achieved on the multidisciplinary panel (63 percent versus 36 percent).

Depending on the criteria for assessment, the RAND field studies have yielded varying levels of appropriateness of chiropractic intervention. These have been grafted onto the recommendations of the two expert panels described above. For one site (San Diego), the level of appropriateness varied between 38 percent and 74 percent and the level of inappropriateness ranged from 19 percent and 7 percent, depending upon whether the criteria of the multidisciplinary or the all-chiropractic panel were applied. Data from other geographic areas of the United States will be required before inferences for the national population can be drawn, and it has been demonstrated that such a study is feasible.[51]

Meta-analyses and Trial Ratings for Low Back Pain

Simply defined, meta-analyses are structured, systematic integrations of the results of different randomized clinical trials. Effect sizes are calculated from pooled results with a variety of statistical procedures. Sometimes, the findings of pooled trials are weighted according to the quality of each investigation's design.

This is borne out by the scoring mechanism illustrated in Table 10-4 taken from Anderson's meta-analyses addressed to the concept of spinal manipulation therapy in the treatment of low back pain. In Anderson's study of 23 randomized clinical trials, in most cases spinal manipulation therapy was compared to alternative therapies rather than true no-treatment placebos, thus obscuring the effectiveness of spinal adjustments. Even so, spinal manipulation therapy consistently proved more effective in the treatment of low back pain than any of the comparison treatments.[15]

Shekelle's meta-analysis, noteworthy in that it represents the first time a chiropractor (Adams) has authored an article in the *Annals of Internal Medicine*, retrieved 58 articles representing 25 trials and supported the short-term benefit of spinal manipulation in some patients, particularly those with uncomplicated, acute low back pain. Data at the time of this publication were judged insufficient to evaluate the efficacy of spinal manipulation for chronic low back pain.[16]

Figure 10–2 illustrates Koes's more recent ranking of 69 randomized clinical trials on low back pain. It vividly demonstrates both increasing frequencies and rising overall methodological scores over the past 30 years. For those trials involving chiropractic intervention, frequent strengths were adequate follow-up periods, avoidance of cointerventions, and avoidance of dropouts. Frequent weaknesses were found in randomization procedures, sample sizes, and blinded assessments of outcomes, the latter being virtually impossible to perform in a trial involving manual therapy.[52] In a meta-analysis of 51 literature reviews of spinal manipulation therapy, Assendelft recently concluded that, although the overall methodologic quality was low, 9 of the 10 methodologically best reviews reached positive conclusions regarding spinal adjustments.[53]

In summary, the vast preponderance of clinical trials, cohort studies, appropriateness assessments, literature reviews, and meta-analyses all conclude that spinal manipulation therapy is an effective treatment for low back pain, perhaps uniquely so.

Lumbar Disc Herniation Research

The options for treating disc herniations are surgery or conservative care, the latter often involving spinal manipulation. With no controlled trials directly comparing these two options, it is perhaps worth beginning this discussion with the statement by a leading orthopedic surgeon that, during his 30-year career, he never encountered a patient with a disc herniation that was aggravated by manipulation.[54] Single controlled trials exist in the literature for discetomy[55] and manipulation.[56]

The only randomized trial to date involving 51 cases of myelographically confirmed disk herniations compared rotational mobilization to conventional physical therapy (e.g., diathermy, exercise, and postural education). The manipulation group demonstrated greater improvement in range of motion and straight leg raising compared to the physical therapy cohort, leading Nwuga[56] to conclude that manipulation was superior to conventional treatment.

Further support for manipulation in the treatment of disc herniations is provided from several prospective studies.[57–61] The largest involved 517 patients diagnosed with lumbar disc protrusion, 77 percent of these having a favorable response from pain after manipulative therapy.[60] A literature review by Cassidy et al.[62] suggests that an additional 14 of 15 patients with lumbar disc herniations experienced significant relief from pain and clinical improvement after a 2- to 3-week course of side posture manipulation.

The safety of rotational manipulation in the treatment of lumbar disc herniations is supported in the literature review by Cassidy et al.,[62] which disputes the assertion by Farfan that rotational stress causes disc failure. This is because Farfan's work demonstrates that in rotation, normal discs with-

Table 10-4. Methodology Quality Coding Document for Meta-analysis

Study #

Discussion of Research Question/Hypothesis

____ (3) Yes

____ (0) No

Randomization Performed

____(12) Adequate randomization

____ (6) Partial—not adequately described

____ (0) Inadequate or no randomization

Analysis of Randomization Efficacy

____ (6) Adequate—table showing distribution of major prognostic factors

____ (3) Partial—reported successful but no data

____ (0) No information

Selection Description/Discussion of Inclusion/Exclusion Criteria

____(12) Adequate = reproducible (pt. source, inclusion/exclusion, diagnosis)

____ (6) Partial—2 of 3 above

____ (0) Inadequate—1 of 3 above

Patient Characteristics

____ (6) Standard reporting (e.g., age, sex) + other possible

____ (3) Standard

____ (0) Substandard (not even minimal characteristics)

Blinding of Patients

____(12) Yes

____ (6) Unsuccessful or results not stated

____ (0) No

Blinding of Evaluators

____(12) Yes (successful)

____ (6) Partial (blinding not rigorous or not completely successful)

____ (0) No

Description of Interventions

____(12) Adequate—clear/reproducible + definitions

____ (6) Partial—some description/not well defined

____ (0) Inadequate—broad description/no definition

Intervention Controls

____(12) No contamination/ideal control

____ (6) Some contamination (confounding variables) but minor

____ (0) Significant contamination/results in question

Discussion of TX Number, Frequency, Duration

____(12) Protocol + actual numbers for all

____ (9) Protocol + actual numbers for 2 of 3

____ (6) Protocol + actual numbers for 1 of 3

____ (3) Protocol only/no actual

____ (0) No actual/protocol insufficient to reproduce

Outcome Measures

____(12) Subjective + objective + other (e.g., MMPI)

____ (6) Subjective + objective

____ (3) Objective only

____ (0) Subjective only

Compliance

____ (6) Exact report of data

____ (3) Qualitative description

____ (0) Not mentioned

Discussion of Bias

____ (6) Yes

____ (0) No

Withdrawals

____ (6) Mentioned

____ (3) Mentioned, disregarded in analysis or unclear how they were handled

____ (0) Not mentioned

Discussion of Alpha/Beta Errors

____ (6) Yes (explicit)

____ (3) Brief mention of small sample size

____ (0) No

Total Score____

Denominator for percentage calculation will be based on only those questions applicable to paper evaluated. If all questions apply, then 135 points are possible.

From Anderson et al.,[15] with permission.

stand an average of 23 degrees and degenerated discs an average of 14 degrees before failure.[63] However, posterior facet joints limit rotation to only 2 to 3 degrees and would have to fracture to allow further rotation to occur,[64] and any disc failures produced experimentally by torsion are caused by peripheral tears in the annulus, rather than prolapse or herniation.[64]

NECK PAIN RESEARCH

The RAND Appropriateness Study: Manipulation and Mobilization of the Cervical Spine

As it had for the low back pain study, the RAND Corporation conducted both a literature review and a

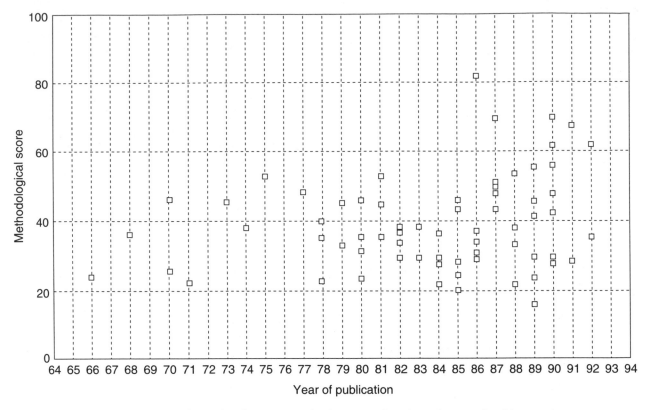

Figure 10-2. Relationship between methods score of trials and year of publication. (From Shekelle et al.,[51] with permission.)

multidisciplinary panel appropriateness study for cervical spine, headache, and upper extremity disorders. With regard to the cervical spine, the RAND literature review suggested that short-term pain relief and enhancement of the range of motion might be accomplished by manipulation or mobilization in the treatment of subacute or chronic neck pain; literature describing acute neck pain was regarded as extremely scanty (Table 10-5).

For subacute and chronic neck pain, the trial receiving the highest rating indicated that, for neck and back complaints together, improvements in severity of the main complaint were larger with manipulative therapy rather than physiotherapy; for neck complaints only, the mean improvement in the main complaint as shown by the Visual Analog Scale (VAS) was slightly better for manipulative rather than physical therapy.[65,66] Cassidy's trial, studying 100 subjects with unilateral neck pain with referral

into the trapezius, revealed that immediately after the intervention, 85 percent of the manipulated group and 69 percent of the mobilized group reported pain improvement. The decrease in pain intensity was more than 1.5 times greater in the manipulated group.[67] The literature regarding upper extremities, headache, and complications is referred to in the appropriate sections below.

As in the earlier low back study,[49] the appropriateness of chiropractic cervical spinal manipulation was assessed by an expert multidisciplinary panel, rating an array of more than 1,400 clinical scenarios for appropriateness of chiropractic intervention. In the final ratings, panelists rated 41 percent of all conditions as appropriate and 43 percent as inappropriate for chiropractic with disagreement on only two percent of all conditions. Unlike the previous low back pain study,[49] the frequency with which indications occurred in the patient population was unknown.[68,69]

Table 10-5. RAND Cervical Spine Appropriateness Study: Summary of Literature Review

Anatomical Complaint	Published Research	Overall Conclusions
Acute neck pain	0 RCTs	Limited mobilization literature published:
	0 case series	May be useful; cf rest/cervical collar
		Exercise instruction may be useful
Subacute/chronic neck pain	5 RCTs manipulation/ 1 RCT mobilization	Short-term pain relief?
	7 additional studies	Range of motion enhancement?
Muscle tension headache	4 RCTs manipulation/ 1 RCT mobilization	Short-term relief likely
	9 additional studies	
Migraine headache	1 RCT	Literature too limited
	5 additional studies	
Shoulder/arm/hand pain	1 RCT	Literature too limited
Thoracic, outlet syndrome/ carpal tunnel syndrome/ temporomandibular joint	2 case series	
disorders	0 RCTs	Clinical improvement?
	Isolated case reports	

Abbreviation: RCT, randomized clinical trial. (From Kirkaldy-Willis and Cassidy,[54] with permission.)

Whiplash Research

The problem facing both diagnosticians and patients with whiplash is that most moderate to severe cases are invisible upon standard medical examination.[25] As elusive as the "smoking gun" might be in evaluating this condition, it involves a broader array of soft tissue, neurologic, and temporomandibular joint problems than presumed only a decade ago.[25] In Quebec alone, the fact that whiplash in 1989 accounted for 20 percent of all traffic injury insurance claims with an average compensation period of 108 days[70,71] led a multidisciplinary task force to conclude that neck pain is to the automobile what low back pain is to the workplace.[26]

The elusiveness of a definitive, reproducible pathology for whiplash-associated disorders has often led the legal and insurance communities as well as the medical to erroneously conclude that there is no physical or organic basis for the symptoms of whiplash-associated disorders. This has produced charges of malingering or litigation neurosis on the part of the patient, leading to the overlaying of psychosocial factors which have only compounded the problem. An excellent index of increased scien-

tific and societal concern about whiplash is the fact that Foreman and Croft, in the 1995 revision of their 1988 text on whiplash-associated disorders have increased the number of references cited from 600 to more than 1,250.[25]

Also known as cervical acceleration/deceleration syndrome,[25] whiplash has often been misunderstood as having the spontaneous recovery rate of 90 percent often associated with back pain victims.[2] In a review of the literature, Bannister and Gargan[72] document recoveries from cervical injury cited in 12 published studies ranging from 12 percent to 86 percent, averaging 57 percent. Stabilization or resolution of pain occurs with an unweighted average of 7.3 months.[72] Even more dramatic evidence is provided in Croft's review of 15 additional studies, in which he documents the persistence of symptoms following whiplash-associated disorders injuries for periods exceeding 18 years.[73]

From a morphologic point of view, immobilization of the neck following the soft tissue trauma that accompanies whiplash-associated disorders is indefensible. Severe soft tissue injury (rupture of muscles, joint capsules, and synovial folds) can be expected around the cervical spines of accident victims.[74] Consequently, scar formation, cross-linking of collagen fibers, and adhesions can develop in traumatized soft tissues not rehabilitated soon after injury. Specifically:

1. Healing without proper motion will cause a disorganized matrix to appear, with adhesions and unnecessary scar formation.[75,76]
2. Early exercise and joint motion in rehabilitation produces a better collagen concentration, which is superior to scar tissue.[77]
3. Improved tensile strength is observed in the collagen deposit when proper rehabilitation takes place after injury.[78,79]
4. If venous blood supply to paraspinal muscles is depressed for two hours (which might be anticipated in some soft tissue injuries), irreversible muscle damage occurs.[80] With decreased vascularization, rapid degeneration of the muscle spindles occurs with subsequent revascularization changing their shape and neural innervation.[81]

Regarding manual therapy in the management of whiplash patients, two substantial studies have been reported in the literature. One demonstrated that, in subjects displaying significant cervical lateral flexion passive end-range asymmetries and who have a history of neck trauma and frequent episodic neck stiffness, a single unilateral lower cervical adjustment delivered to the side of most restricted end range of motion is capable of reducing the magnitude of asymmetry, but only transiently (for periods less than 48 hours).[82] The Cassidy study on neck pain described earlier likewise produced at least short-term increases of neck ranges of motion for patients presenting with unilateral neck pain with referral into the trapezius muscle, after these individuals were subjected to either manipulation or mobilization. The decrease in pain intensity was more than 1.5 times greater in only the manipulated group.[67]

The abundance of literature on the etiology, diagnosis, treatment, and sociology of whiplash led the Quebec Task Force to collect 10,382 titles and abstracts, of which 1204 met the criteria for preliminary screening before 294 (0.03 percent of the initial sample) were ultimately rated; 21 percent of the latter (0.006 percent of the initial sample) were ultimately accepted.[26] Of the 10 randomized controlled trials pertaining to whiplash-associated disorders that were accepted by the Quebec Task Force only one, Cassidy's,[67] addressed spinal manipulation.

The conclusions of the Quebec Task Force can be summed up as follows[26]

1. New classification of whiplash-associated disorders: These disorders were classified on two scales. The first, based on clinical presentation specified five grades based on the presence of musculoskeletal signs (decreased range of motion and point tenderness), neurologic signs (decreased or absent deep tendon reflexes, weakness, and sensory deficits), or fracture/dislocation. The second scale specified five grades based on the duration of the injury, ranging from 4 days to more than 6 months.
2. Management advice and algorithm: Even though mobilization and manipulation are distinguished from each other, they were both classified as active treatments. In the precise language of the Task Force, the "consensus is that manipulation treatments by trained persons for the relief of pain and facilitating early mobility can be used in whiplash associated disorders. All such treatments should ... discourage extended dependence upon the health professional ... Long-term, repeated manipulation without multidisciplinary evaluation is not justified."
3. Directives for education and research: In defining the skills and knowledge need for the effective management of whiplash-associated-disorder patients, the Quebec Task Force concluded that the primary practitioner involved "must possess the qualities of a clinical anatomist," as well as possessing a fundamental knowledge of rehabilitation of the musculoskeletal system in addition to clinical epidemiology. Research was found to be extremely scanty, with therapeutic interventions requiring immediate further investigation including manipulation and specific physiotherapeutic methods. The Task Force praised the research both David Cassidy in Saskatchewan and Ake Nygren in Sweden as ideals for international, interdisciplinary research.

The work of the Quebec Task Force has not gone uncriticized. Croft[83] raises several objections to the Task Force Guidelines, including the following:

1. Near total elimination of relevant literature: The fact that 99.994 percent of all articles were eliminated before consideration raises a strong possibility that instructive as well as useless data were discarded.
2. Arbitrary recommendations: In the resulting absence of literature to consider, the Task Force gave its own opinion equal weight with primary research data, lending a misleading sense of robustness to its recommendations.
3. Propagation of the myth that most patients with whiplash-associated disorders recover in 6 to 12 weeks: Upon closer examination, this time course has no basis in primary research; in fact, considerable data already cited contradicts this impression and paints a far bleaker picture.[72–81]
4. The undertaking was sponsored by an insurance industry: Societe d'assurance automobile du Quebec (SAAQ) as the supporting organization of the entire project would be expected to have an "obvious and serious" interest in its outcome, possibly compromising the objectivity of the literature research, evaluation, and ultimate recommendations of the Task Force.

Clearly, there is a major need for more data from both clinical trials and case series addressed to this very complex and elusive condition. One encouraging note is that Cassidy's group is conducting a 5-year study addressed to both the incidence and management of whiplash injuries, including controlled trials to assess both the clinical and cost-effectiveness of chiropractic and other interventions.[84]

HEADACHE RESEARCH

The treatment of headaches with spinal manipulation has generated a proliferation of research designs in the peer-reviewed literature (Table 10-6). At least six randomized clinical trials examining the effects of spinal adjustment upon various types of headaches have been published.[85–90] Still others, including a migraine study[91] that compares the outcomes of chiropractic and medical management, are in progress at medical or research centers around the world. The pilot for yet another randomized trial appeared in the literature in 1994.[92]

Published studies have generally classified headaches into three major groups, as recommended by the International Headache Society.[93]

Tension Headache

The most dramatic of the trials pertaining to tension headaches[85] was published in 1995. A group of 70 patients who received chiropractic care over a 6-week period showed parity with a cohort of 56 patients who were administered amitriptyline (a leading medical intervention for headache treatment) over the same period, in terms of four primary outcome measures (headache frequency, total headache pain, over-the-counter medication use, and global health). Most significantly, during the 4-week follow-up period, these same four outcome measures showed a statistically and clinically significant difference in the patient groups favoring spinal manipulation. Essentially, the chiropractic patients sustained the improvements achieved during the treatment phase, while the headaches of those treated medically returned when the medication was withdrawn.

This prolonged endurance of positive outcome measures seen with chiropractic patients compared to medically treated ones is reminiscent of the randomized trials pertaining to low back pain, where the superior effects of chiropractic intervention were apparent for up to 3 years following treatment, as discussed earlier.[38] The superior effects of chiropractic management in the treatment of tension headaches is supported by two other randomized controlled trials,[86,87] although sample sizes were smaller so as to blunt the statistical analyses. In addition, a case series analysis demonstrated headache frequency decreasing from 6.4 episodes to 3.1 episodes/week with an accompanying drop in duration from 6.7 hours to 3.9 hours/episode.[92] Finally, an earlier retrospective series of 332 patients examined by Droz likewise indicated a positive response to spinal adjustment.[95]

Cervicogenic Headache

Studies pertaining to cervicogenic headache are equally compelling. The results of a 1995 randomized controlled trial suggest that chiropractic treatment produces a consistent reduction in the use of analgesics, headache intensity, and number of

Table 10-6. Headache Outcomes Research Employing Spinal Manipulation

Headache Type	Investigator	No. of pts	Arms	Outcomes	Design
Tension[85]	Boline	126	SMT Amiltriptyline	Frequency Total pain OTC Global health	RCT
Tension[86]	Bitterli		SMT No treatment		RCT
Tension[87]	Hoyt	22	Palpation Palpation + SMT No treatment	Intensity EMG	RCT
Cervicogenic[88]	Nilsson	40	SMT Laser/massage	Analgesic use Frequency Intensity	RCT
Migraine[89]	Parker	85	Mobilization SMT by DC SMT by MD	Frequency Intensity Duration	RCT
Postraumatic[90]	Jensen	19	SMT Cold packs	Pain index Range of motion Adj symptoms	RCT
Migraine[91]	Nelson	209	SMT Amiltriptyline SMT + Amiltriptyline	Frequency Intensity OTC use Functional capacity	RCT
Cervicogenic[92]	Whittingham	26	SMT Toggle	Analgesic use Frequency Intensity	Pilot CS
Tension[94]	Mootz	11	SMT/Packs/TP	Frequency Intensity Duration	CS
Tension[95]	Droz	332	SMT	Pain	R
Cervicogenic[96]	Vernon	33	SMT	Frequency Intensity Duration	PS
Migraine[97]	Wight	87	SMT	Pain	CS
Cervical migraine[98]	Stodolny	31	SMT	Pain Range of Motion Dizziness	PS
Chronic[99]	Turk	100	SMT	Analgesic use	PS

Abbreviations: CS, case study; DC, doctor of chiropractic; EMG, electromyography; MD, medical doctor; OTC, over the counter; PS, prospective series; RS, retrospective study; RCT, randomized clinical trial; SMT, spinal manipulation therapy.

headaches per day in the chiropractic group, but not in a control group receiving massage and low-level laser treatment.[88] Elsewhere, a consecutive time series showed in a group of 26 patients receiving chiropractic manipulation that several headache scores improved dramatically. Specifically, headache duration was reduced to 23 percent of its original value, headache intensity diminished to 40 percent of its original value, and headache frequency dropped to 39 percent of what it had been preceding treatment.[92] These results represent a confirmation of Howard Vernon's prospective and retrospective findings of 14 years ago, also demonstrating a decrease of frequency, duration, and severity of cervicogenic headaches following spinal manipulation.[96]

Migraines and Unclassified Headaches

Three studies relating to migraine headache also suggest a positive response to chiropractic spinal adjustments, as demonstrated by reductions of frequency, intensity, and duration[89] or of pain,[97,98] motion restriction, or dizziness.[98] Studies of unclassified headache responses to manipulation are also shown in Table 10-6. In an examination of 100 patients with chronic headaches treated by manipulation, Turk and Ratkolb[99] demonstrated an absence of headaches in 25 percent and an improvement in 40 percent of the patients 6 months after completing treatment. The remaining 35 percent reported improvement which lasted for approximately 1 month. Comparing cold packs with mobilization, Jensen showed a reduction of post-traumatic headache pain by 43 percent in the manual therapy population compared to the cold therapy group at 2 weeks following treatment.[90]

Vernon[100,101] has also recently provided comprehensive overviews of the effectiveness of chiropractic intervention in the management of headache.

CARPAL TUNNEL SYNDROME RESEARCH

Compression of the median nerve in the vicinity of the wrist may lead to unilateral or bilateral paresthesia in the fingers, with or without pain in the wrist, palm, and/or forearm proximal to the area of compression. This condition, known as carpal tunnel syndrome (CTS), presents a variety of symptoms and is commonly confused with tendinitis. One of its major causes is the protracted strain on an extended or flexed wrist caused by repetitive stress, often found in the workplace and therefore having the potential to affect a significant population.

The rationale for manipulation is to take pressure off the transverse carpal ligament and add adjustments of the lunate to help decompress the tunnel. This represents a departure from traditional spinal adjustment; in its application to the extremities instead, it provides a conservative, noninvasive alternative to surgery.[102]

Case control studies supporting chiropractic intervention in the management of this condition suggest that, in 38 subjects, an array of dietary, exercise, and manipulative interventions result in statistically significant improvements in several

strength measures of up to 25 percent over pretreatment values[103]; also, improved objective, pain, and distress measures were observed in 22 returning subjects to persist for at least six months post-treatment.[104]

A single randomized control trial of 23 patients comparing traditional conservative therapy to traditional conservative therapy plus osteopathic manipulation showed that, in the latter group, electromyography and nerve conduction studies as well as pain improved dramatically as compared to the former cohort of patients. Crossovers into the osteopathic manipulation therapy group likewise displayed the same improvements following the application of osteopathic manipulation therapy.[105]

Osteopathic manipulation has also been shown to be effective in two case series studies by Benjamin Sucher. The first, involving four patients with CTS, showed both clinical improvement and changes in MRI where the anteroposterior and transverse dimensions of the carpal canal increased significantly after treatment. Electromyography and nerve conduction study measurements documented improvement consistent with the clinical recovery.[106] Both clinical and electrical improvement were subsequently observed in a larger group of 16 patients with CTS.[107]

A full-scale clinical trial[108] is currently underway that seeks to more rigorously assess the effect of chiropractic extremity adjusting upon CTS. At least 45 subjects will receive either conservative medical treatment, consisting of NSAIDs plus 24-hour wrist bracing, or chiropractic treatment, including manipulation, ultrasound, and 24-hour wrist bracing. Evaluations are scheduled immediately before, during, and after the 9-week treatment period.

Research on CTS is still in its preliminary stages. However, because CTS occurs on an epidemic scale in the workplace (see Ch. 18), with more than 2.6 million adults in the United States self-reporting this condition in 1988,[109] CTS is a significant problem of potential importance to the chiropractor as well as to the osteopath.

SAFETY

As with any therapeutic intervention, contraindications exist for chiropractic, however rare. Two primary complications have been reported:

- *Cauda equina syndrome:* following manipulation in patients with lumbar disc herniation, consisting of neurogenic bowel and bladder disturbances, saddle anesthesia, bilateral leg weakness, and sensory changes.
- *Cerebrovascular accidents (CVAs):* as a result of cervical manipulations. The research accompanying each of these conditions is reviewed briefly below (for a more extensive discussion, see Ch. 14).

The symptoms of cauda equina syndrome have been extensively described[110,111]; a review of the world's medical literature indicates that 16 of the 26 reported cases of manipulation-related cauda equina syndrome occurred with the far more vigorous manipulation applied under anesthesia. Of the remaining 10 cases, only 4 have been reported in North America.[112] Estimates of the frequency of cauda equina syndrome range from 2 per million[113] to 1 per 12 million adjustments.[114]

As established by researchers from both the medical and chiropractic professions, the risk of cerebrovascular accidents is as low as one case per million treatments,[114] ranging upwards to 2 to 4 per million.[115,116] The more recent data from the RAND Corporation suggests the rate of vertebrobasilar accident or other complications (e.g., cord compression, fracture, or hematoma) to be 1.46 per million manipulations, with the rates of serious complications and death from cervical spine manipulation estimated to be 0.64 and 0.27 per million manipulations, respectively.[68]

The mechanism of CVAs involves the vertebral and carotid arteries in the upper cervical spine. Following cervical manipulation, the most common site of injury to the vertebral arterial system appears to be in the vicinity of the atlanto-occipital joint, where the vertical artery bends into a horizontal configuration.[117] Brain stem ischemia is produced by trauma to the arterial wall, producing either vasospasm or damage to the arterial wall itself. Vasospasm may trigger a cascade of events leading to fibrin deposition and resulting thrombus formation; injuries to the arterial wall could involve tearing, dissection, or branch occlusion.[118] Because stretching, shearing, or crushing are the forces leading to these arterial problems, they are suspected to be the main culprits

generating CVAs produced under certain circumstances involving the rotation and/or extension of the head. Any head movement that produces occlusion of a vertebral artery in cases where the flow in the contralateral artery is already compromised has the potential to lead to a CVA.

In his exhaustive report, Terrett[118] concluded that "until more reliable screening procedures are developed, the chiropractic profession should lead the field of manual medicine by abandoning those techniques which appear to carry the greatest risk." Since it is in the rotated position that the greatest stress to the vertebral artery is imparted, thrusting maneuvers on the cervical spine to produce yet more axial rotation might appear to carry additional risk, as they further stretch the vertebral artery. Indeed, sustained rotation at 45 degrees or 90 degrees influences blood velocity in the extracranial vessels, which may have relevance in patients with abnormal blood flow who are candidates for cervical manipulation.[119] However, a more recent analysis of four patients by magnetic resonance angiography showed that no stenosis or extrinsic compression of the basovertebral system was noted prior to or following 45-degree right rotation with 10-degree hyperextension.[120]

COST-EFFECTIVENESS

An integral part of evaluating the future of any health care modality is its cost. In this regard, chiropractic has been found to be distinctly advantageous in the treatment of musculoskeletal disorders. In comparing patients matched for severity, the research of Stano is perhaps the most elegantly designed.[121]

The purpose of Stano's most recent study is to compare health insurance payments for patient episodes of care for common lumbar and low back conditions initiated by either chiropractic or medical treatment. This complements a preponderance of studies derived from worker's compensation data[17,121–124] and a nationwide longitudinal survey of medical care usage and costs for 6,000 randomly selected households[125] as well as Stano's earlier paper based on health insurance data.[126] Most reports conclude that costs associated with both treatment and lost time from work for medical patients are strikingly higher than those for the patients of chiropractors.

In contrast, are two recent studies which come to the opposite conclusion, suggesting that chiropractic services are more, rather than less, expensive than medical treatments for back conditions. Both studies appeared recently in prominent medical journals[127,128] attracting the attention of third-party payors faced with the prospect of including chiropractic services in managed care plans. However, these two studies are fraught with weaknesses that have been addressed in detail[129]:

1. The effects of severity of illness are virtually ignored.
2. The degree of recovery does not receive adequate attention.
3. Matching of services with provider type may be irregular.
4. Compliance has been disregarded.
5. Types of medication and their side effects are not specified.
6. The calculation of charges is neither precise nor balanced among provider types.
7. Episodes are poorly defined or contained.

Common weaknesses in other cost analyses have also been discussed in the literature.[125]

The key conceptual breakthrough in Stano's recent report is the "bundling" of episodes (e.g., the more careful inclusion of all relevant treatment costs truly associated with either the medical or the chiropractic care of patients). This is accomplished by first assigning one or more of nine commonly used International Classification of Disease (ICD) codes to those patients initially complaining of such conditions, out of a cohort of 43,476 patients whose insurance claims information was kept on file in a primary database developed by MEDSTAT Systems, Inc. These conditions, called *trigger codes*, launch an episode of care judged to be terminated if a disease-free period (called a "clean window") exceeds the number of days that elapsed between the last treatment and the next one. The importance of correctly identifying these episodes and distinguishing them from recurring conditions cannot be overstated, as it has led to the downfall of previous studies that have achieved prominence.[127,128]

In addition to identifying the first-contact (initiating) provider, Stano's program tracked various categories of total inpatient and outpatient payments over each episode. It showed a distinct advantage over other studies[127,128] by factoring in key patient demographic and insurance characteristics, as well as case-mix severity differences missing from the previous work[127,128] and that have been cited as key components that should have been included.[129] Finally, it should be recognized that Stano has used a huge database. He has randomly sampled from a database of 434,763 patients and run his actual cost comparison for the nine ICD codes identified in a total of 6,799 patients.

Stano's conclusions are straightforward and dramatic. When all episodes of care are considered, the mean total costs are $1,000 for each medical episode and $493 per chiropractic episode, yielding a statistically significant difference at the one percent level of confidence. Differences in the same direction and of similar statistical significance are obtained if (1) 1-day as well as total, and (2) outpatient as well as inpatient episodes, are compared. For example, outpatient costs across all conditions combined are $554 per medical and $425 per chiropractic episode. Outpatient costs are lower for most of the nine categories of episodes initiated by chiropractors and substantially lower for some conditions. For intervertebral disc disorders, for instance, outpatient costs for chiropractic services are anywhere from 49–64 percent of those charged by medical practitioners treating the same conditions.

Two serendipitous observations are worth noting in this study. First, Stano observed that over a third of all patients in the nine ICD codes sampled initiated their care with chiropractors, indicating that chiropractors as a first-contact resource by patients with neuromusculoskeletal conditions cannot be ignored by third-party managers of health care. Secondly, the length of care provided by chiropractors was greater than that offered by medical physicians, even though the chiropractors' costs were lower. The latter observation has major implications regarding the role of chiropractors in offering primary care in a patient-centered paradigm.[130]

A minor limitation of Stano's study is that the database used was capable of providing only limited categorical values for each patient's coinsurance and deductible expenses. Therefore, the study could not provide precise values for these variables, although there is no obvious evidence to suggest that its results were biased in the comparison of expenses across the two provider groups. In other studies involving worker's compensation, the cost advantages of chiropractic are dramatically shown by the results in Table 10-7.[17,123-124,131-137] From the perspective of number of days lost from work, cost from compensation, and cost of health care expenses, the beneficial economic impact of chiropractic intervention for low back pain is plainly evident from most instances.

FUTURE PERSPECTIVES

The clinical efficacy and cost-effectiveness of chiropractic management of musculoskeletal conditions make it clear why the recognition extended to this modality by the United States government[2] was granted. Similar endorsement was given to spinal manipulation for the treatment of back pain by the British government.[138] Major documents that reviewed and summarized this research not only served as steppingstones toward this recognition[139,140] but also served as practice guidelines[140] unequaled in other health care professions.

One cannot conclude this review of musculoskeletal research without citing the muscular elements that have recently been identified as links to other body tissues. A connective tissue bridge has now been identified between the rectus capitus posterior minor muscle and the dorsal spinal dura at the atlanto-occipital junction.[141] With muscles of this nature thus having been shown to directly influence the dura mater (a pain-sensitive structure), alternative mechanisms may be proposed for the pain generation of cervical headaches.[142] Similarly, the tensor veli palatini muscle has been shown to control the eustachian tube and would thus be implicated in the causation of otitis media infections where middle ear fluid fails to drain properly.[143-145] Both muscles regulating eustachian tube and upper neck function, the malfunction of which directly leads to ear infections or headache, are innervated by the trigeminal nerve.[142] Thus, one could easily visualize how aberrant neuromuscular activity could directly lead to malfunctions in several areas of the body in addition to the back. The implications of these findings for chiropractic health management cannot be overstated.

The conduct and outcomes of contemporary musculoskeletal disorders research have the poten-

tial not only to midwife an emergent paradigm for the future of chiropractic manipulation, but to contribute as well to the evolution of the broader health care field. Only from blending the incremental results from many different types of research conducted by investigators with a variety of backgrounds will the needs of present and future patients truly be served.

Terminology

whiplash
alternative therapy
acute/subacute/chronic
tension headache
cervicogenic headache
migraine headache
meta-analysis

Review Questions

1. What were the major events in chiropractic research prior to 1950?

2. What is the significance of the 1975 Conference on Research sponsored by the National Institute of Neurological Diseases and Stroke?

3. What is the difference between a clinical trial and a prospective study?

4. What is the difference between the appropriateness and utilization portions of the recent study on back pain by the RAND Corporation?

5. What were the strengths and weaknesses of the 69 randomized clinical trials involving a chiropractic component cited by Koes?

6. What were the accomplishments of the Quebec Task Force, and what were its weaknesses as discussed by Croft?

7. Why is disc herniation unlikely to be caused by rotational manipulation?

8. From a morphologic point of view, immobilization of the neck following soft tissue trauma accompanying whiplash-associated disorders is indefensible. Why?

9. What is the incidence of CVAs, and what is their mechanism?

10. Name at least 3 major classes of headache as defined by the International Headache Society.

Table 10-7. Cost Comparison Analysis: Chiropractic Versus Medical Care

	1991 Utah[17]	1991 Oregon[131–133]	1989 Iowa[134]	1988 Florida[123]	1983 West Virginia[135]	1980 Oregon[136]	1977 Wisconsin[137]
Similar diagnoses in patient populations	ICD9-Codes back only	Categories of injury, back only	Strain/sprain, back only	DRG/Medical back diagnoses	Strain/sprain 2/3 cases, others not matched, back/neck	Strain/sprain, non-acute, non-surgical, back only	Strain/sprain, back only
Number of days lost from work (compensation time)	2.4—DC 20.7—MD	Not available	11.76—DC 14.08—MD	39—DC 58—MD	57.8—DC 38.8—MD	18.8—DC 41.6—MD	13.2—DC 21.8—MD
Cost from compensation	$68.38—DC $688.39—MD	Not available	$263.00—DC $617.00—MD	Not available	$1,887—DC $1,100—MD	$276.00—DC $699.00—MD	$285.00—DC $442.00—MD
Cost of health care expenses	$526.80—DC $684.15—MD	$1,712—DC $1,112—MD	$222.70—DC $351.90—MD	$1,204—DC $2,352—MD	$1,275—DC $610—includes surgery—MD	$181.00—DC $327.00—MD	$145.00—DC $267.00—MD
Cost per visit	$40—DC $133—MD	$41.70—DC $111.20—MD	Not available	Not available	Not available	$9.36—DC $12.39—MD	$9.36—DC $12.90—M.D.
Number of visits	12.9—DC 4.9—MD	41—DC 10—MD	Not available	Not available	Not available	11.8—DC 10.7—MD	14.1—D.C 18.3—M.D.
Length of treatment	34.3 days—DC 54.5 days—MD	53 weeks—DC 19 weeks—MD	Not available	Not available	Not available	53.24 days—DC 97.3 days—MD	14.1 days—DC 18.3 days—MD
Previous history of injury	Not available	2,184 patients w/ previous injury—DC 1,224 w/ previous injury—MD	Not available	Not available	Not available	13.6 more days compensation with injury—DC 36 more days of compensation time with previous injury—MD	Not available
Additional risk factors	Older—DC population	More chronic obese females, more extremity diagnosis and multiple diagnosis—DC	Not available	Not available	Multiple diagnosis, more chronic patients—DC	Age 39—DC Age 36—MD	Not available
Gender differences	Equal distribution	Females considered as more chronic patients More female patients—DC	$192/female—DC $1,756/female—MD	Not available	Not available	10% female—DC	Not available

181

Concept Questions

1. What are the limitations of the randomized clinical trial, and what types of research offer data that helps to answer these deficiencies?

2. Discuss the weaknesses of the two studies cited which suggest that chiropractic interventions are more, rather than less, expensive for medical treatments for back conditions.

References

1. Goldstein M (ed): Monograph No. 15. The research status of spinal manipulation, U.S. Department of Health, Education, and Welfare, Washington, DC, 1975

2. Bigos S, Bowyer O, Braen G et al: Acute low back pain in adults. Clinical practice guideline No. 14. AHCPR Publ No. 95-0642. Agency for Health Care Policy and Research, Public Health Service, U.S. Department of Health and Human Services, Rockville, MD, 1994

3. Bergquist-Ullman M, Larsson U: Acute low back pain in industry. A controlled prospective study with special reference to therapy and confounding factors. Acta Orthop Scand 170:1, 1977

4. Postacchini F, Facchini M, Palier P: Efficacy of various forms of conservative treatment in low back pain. A comparative study. Neuroorthopedics 6:28, 1988

5. Brodin H: Inhibition-facilitation technique for lumbar pain treatment. Int J Rehabil Res 7:328, 1984

6. Coxhead CE, Meade TW, Inskip H, North WRS, Troup JDG: Multicentre trial of physiotherapy in the management of sciatic symptoms. Lancet 8229:1065, 1981

7. Farrell JP, Twomey LT: Acute low back pain. Comparison of two conservative treatment approaches. Med J Aust 1:160, 1982

8. Gibson T, Grahmam R, Harkness J, Woo P, Blagrave P, Hills R: Controlled comparison of short-wave diathermy treatment with osteopathic treatment in nonspecific low back pain. Lancet 8440:1258, 1985

9. Glover JR, Morris JG, Khosla T: Back pain: a randomized clinical trial of rotational manipulation of the trunk. Br J Ind Med Jan 31:59, 1974

10. Godfrey CM, Morgan PP, Schatzker J: A randomized trial of manipulation for low back pain in a medical setting. Spine 9:301, 1984

11. Hadler NM, Curtis P, Gillings DB, Stinnett S: A benefit of spinal manipulation as adjunctive therapy for acute low-back pain: a stratified controlled trial. Spine 12:703, 1987

12. MacDonald RS, Bell CM: An open controlled assessment of osteopathic manipulation in nonspecific low-back pain. Spine 15:364, 1990 [published erratum appears in Spine 16:104, 1991]

13. Matthews JA, Mills SB, Jenkins VM et al: Back pain and sciatica: controlled trials of manipulation, traction, sclerosant and epidural injections. Br J Rheumatol 26:416, 1987

14. Waterworth RF, Hunter IA: An open study of diflunisol, conservative and manipulative therapy in the management of acute mechanical low back pain. NZ Med J 98:372, 1985

15. Anderson R, Meeker WC, Wirick BE et al: A meta-analysis of clinical trials of spinal manipulation. J Manipul Physiol Ther 15:181, 1992

16. Shekelle PG, Adams AH, Chassin MR, Hurwitz EL, Brook RH: Spinal manipulation for low-back pain. Ann Intern Med 117:590, 1992

17. Jarvis KB, Phillips RB, Morris EK: Cost per case comparison of back injury claims of chiropractic versus medical management for conditions with identical diagnostic codes. J Occup Med 33:847, 1991

18. Wardwell WI: Chiropractic: History and Evolution of a New Profession. Mosby–Year Book, St. Louis, 1992

19. Bernard C: An Introduction to the Study of Experimental Medicine. Translated by H.C. Greene. Macmillan, New York, 1927

20. Fishbein M: The Medical Follies. Boni and Liveright, New York, 1925

21. Canterbury R, Krakos G: Thirteen years after Roentgen: the originals of chiropractic radiology. Chiro Hist 6:25, 1986

22. Dye AA: The Evolution of Chiropractic: Its Discovery and Development. Author, Philadelphia, 1939

23. Thompson EA: Text on chiropractic spinography. Palmer School of Chiropractic, Davenport, IA, 1919

24. Crowe HE: Injuries to the cervical spine. Presented at the Western Orthopedic Association, San Francisco, 1928

25. Foreman SM, Croft AC: Whiplash Injuries: The Cervical Acceleration/Deceleration Syndrome. 2nd Ed. Williams & Wilkins, Baltimore, 1995

26. Spitzer WO, Skovron ML, Salmi LR et al: Scientific Monograph of the Quebec Taskforce on Whiplash

Associated Disorders: Refining "whiplash" and its management. Spine 20:1S, 1995

27. Illi FWH: The vertebral column, life line of the body. National College of Chiropractic, Chicago, 1951

28. Smith OG, Langworthy SM, Paxon M: Modernized chiropractic. Solon M. Langworthy, Cedar Rapids, IA, 1906

29. Gillet H: Clinical measurements of sacro-iliac mobility. Ann Swiss Chiro Assoc 6:9, 1976

30. Gillet H: Spinal and related fixations. Dig Chiro Econ; summary lesson 1:25, lesson 2:22, lesson 3:26, 1964

31. Goldstein M: Foreword. p. xi. In Korr IM (ed): The Neurobiologic Mechanisms in Manipulative Therapy. Plenum, New York, 1978

32. Report of the U.S. Preventive Services Task Force. Williams & Wilkins, Baltimore, 1989

33. Jayson MIV: A limited role for manipulation. BMJ 293:1454, 1986

34. Chapman-Smith D: Manipulation for chronic back pain: strong new evidence of long-term results. Chiro Rep 6:1, 1992

35. Bronfort G: Chiropractic treatment of low back pain. A prospective survey. J Manipul Physiol Ther 9:99, 1986

36. Kirkaldy-Willis WH, Cassidy JD: Spinal manipulation in the treatment of low back pain. Can Fam Phys 31:535, 1985

37. Meade TW, Dyer S, Browne W et al: Low back pain of mechanical origin: randomised comparison of chiropractic and hospital outpatient treatment. BMJ 300:1431, 1990

38. Meade TW, Dyer S, Browne W et al: Randomised comparison of chiropractic and hospital outpatient management for low back pain: results from extended follow-up. BMJ 11:349, 1995

39. Koes BW, Bouter LM, van Mameren H et al: The effectiveness of manual therapy, physiotherapy, and treatment by the general practitioner for nonspecific neck and back complaints: A randomized clinical trial. Spine 17:28, 1992

40. Pope MH, Phillips RB, Haugh LD et al: A prospective randomized three-week trial of spinal manipulation, transcutaneous muscle stimulation, massage and corset in the treatment of subacute low back pain. Spine 19:2571, 1994

41. Blomberg S, Svarsudd K, Mildenberger F: A controlled multicentre trial of manual therapy in low back pain: initial status, sick leave and pain score during follow-up. Orthop Med 16:1, 1994

42. Triano J, McGregor M, Hondras MA, Brennan PC: Manipulative therapy versus education programs in chronic low back pain. Spine 20:948, 1995

43. Waagen GN, Haldeman S, Cook G et al: Short-term trial of chiropractic adjustments for the relief of chronic low back pain. Manual Med 2:63, 1986

44. Farrel JP, Twomey LT: Acute low back pain: comparisons of two conservative treatment approaches. Med J Aust 1:160, 1982

45. Hadler NM, Curtis P, Gillings DB: A benefit of spinal manipulation as adjunctive therapy for low back pain: a stratified controlled trial. Spine 12:703, 1987

46. Hoehler FK, Tobis JS, Buerger AA: Spinal manipulation for low back pain. JAMA 245:1835, 1981

47. Glover JR: Back pain: a randomized clinical trial of rotation manipulation of the trunk. Br J Ind Med 31:59, 1974

48. Shekelle PG, Adams AH, Chassin MR et al: The appropriateness of spinal manipulation for low back pain: Project overview and literature review. Monograph No. R-4025/1-CCR/FCER. RAND: Santa Monica, CA, 1991

49. Shekelle PG, Adams AH, Chassin MR et al: The appropriateness of spinal manipulation for low back pain: indications and ratings by a multidisciplinary expert panel. Monograph No. R-4025/2-CCR/FCER. RAND: Santa Monica, CA, 1991

50. Shekelle PG, Adams AH, Chassin MR et al: The appropriateness of spinal manipulation for low back pain: indications and ratings by an all-chiropractic expert panel. Monograph No. R-4025/3-CCR/FCER. RAND: Santa Monica, CA, 1992

51. Shekelle PG, Hurwitz EL, Coulter I et al: The appropriateness of chiropractic spinal manipulation for low back pain: a pilot study. J Manipul Physiol Ther 18:265, 1995

52. Koes BW, Bouter LM, van der Heijden GJMG: Methodological quality of randomized clinical trials on treatment efficacy in low back pain. Spine 20:228, 1995

53. Assendelft WJJ, Koes BW, Knipschild PG, Bouter LM: The relationship between methodological quality and conclusions in reviews of spinal manipulation. JAMA 274:1942, 1995

54. Kirkaldy-Willis WH, Cassidy JD: Manipulation. p. 287. In Kirkaldy-Willis WH (eds): Managing Low Back Pain. Churchill Livingstone, New York, 1988

55. Weber H: Lumber disc herniation. A controlled prospective study with 10 years of observation. Spine 8:131, 1983

56. Nwuga VCB: Relative therapeutic efficacy of vertebral manipulation and conventional treatment in back pain management. Am J Phys Med 61:273, 1982

57. Henderson RS: The treatment of lumbar disk intervertebral disk protrusion: an assessment of conservative measures. BMJ 2:597, 1952

58. Mensor MC: Non-operative treatment, including manipulation, for lumbar intervertebral disc syndrome. J Bone Joint Surg 37A:925, 1955

59. Chrisman OD: A study of the results following rotary manipulation in the lumbar intervertebral disc syndrome. J Bone Joint Surg 46A:517, 1964

60. Kuo PP-F, Loh Z-C: Treatment of lumbar intervertebral disc protrusions by manipulation. Clin Orthop 215:47, 1987

61. d'Ornano J, Conrozier T, Bossard D et al: Effects des manipulations vertébrales sur al hernie discale lombaire. Rev Med Orthop 9:21, 1990

62. Cassidy JD, Thiel HW, Kirkaldy-Willis KW: Side posture manipulation for lumbar disc herniation. J Manipul Physiol Ther 16:96, 1993

63. Farfan HF, Cossette JW, Robertson GH et al: The effects of torsion on the lumbar intervertbral joints: the role of torsion in the production of disc degeneration. J Bone Joint Surg 52A:468, 1970

64. Adams MA, Hutton WC: Mechanics of the intervertebral disc. p. 39. In Ghosh P (ed): The Biology of the Intervertebral Disc. Vol. II. CRC Press, Boca Raton, FL, 1988

65. Koes BW, Bouter LM, van Mameren H et al: A randomised clinical trial of manual therapy and physiotherapy for persistent back and neck complaints: subgroup analysis and relationship between outcome measures. J Manipul Physiol Ther 16:211, 1993

66. Koes BW, Bouter LM, van Mameren H, Essers AH et al: A blinded randomised clinical trial of manual therapy and physiotherapy for chronic back and neck complaints. J Manipul Physiol Ther 15:16, 1992

67. Cassidy JD, Lopes AA, Yong-Hing K: The immediate effect of manipulation versus mobilization on pain and range of motion in the cervical spine: A randomized controlled trial. J Manipul Physiol Ther 15:570, 1992

68. Coulter I, Hurwitz E, Adams A et al: The appropriateness of spinal manipulation and mobilization of the cervical spine: literature review, indications and ratings by a multidisciplinary expert panel. Monograph No. DRU-982-1-CCR. RAND: Santa Monica, CA, 1995

69. Coulter I, Shekelle PG, Mootz RD, Hansen DT: The use of expert panel results: The RAND panel for appropriateness of manipulation and mobilization of the cervical spine. Top Clin Chiro 2:54, 1995

70. Girard N: Statistiques déscriptives sur la nature des blessures. Quebec. Régie de l'assurance automobile du Québec. Direction des services medicaux et de la réadaption. Internal document. Quebec, 1989

71. Giroux M: Les blessures a la colonne cervicale: Importance du probleme. Le Medicin du Quebec, Montreal, September 22–26, 1991

72. Bannister G, Gargan M: Prognosis of whiplash injuries: a review of the literature. Spine 7:557, 1993

73. Croft AC: A proposed classification of cervical acceleration-deceleration (CAD) injuries with a review of prognostic research. Palmer J Res 1:10, 1994

74. Jonsson H Jr, Bring G, Rausching W et al: Hidden cervical spine injuries in traffic accident victims with skull fractures. J Spinal Disord 4:251, 1991

75. Akeson WH, Ameil D, Mechanic CL et al: Collagen cross-linking alterations in joint contractures. Changes in the reducible cross-links in periarticular connective tissue after nine weeks of immobilization. Connective Tissue Res 5:15, 1977

76. Frank C, Woo SL-Y, Amiel D et al: Medical collateral ligament healing a multidisciplinary assessment in rabbits. Am J Sports Med 11:379, 1983

77. Long ML, Frank C, Schachlan NS et al: The effects of motion on normal healing ligaments, abstracted. Proc Orthop Res 7:43, 1982

78. Fronek J, Frank C, Amiel D et al: The effects of intermittent passive movement (IPM) in the healing of medical collateral ligament, abstracted. Proc Orthop Res Soc 8:31, 1983

79. Gelberman RH, Manske PR, Akeson WH et al: Flexor tendon repair. J Orthop Res 4:119, 1986

80. Crock H: Low back surgery. International Chiropractic Conference, London, 1987

81. Baker D: Development and regeneration of mammalian muscle spindles. Scient Progr 69:45, 1984

82. Nansel D, Peneff A, Cremata E, Carlson J: Time course considerations for the effects of unilateral lower cervical adjustments with respect to the amelioration of cervical lateral flexion passive end-range asymmetry. J Manipul Physiol Ther 13:297, 1990

83. Croft A: Whiplash outcome: do most patients recover in 6–12 weeks? Dynam Chiro 14:14, 1996

84. Chapman-Smith D: Redefining whiplash and its management. Chiro Rep 9:1, 1995

85. Boline P, Kassak K, Bronfort G et al: Spinal manipulation vs. amiltriptyline for the treatment of chronic tension-type headaches: a randomized clinical trial. J Manipul Physiol Ther 18:148, 1995

86. Bitterli J, Graf F, Robert F et al: Zur objektivierung der manualtherapeutischen beeinflussbarket des spondylogenen korpschemerzes [Objective criteria for the evaluation of chiropractic treatment of spondylotic headache]. Nervenart 48:259, 1977

87. Hoyt WH, Shaffer F, Bard DA et al: J Am Osteopath Assoc 78:322, 1979

88. Nilsson N: A randomized controlled trial of the effect of spinal manipulation in the treatment of cervicogenic headache. J Manipul Physiol Ther 18:435, 1995

89. Parker G, Tupling H, Pryor D: A controlled trial of cervical manipulation for migraine. Aust NZ J Med 8:589, 1978

90. Jensen IK, Nielsen FF, Vosmar L: An open study comparing manual therapy with the use of cold packs in the treatment of post-traumatic headache. Cephalalgia 10:243, 1990

91. Nelson C, Boline P: Comparison among medication, chiropractic therapy, and a combined therapy in the prophylaxis of migraine headache: a pilot study and a full-scale multidisciplinary trial. Foundation for Chiropractic Education and Research, Arlington, VA, Grant #92-03-06, research in progress, 1996.

92. Whittingham W, Ellis WB, Milyneux TP: The effect of manipulation [toggle recoil] for headaches with upper cervical joint dysfunction: a pilot study. J Manipul Physiol Ther 17:369, 1994

93. International Headache Society: Classification and diagnostic criteria for headache disorders, cranial neuralgias and facial pain. Cephalalgia 8, Suppl 7: 1988

94. Mootz RD, Dhami MSI, Hess JA et al: Chiropractic treatment of chronic episodic tension type headache in male subjects: a case series analysis. J Can Chiro Assoc 38:152, 1994

95. Droz JM, Crot F: Occipital headaches: statistical results in the treatment of vertebrogenic headache. Ann Swiss Chiro Assoc 8:127, 1985

96. Vernon HT: Spinal manipulation and headaches of cervical origin. J Manipul Physiol Ther 5:109, 1982

97. Wight JS: Migraine: a statistical analysis of chiropractic treatment. Chiro J 12:363, 1978

98. Stodolny J, Chmielewski H: Manual therapy in the treatment of patients with cervical migraine. Manual Med 4:49, 1989

99. Turk Z, Ratkolb O: Mobilization of the cervical spine in chronic headaches. Manual Med 3:15, 1987

100. Vernon HT: The effectiveness of chiropractic manipulation in the treatment of headache: an exploration of the literature. J Manipul Physiol Ther 18:611, 1995

101. Vernon HT: Spinal manipulation and headaches: an update. Top Clin Chiro 2:34, 1995

102. Karpen M: Treating carpal tunnel syndrome. Alt Comp Ther 1:284, 1995

103. Bonebrake AR, Fernandez JE, Marley RJ et al: A treatment for carpal tunnel syndrome: evaluation of objective and subjective measures. J Manipul Physiol Ther 13:507, 1991

104. Bonebrake AR, Fernandez JE, Dahalan JB, Marley RJ: A treatment for carpal tunnel syndrome: results of a follow-up study. J Manipul Physiol Ther 6:125, 1993

105. Strait BW: Osteopathic manipulation for patients with confirmed mild, modest and moderate carpal tunnel syndrome. J Am Osteo Assoc 94:673, 1994

106. Sucher BM: Myofascial manipulative release of carpal tunnel syndrome. Documentation with magnetic resonance imaging. J Am Osteo Assoc 93:1273, 1993

107. Sucher BM: Palpatory diagnosis and manipulative management of carpal tunnel syndrome. J Am Osteo Assoc 94:647, 1994

108. Davis TP, Kassak KM: Outcomes of chiropractic and allopathic care in the treatment of carpal tunnel syndrome. Foundation for Chiropractic Education and Research, Arlington, VA, Grant #92-10-03, research in progress, 1996

109. Tanaka S, Wild DK, Seligman PJ et al: The US prevalence of self-reported carpal tunnel syndrome: 1988 National Health interview survey data. Am J Publ Health 84:1846, 1994

110. Kleynhans AM: Complications of and contraindications to spinal manipulative therapy. p. 359. In Haldeman S (ed): Modern Developments in the Principles and Practice of Chiropractic. Appleton & Lange, Norwalk, CT, 1980

111. Laderman JP: Accidents of spinal manipulations. Ann Swiss Chiro Assoc 7:161, 1981

112. Haldeman S, Rubinstein SM: Cauda equina syndrome in patients undergoing manipulation of the lumbar spine. Spine 17:1469, 1992

113. Terrett AGL, Kleynhans AM: Complications from manipulations of the low back. Chiro J Aust 22(4):129, 1992

114. Hosek RS, Schram SB, Silverman H et al: Cervical manipulation, letter JAMA 245:22, 1981

115. Hamann G, Haas A, Kujat C et al: Cervico-cephalic artery dissections due to chiropractic manipulations. Lancet 341:114, 1993

116. Dvorak J, Orelli F: How dangerous is manipulation of the cervical spine? Manual Med 2:1, 1985

117. Thiel HW: Gross morphology and pathoanatomy of the vertebral arteries. J Manipul Physiol Ther 14:133, 1991

118. Terrett AGJ: Vascular accidents from cervical spine manipulation: the mechanisms. J Aust Chiro Assoc 17:131, 1987

119. Refshaugh KM: Rotation: a valid premanipulative dizziness test? Does it predict safe manipulation? J Manipul Physiol Ther 17:15, 1994

120. Esposito V, Esposito C, Cianciulli A, Goldberg N: Spinal manipulative therapy: no evidence for neurovascular trauma. Int J Neurol 86:1, 1996

121. Stano M: The economic role of chiropractic: further analysis of relative insurance costs for low back care. J Neuromusculoskel Syst 3:139, 1995

122. Ebrall P: Mechanical low-back pain: a comparison of medical and chiropractic management within the Victorian Workcare scheme. Chiro J Aust 22:47, 1992

123. Wolk S: An analysis of Florida workers' compensation medical claims for back-related injuries. Am Chiro Assoc J 27:50, 1988

124. Johnson MR, Ferguson AC, Swank LL: Treatment and cost of back or neck injury: a literature review. Res Forum 65:68, 1985

125. Dean H, Schmidt R: A Comparison of the Cost of Chiropractors Versus Alternative Medical Practitioners. Virginia Chiropractic Assoc, Richmond, VA, 1992

126. Stano M: A comparison of health care costs for chiropractic and medical patients. J Manipul Physiol Ther 16:291, 1993

127. Carey TS, Garrett J, Jackman A et al: North Carolina Back Pain Project. N Engl J Med 333:913, 1995

128. Shekelle PG, Markovich M, Louie R: Comparing the costs between provider types of episodes of back care. Spine 20:221, 1995

129. Rosner A: Spine 20:2595, 1995 (Letter)

130. Bowers LJ, Mootz RD: The nature of primary care: the chiropractor's role. Top Clin Chiro 2:66, 1995

131. Nyiendo J, Lamm L: Disability low back Oregon Workers' compensation of claims. Part I. Methodology and clinical categorization of chiropractic and medical cases. J Manipul Physiol Ther 14:177, 1991

132. Nyiendo J: Disability low back Oregon Workers' compensation of claims. Part II. Time loss. J Manipul Physiol Ther 14:231, 1991

133. Nyiendo J: Disability low back Oregon Workers' compensation of claims. Part III. Diagnostic and treatment procedures and associated costs. J Manipul Physiol Ther 14:287, 1991

134. Johnson MR: A comparison of chiropractic, medical and osteopathic care for work-related sprains/strains. J Manipul Physiol Ther 12:335, 1989

135. Greenwood JG: Report on work-related back and neck injury cases in West Virginia: issues related to chiropractic and medical costs. Publication of the West Virginia Workers' Compensation Fund, Charleston, WV, 1983

136. Bergmann BW, Cichoke AJ: Cost-effectiveness of chiropractic treatment of low-back injuries. J Manipul Physiol Ther 3:143, 1980

137. Duffey DJ: A Study of Wisconsin Industrial Back Injury Cases. University of Wisconsin Market Research, Madison, 1978

138. Rosen M: Back pain. Report of a Clinical Standards Advisory Group Committee on Back Pain. HMSO, London, 1994

139. Manga P, Angur D, Papadopoulos C, Swan W: The effectiveness and cost-effectiveness of chiropractic management of low-back pain. Kenilworth, Richmond Hill, ON, 1993

140. Haldeman S, Chapman-Smith D, Peterson DM Jr: Guidelines for chiropractic quality assurance and practice parameters. In Proceedings of a Consensus Conference Commissioned by the Congress of Chiropractic State Associations, held at the Mercy Conference Center, Burlingame, CA, January 25–30, 1992. Aspen, Gaithersburg, MD, 1993

141. Hack GD, Koritzer RD, Robinson WL, Hallgren RC, Greenman PE: Anatomic relation between the rectus capitus posterior minor muscle and the dura mater. Spine 20:2484, 1995

142. Haldeman S: Point of view. Spine 20:2486, 1995

143. Bluestone CD: Update on antimicrobial therapy for otitis media and sinusitis in children. Cutis 36:7, 1985

144. Warwick R, Williams P: Gray's Anatomy. 35th British Ed. WB Saunders, Philadelphia, 1973

145. Harker LA: Middle ear disease from eustachian tube malformation. Alaska Med 14:90, 1972

11

Visceral Disorders Research

Charles Masarsky
Marion Weber

This is a paradoxical time for chiropractic somatovisceral research. Mainstream research organizations such as the Foundation for Chiropractic Education and Research now actively support research on a wide range of visceral disorders. At the same time, a small sector of the profession wishing to restrict chiropractic to the care of acute, uncomplicated musculoskeletal pain in adults is increasingly vocal and visible.[1] This is due in part to the managed care revolution, which has convinced some that chiropractic's scope should be defined by the limits of its third-party insurance coverage.

If chiropractic is not to surrender its identity to such external forces, the implications of recent somatovisceral research findings must be clearly understood, first by the profession and then by the general public. The profession's future depends on the scientific study of chiropractic's role in maintaining wellness. While wellness and general health can be studied in any patient, whole-person benefits are less obvious in sprain/strain cases. Research at the somatovisceral interface may provide a window into wellness.

Enhanced understanding of the autonomic effects of somatic dysfunction in general, and of the vertebral subluxation complex (VSC) in particular, can improve chiropractic assessment methods. To the extent that measurement of autonomic tone becomes a routine step in evaluating VSC, every patient examination can serve as a lesson in the whole-person benefits of chiropractic care. This is no radical departure; the assessment of autonomic tone has a solid pedigree in chiropractic history (Fig. 11-1).

HISTORICAL PERSPECTIVES

The earliest method of chiropractic analysis was nerve tracing, the use of digital pressure to follow a line of hypersensitive tissue from an uncomfortable body part to the spine or vice versa. A nerve trace to a particular spinal segment was held to represent disturbed tone in the indicated spinal nerve. The chiropractor would suspect disturbed neurologic tone as a cause of dysfunction in all tissues—somatic or visceral—innervated by the indicated nerve. Originating a nerve trace from a nauseous stomach or painful kidney was held to be as legitimate as tracing from a sore shoulder or painful hip.[2]

Nerve-tracing data, correlated with autonomic neuroanatomy, was systematized into the Meric system of chiropractic analysis. This development was already under way when Mabel Palmer published *Chiropractic Anatomy* in 1918 and had reached maturity by the time R.W. Stephenson published his *Chiropractic Textbook* in 1927. In Meric analysis, a clinical problem is considered in terms of the *zone* (the body

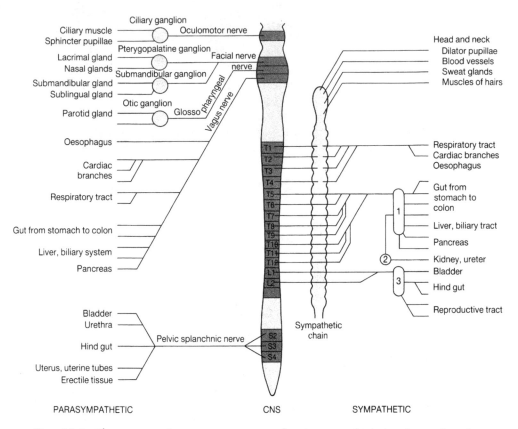

Fig. 11-1. The autonomic nervous system, showing at which levels, and within which cranial and spinal nerves, autonomic fibers link with the central nervous system. (1, coeliac ganglion; 2, renal ganglion; 3, pelvic ganglion. (From Rogers,[68] with permission.)

section innervated by a particular pair of spinal nerves) in which it occurs. All tissue of a particular type within a zone is termed a *mere*. For example, a zone's muscle tissue is its *myomere;* its visceral tissue is its *viscemere.*

When a patient presented with stomach complaints, the Meric chiropractor would recognize the involved organ as part of the viscemere corresponding to the fifth through eighth thoracic vertebrae. The results of nerve tracing and the palpation of paraspinal "taut and tender fibers" would indicate the precise subluxated vertebra. If these results were ambiguous, a radiographic examination would serve as the tie-breaker.[3]

By the early 1920s, many chiropractors used the back of the hand to palpate for "hot boxes"—areas of increased temperature along the spine. Fasci-

nated by this analytic method, Dossa D. Evins, a 1922 graduate of the Palmer School of Chiropractic, developed the neurocalometer, the first chiropractic heat-reading instrument. It consisted of two thermocouple probes and a galvanometer, which indicated left-to-right thermal asymmetry as the examiner glided the instrument up or down the spine. Persistent thermal asymmetry was taken to be a sign of disturbed vasomotor tone, consistent with the presence of VSC.[4]

In chiropractic's early years, assessment of autonomic tone was an integral part of chiropractic analysis. This took the form of nerve tracing, Meric analysis, and vasomotor analysis by instrument or by hand. The goal of this autonomic assessment was not to determine whether a patient could be cured of hypertension, asthma, constipation, or other visceral disorders. Rather, it was an essential part of characterizing a patient's state of disturbed tone (or "dis-ease").

The traditional viewpoint was that VSC can disturb the tone of any neurologically controlled function. Given this assumption, chiropractic analysis logically was not limited to muscular or ligamentous tone, encompassing instead all aspects of physiologic tone: sympathetic tone, parasympathetic tone, vasomotor tone, bronchial tone, alimentary tone, and so forth.

Contemporary somatovisceral research is best understood in the spirit of this traditional viewpoint. Our hope is that this research will encourage the modern evolution of D.D. Palmer's "science of tone."

RECENT SOMATOVISCERAL RESEARCH

Our discussion is limited to areas in which at least one controlled experimental study or controlled clinical trial has been published. Most somatovisceral studies are descriptive rather than experimental, due in large measure to historically low levels of funding for such research. Therefore, each summary of controlled studies is followed by a discussion of major descriptive research, as well as implications for chiropractic assessment.

PELVIC ORGANIC DYSFUNCTION

Controlled Experimental and Clinical Studies

To date, dysmenorrhea and nocturnal enuresis are the only pelvic organic dysfunctions subjected to controlled study in the chiropractic scientific community. In a 1979 study, Thomason et al.[5] studied the responses of women suffering from menstrual pain and dysfunction. Among women given lumbar side-posture adjustments, 88 percent demonstrated significant symptomatic improvement, as assessed by a menstrual symptom questionnaire, whereas none of the women in a control group or in a sham adjustment group were able to report significant improvement.

A more recent study, by Kokjohn et al.,[6] used both symptomatic measurements and serum prostaglandin levels as outcome measures. Citing previous biomedical research implicating elevated serum

levels of prostaglandins as an important cause of symptoms of dysmenorrhea, Kokjohn's team theorized that chiropractic adjustments might reduce these levels. However, there was no statistically significant difference in serum prostaglandin levels between women receiving side-posture adjustments and women in the control or sham adjustment groups. Nevertheless, symptomatic improvement in the experimental group was approximately twice that of the control group, a statistically significant outcome that confirmed Thomason's findings.

Leboef et al.[7] presented a study on nocturnal enuresis, in which the bedwetting children served as their own controls. Baselines were established by monitoring the children for 2 to 4 weeks before the administration of chiropractic adjustments. On the basis of parental records, no significant difference was found between the baseline and intervention periods. These investigators did not note which spinal levels were adjusted, nor the methods used to determine these levels, a serious descriptive flaw.

A contrasting view is provided in a more recent study by Reed et al.,[8] in which, after a 2-week baseline period the children were divided into two groups—one receiving sham adjustments administered with an Activator instrument set on zero tension, and the other receiving actual adjustments, generally in the upper cervical and pelvic areas. The group receiving actual adjustments experienced a statistically significant 17.9 percent decrease in the frequency of wet nights, compared to a slight increase in wet night frequency among the group receiving sham adjustments.

Major Descriptive Research

Further evidence of the effects of VSC and its chiropractic correction on pelvic organic dysfunction come from case studies and case series. Liebl and Butler[9] demonstrated substantial improvement in a patient suffering from dysmenorrhea, based on a daily symptom-intensity diary. Well-described cases of improvement in nocturnal enuresis were presented by Gemmell and Jacobson[10] and more recently by Blomerth.[11]

Perhaps the most compelling body of case studies and case series in this literature has been presented by Browning,[12,13] whose work demonstrates a relationship between pelvic pain and organic dysfunction and spinal nerve root irritation at the S2 to S4 levels. The dermatomes corresponding to these levels, which are most readily tested at the buttocks, are often overlooked in clinical examination. Straight-leg raising enhanced by suprapubic pressure will often provoke intrapelvic pain in these patients, as will digital pressure at the L5-S1 intervertebral space. These sensory signs provide the practitioner with useful outcome measures for patients presenting with this dysfunction.

Particularly interesting among Browning's cases was a woman who had undergone appendectomy, left oophrectomy and partial hysterectomy, three bowel surgeries, and four bladder surgeries over a period of 18 years.[14] These procedures failed to resolve her many pelvic pain and organic dysfunction complaints, and she presented to Browning with pelvic pain, rectal bleeding, diarrhea, bladder discomfort, pain on intercourse, and anorgasmy. Noting signs of S2–S4 irritation, Browning began a course of lumbosacral flexion-distraction adjustments. Within 4 weeks, the symptom complex was noticeably responding, and complete resolution was obtained by 30 weeks. A fascinating aspect of this patient's history was the conspicuous absence of low back pain.

Implications for Chiropractic Assessment

While current research literature does not indicate that chiropractic adjustments offer a cure for any pelvic organic disorder, these disorders can indicate disturbed tone related to VSC.

Monitoring pelvic organic symptoms through patient diaries, questionnaires, and other methods, may be seen as a modern development in the spirit of traditional Meric analysis. Browning's provocation of intrapelvic pain with lumbosacral digital pressure is a modernized form of nerve tracing. Along with other sensory tests he offers for monitoring the S2–S4 nerve roots, Browning makes a strong case for moving beyond low back pain as the sole rationale for adjusting the low back.

RESPIRATORY DISORDERS

Controlled Experimental and Clinical Studies

Asthma and chronic obstructive pulmonary disease (COPD) have attracted significant attention within the chiropractic and osteopathic research communities. Of historic and scientific interest is a paper presented by Miller[15] at an early interdisciplinary conference on spinal manipulation at the National Institutes of Health. In this study, 44 COPD patients underwent osteopathic examination. Signs of somatic dysfunction noted in this examination included asymmetry of paraspinal muscle tension, loss of intersegmental mobility, "skin drag" (palpatory assessment of asymmetry or local alteration in friction offered to the examiner's finger as it moves along the patient's paraspinal skin), and "red reflex" (visual assessment of asymmetry or unusual intensity in reactive skin hyperemia). On the basis of this evaluation, the greatest number of abnormal findings were in the thoracic spine, particularly at T2–T5.

Miller's patients were randomly assigned to treatment and control groups. Both groups received standard medical interventions (including bronchodilators, postural drainage, and breathing exercises), while the treatment group also received osteopathic manipulation, consisting of two visits per week (duration of care was not mentioned). Lung volumes were measured, and patients filled out a questionnaire on respiratory symptoms.

The lung volume results were inconclusive; both groups improved, with no significant difference between groups. However, more patients in the treatment group reported the ability to walk greater distances, as well as fewer colds, less coughing, and less dyspnea, than before treatment.

In a more recent paper, Nielsen et al.[16] reported on a randomized clinical trial of chiropractic care for adult asthma patients. Although no significant differences were found between sham adjustments and actual chiropractic intervention, the sham procedure may not have been as biologically inert as these investigators had anticipated. The sham maneuver consisted of a gentle, apparently specific manual pressure, with the patient positioned on a drop table. While this light pressure was applied with one hand, the drop mechanism was simultaneously released with the other. Since the patient sample as a whole experienced improvement in asthma symptom severity as well as nonspecific bronchial hyperreactivity (a measure of resistance to histamine-induced bronchial obstruction) by the end of the study, both the sham adjustment and the adjustment may have elicited healing effects.

Developing a truly inert sham procedure is a challenge for chiropractic researchers and investigators of other nonpharmaceutical healing arts, such as acupuncture. Because supposedly sham manual interventions may have unexpected positive or negative consequences, analysis of the data must be particularly careful and thorough.

Major Descriptive Research

The case of a COPD patient under chiropractic care was reported by Masarsky and Weber.[17] Following a 2-week baseline period, diversified chiropractic adjustments were administered at various levels, usually including the upper cervical and upper thoracic regions. The frequency of visits was three times weekly for more than 14 months. Intersegmental traction, vitamin C supplementation, cranial adjustments, and soft tissue work were also included in the chiropractic regimen. Outcome measures included lung volumes (forced vital capacity [FVC] and forced expiratory volume$_1$ [FEV$_1$]), a 10-point severity scale, with 1 mildest and 10 most extreme, for coughing, dyspnea, and fatigue, and a daily count of laryngospasms. Up to three laryngospasms per week had been the norm for this patient for 17 years.

Mean scores during the last 7 months of this study were compared to the mean baseline scores. Forced vital capacity increased by more than 1L, and forced expiratory volume in 1 second (FEV$_1$) increased by more than 0.3 L. Coughing intensity, dyspnea, and fatigue all decreased sharply. The patient reported no laryngospasms during the final 5 months of the study. Improved lung volumes lagged behind the subjective improvements by several months.

Peet et al.[18] reported similarly encouraging results with a group of eight pediatric patients with medically diagnosed asthma. Following 10 adjustments according to Chiropractic Biophysics Technique (CBP) protocols, this patient group demonstrated an average increase in peak flow of 25 percent. The parents of seven of the eight children also reported a decrease in medication use. Another instructive case involving pediatric asthma was presented by Bachman and Lantz.[19] Following three Gonstead adjustments at T3, T12, and the sacrum, the 34-month-old patient experienced 8 weeks of freedom from symptoms. During the previous year, the patient had weekly asthma attacks, 20 of them severe enough to require visits to the emergency department. An exacerbation at 8 weeks followed a fall from a step ladder; this time the asthma symptoms were accompanied by nocturnal enuresis. Both sets of symptoms resolved after three more adjustments at the same levels. After a full year of freedom from symptoms, the boy fell from a horse and experienced a return of both asthma and enuresis. A single adjustment resolved this exacerbation; Bachman and Lantz report no recurrence after 2 years of follow-up evaluation.

Following a retrospective study of the files of 79 patients with medically diagnosed bronchial asthma, Nilsson and Christiansen[20] reported that patients likely to have a good response to chiropractic care tend to have less severe asthma symptoms at presentation, and an earlier age of onset, than do those patients with a poor response.

Masarsky and Weber[21] reported on six cases of dyspnea that resolved upon correction of VSC and related somatic dysfunctions. We have coined the term "somatic dyspnea" to refer to such clinical situations. All six patients demonstrated mid-thoracic fixations on motion palpation, leading us to suspect restriction of rib excursion and/or disturbance to the sympathetic nerve supply to the lungs and bronchi. One patient reported a clear-cut association between a C2-C3 correction and relief from the dyspnea she had experienced, suggesting a connection to the phrenic nerve. The most common extravertebral dysfunction associated with somatic dyspnea was at the temporomandibular joint. Somatic dyspnea is a subjective symptom; it is not always accompanied by measurable depression of lung volumes. However, the improved subjective ease of breathing is often rapid and dramatic.

Implications for Chiropractic Assessment

Breathing is a musculoskeletal act. More than most bodily functions, breathing straddles the somatovisceral interface. Even if researchers never provide direct evidence that the chiropractic adjustment can improve the lung tissue of pulmonary patients, the profession has a role in managing such patients on a musculoskeletal basis alone.

While objective measures, such as lung volumes, and subjective measures, such as respiratory symptom severity, do not directly demonstrate the presence of VSC, such measures do help demonstrate the tone of skeletal and smooth respiratory muscles. As reflections of tone, respiratory observations and measurements can be useful to the chiropractor in assessing clinical outcome.

It is important to note that subjective easing of dyspnea was observed in the Miller COPD study, while significant improvement in lung volumes was not. This is consistent with our COPD case, in which lung volumes did not improve until several months after symptomatic improvement had begun. Also consistent is our observation that somatic dyspnea is not always accompanied by depressed lung volumes. We theorize that VSC may increase the work of breathing before frank obstruction develops. By the same token, correction of VSC may reduce the physiologic cost of deep breathing before any measurable improvement in volume occurs, especially in cases of chronic pulmonary disease. Therefore, unlike pain, at the current state of the art dyspnea may be an early clinical indicator, while objective respiratory measurements may be lagging indicators.

CARDIOVASCULAR DISORDERS

Controlled Experimental and Clinical Studies

The only recent controlled clinical trial in the cardiovascular area is the hypertension study by Yates et al.[22] Twenty-one patients with elevated blood pressure were randomly assigned to active treatment (adjustments in the T1 to T5 region, based on Activator protocols), placebo treatment (sham adjustments with the Activator instrument set on zero tension), and control (no intervention) groups. Noting that previous studies may have been confounded by elevated initial readings due to anxiety, Yates and colleagues used a standard psychological questionnaire before and after the intervention. They found a statistically significant decrease in both systolic and diastolic blood pressure in the active treatment group, but not in the placebo-treated or control groups. Since the active and control groups did not differ on anxiety reduction, this was ruled out as an explanation for the difference between groups. These findings support the hypothesis that blood pressure reduction in hypertensives

is a bona fide physiologic effect of the chiropractic adjustment.

Major Descriptive Research

Plaugher and Bachman[23] published an instructive case study involving a 38-year-old man with a 14-year history of hypertension. He also reported side effects due to his two medications, including bloating sensations, depression, fatigue, and impotency. Low back pain was also reported as an incidental issue.

Examination according to Gonstead protocols revealed evidence of VSC at various levels, particularly in the mid-cervical, upper thoracic, and middle thoracic regions. Adjustments were administered once per week. After three visits, the patient's medical doctor was able to stop one medication altogether and reduce the dosage of the other. All medication was discontinued after seven visits. After this, the frequency of visits was reduced to twice per month. Follow-up at 18 months showed that blood pressure stabilized within normal limits without medication. Bloating, depression, fatigue, and low back pain abated, while normal sexual function returned. Publication is pending on a controlled clinical trial of chiropractic care for hypertensive patients, recently completed by a research team directed by Plaugher.

Peterson[24] recently reported reduction of serum cholesterol levels by more than 22 percent in two patients following a single chiropractic adjustment each. These adjustments were administered according to neuro-emotional technique (NET) protocols. Spontaneous fluctuations in serum cholesterol levels average 4.8 percent.

Lott et al.[25] reported electrocardiographic improvements in three of four patients following chiropractic adjustments in conjunction with diet and exercise advice. All four patients experienced improvement in blood pressure or heart rate, or both.

Jarmel and colleagues presented an abstract at the Chiropractic Centennial in Washington, D.C., in 1995. Although the full paper awaits publication, the data presented indicate that 1 month of Diversified chiropractic adjustments at various levels of the cervical and upper thoracic spine resulted in fewer cardiac ischemic episodes, fewer premature ventricular contractions, and improved sympathetic-parasympathetic balance among the 11 patients studied. These findings were verified by a medical cardiologist's blind assessment of 24-hour Holter monitor data.

Implications for Chiropractic Assessment

Sophisticated cardiovascular assessments involving serum cholesterol measurements, electrocardiography, and Holter monitoring are not prominent in most chiropractors' clinical routines. However, these high-technology tools can be of great value in the research arena and situations involving chiropractic-medical co-management.

On the low-technology end of the spectrum, pulse rate and blood pressure measurement are commonly employed by chiropractors. While these cannot provide stand-alone demonstrations of the presence of VSC, they strengthen the clinician's suspicion of VSC and add options for outcome assessment.

Plaugher and Bachman[23] note that the combined effects of antihypertensive medication and chiropractic adjustments can temporarily drive a patient's blood pressure below normal levels. This can result in disturbing symptoms, such as vertigo. If this follows a cervical adjustment, the patient may believe the chiropractor was responsible for causing a stroke or some other deleterious process. For this reason, Plaugher and Bachman urge clinicians to monitor blood pressure on a visit-to-visit basis for patients who are taking antihypertensive medication. If blood pressure drops toward hypotensive levels, the patient should seek medical advice regarding reduced drug dosages. Patients should be made aware of this possibility at the first visit, so they will respond to episodes of dizziness without panic.

ALIMENTARY TRACT

Controlled Experimental and Clinical Studies

The only controlled study in the chiropractic research community involving the alimentary tract was presented by medical practitioners of spinal manipulation, Pikalov and Kharin.[26] Sixteen adult patients with endoscopically confirmed duodenal

ulcer received spinal manipulation supplemented with regional mobilization and manual soft tissue therapy. This group was compared to 40 ulcer patients receiving medication. Weekly physical and endoscopic examination were the major outcome measures. Ulcer remission in the experimental group took place an average of 10 days earlier than in the control group. The most frequently manipulated segments were in the T9 to T12 region. (See Ch. 4 for futher details).

Major Descriptive Research

DeBoer et al.[27] demonstrated inhibition of stomach and duodenal smooth muscle activity in rabbits as a result of surgical misalignment of T6. Fallon and Lok[28] presented the case of an infant with medically diagnosed pyloric stenosis, in which screaming and projectile vomiting were clearly abating after four upper cervical adjustments delivered over a period of 8 days. After another six adjustments, complete symptomatic resolution was achieved. This was accompanied by the disappearance of an olive-shaped mass in the right upper abdominal quadrant corresponding to the spasm in the pyloric muscles, as well as improved thermal symmetry at the styloid fossae corresponding to upper cervical VSC.

Infantile colic is the subject of a number of well-described studies. Pluhar and Schobert[29] reported reduced crying, improved sleep, and increased formula consumption following a single adjustment (at T7, T9, and C1) of a 3-month-old girl with a 4-week history of colic. Hyman[30] reported alleviation of colicky crying, of arching of the back, and of flatulence following a single adjustment (T9 and C1) of a 5-week-old boy with a 3-week history of colic. The most impressive descriptive study involving colic to date was published by Klougart et al,[31] in which 38 percent of Denmark's chiropractors participated in a prospective study. According to parental reports, 90 percent of the infants improved within 2 weeks; 23 percent improved after a single adjustment. Klougart and colleagues cite previous research indicating that spontaneous resolution of infantile colic generally takes 12 to 16 weeks. The most commonly adjusted segments were occiput, C1 and C2.

Bowel function has been the subject of several well-documented cases. Falk[32] reported the case of a 40-year-old man, whose chief complaints were low back pain and left sciatica. Concomitant with these problems, the patient reported constipation, a problem he denied experiencing in the past. Side-posture adjustments at L5 resolved these problems. Eriksen[33] reported the case of a 5-year-old girl with a lifetime history of constipation. Despite medication, she was experiencing only one bowel movement per week. This promptly changed to four to six bowel movements per week following Grostic upper cervical adjusting. Wagner et al.[34] reported the case of a 25-year-old woman with a 5-year history of irritable bowel syndrome. Following an initial intervention of two adjustments within 1 week, she received adjustments, primarily at C1 and T12, on a monthly basis. Diarrhea abated after the first adjustment, and she has been free of this and of sharp abdominal pain for 2 years.

Implications for Chiropractic Assessment

Much chiropractic clinical experience relevant to the alimentary tract has been with pediatric patients. Nyiendo and Olsen[35] found that gastrointestinal problems are common primary complaints among pediatric patients attending a chiropractic teaching clinic. These investigators also found that pediatric patients were more likely than adult patients to have nonmusculoskeletal primary complaints. The widespread nerve supply to the alimentary tract makes any symptoms of distress in this system good general indicators of disturbed autonomic tone.

VISUAL SYSTEM

Controlled Experimental and Clinical Studies

The only controlled chiropractic study involving the visual system is the work on pupil diameter by Briggs and Boone.[36] During a 4-day baseline period, 15 subjects had their pupils photographed in a darkened room, using infrared film. Chiropractic analysis was performed during this same period, primarily based on heat-reading instrumentation and the Derefield-Thompson leg check. Eight subjects were found to have signs of cervical subluxation, while seven did not. Following adjustment of the subluxated subjects with toggle-recoil or Diversified methods and light soft tissue massage of the unsubluxated subjects, a fifth pupil measurement was performed. While the

subjects receiving massage demonstrated no post-intervention change in pupillary diameter, there was change in all the adjusted subjects—dilation in some, constriction in others. Briggs and Boone suggest that cervical subluxation creates imbalance in the tone of the sympathetic and parasympathetic innervation to the pupils. As such, pupillary diameter may provide a noninvasive method for studying autonomic balance.

Major Descriptive Research

Gilman and Bergstrand[37] report the case of a 75-year-old man with a 6-month history of total blindness following head trauma. After three upper cervical adjustments, the patient was able to tell the difference between light and darkness. After 11 adjustments administered over a 3-month period, the patient could distinguish colors and experienced a return of the normal pupillary response. After 5 months of care, the patient was able to read again.

Although spontaneous remission of post-traumatic blindness has been reported, it is rare after 6 months. Gilman and Bergstrand suggest that upper cervical VSC may cause retinal vasospasm if there is sufficient irritation to the superior cervical sympathetic ganglia, which innervates most cranial blood vessels.

A fascinating body of ophthalmological clinical research by Gorman and colleagues, published primarily in chiropractic journals, features automated static perimetry as a major outcome measure.[38–41] In this technique, points of light of various intensities are projected at different spots on a hemispheric screen placed over a patient's head. The patient presses a button each time he or she sees a point of light. Computerized mapping of the patient's visual field based on these responses identifies perceptual defects not usually detected by less sensitive techniques.

Gorman has repeatedly noted improved perimetry results following general ("pan-spinal") manipulation, usually performed under anesthesia. Most of these results have been verified by an independent medical ophthalmologist. Patients have included adults and children, traumatic and nontraumatic cases, mildly depressed visual sensitivity and overt bilateral tunnel vision. Concomitant problems, such as neck pain, headache, arm pain, dizziness, fatigue, and abdominal pain, often resolve with the visual problems. Gorman hypothesizes that microischemia of the retina, the optic nerve, or the visual cortex may be related to spinal dysfunction.

Implications for Chiropractic Assessment

Infrared pupillometry and automated static perimetry are not commonly performed in chiropractic offices. However, research to date suggests that the visual system may be sensitive to VSC, via the superior cervical sympathetic ganglia. Further study of the potential role of visual testing in chiropractic analysis is warranted, as is clinical collaboration with optometrists and ophthalmologists.

CENTRAL NERVOUS SYSTEM

Controlled Experimental and Clinical Studies

While not a controlled experiment in the classic sense, the study of hyperactive children by Giesen et al.[42] is a type of controlled clinical study called a "time-series design." In studies of this sort, the subjects serve as their own control group.

During a placebo period, seven hyperactive children were given sham adjustments with an Activator instrument placed on zero tension. During this period, parents kept a diary of the children's activity levels. Electrodermal testing provided a measure of sympathetic arousal, and a motion recorder disguised as a wristwatch was used to measure activity during a simulated homework assignment.

After the placebo period, Gonstead, Diversified, or Upper Cervical Specific adjustments (depending on examination results and doctor–patient comfort) were administered at various levels once per week. Across all measures, and across all seven subjects, improvement was noted from the placebo phase to the end of the treatment phase. This improvement was statistically significant, despite the small number of subjects.

Major Descriptive Research

Well-described cases of hyperactivity and other learning disabilities improving under chiropractic care have been presented by Phillips,[43] Thomas and Wood,[44] Arme,[45] and Araghi.[46] Moreover, the Ken-tuckiana Children's Center in Louisville, Kentucky, has been providing chiropractic care to children with learning disabilities since 1957. In this non-profit setting, chiropractic adjustments are part of a multidisciplinary program, which includes nutritional therapy, counseling, special education, visual therapy, speech therapy, Doman-Delacato patterning, and dental and medical care. Along similar lines, Oklahaven Children's Center in Oklahoma City, Oklahoma, has been providing chiropractic care for learning-disabled children on a sliding scale based on family income since 1962. At Oklahaven, chiropractic care is the only intervention.

Seizure disorders have been discussed in recent publications. Woo[47] and Duff[48] each presented cases of adult women with myoclonic seizures of 17 years and 18 months duration, respectively. Antiseizure medication was ineffective in both cases. Thoracolumbar adjustments in Woo's case and upper cervical adjustments in Duff's case brought about rapid resolution. Goodman[49] described a 5-year-old girl with a 9-month history of grand mal seizures. Dramatic improvement followed upper cervical adjustments.

Hospers[50] presented a series of five cases with complaints, including seizures, hyperactivity, and inability to concentrate. The major outcome measure in her study was computerized electroencephalography (EEG) or "brain mapping." In this procedure, a computer software program analyzes brain activity measured from surface EEG electrodes. The display is in the form of a diagram of the brain, with the percentage of various types of brainwaves written or color-coded over the various lobes. Previous research has identified normal values for each type of brain wave (alpha, beta, delta, theta) from each cerebral lobe for various age groups. Following Life Upper Cervical adjustments (four patients) or Category II pelvic blocking according to Sacro-occipital Technique protocols (one patient), all five patients demonstrated improved brain-mapping results, with concomitant symptomatic relief.

Chiropractic journals have just begun to touch on the subject of multiple sclerosis (MS). Stude and Mick[51] described an MS patient who responded favorably to thoracolumbar adjustments. More recently, Kirby[52] provided a well-described case of an MS patient responding well to upper cervical adjusting, after steroid medication and a low-fat diet provided no relief. Woo[53] reported a case of myelopathy that followed a sports injury. Despite 3 months of steroid therapy, the patient continued to deteriorate. At presentation, this young adult man had lost bladder and bowel control, was unable to stand, and suffered from iatrogenic Cushing's syndrome. After 2 months of adjustments at the C7-T1 level, the patient was able to walk with crutches. At 9 years of follow-up, the patient could run, needed no crutches, and had no bladder or bowel complaints.

Probably the single most spectacular case involving a central nervous system (CNS) disorder was described by Plaugher et al.[54] A 21-year-old man had been comatose for more than 1 year after an auto accident. After three modified Gonstead upper cervical adjustments, the patient woke up, with a concomitant return of pulse rate and blood pressure to normal levels. Adjustments were later performed at L5-S1 and various levels of the thoracic spine. At the time Plaugher's paper was presented, the patient was able to ambulate with the aid of crutches.

Implications for Chiropractic Assessment

If VSC can contribute to disorders of the brain and spinal cord, greater emphasis should be placed on the clinical assessment of these structures. All too often, chiropractic educators relegate such examination steps as the Babinski sign, Hoffmann sign, L'Hermitte sign, clonus, hyperreflexia, and other signs of CNS involvement to written or verbal descriptions only. Direct observation of these phenomena—whether through patient contact or simulation—should be included in chiropractic professional curricula.

Chiropractic clinicians are becoming increasingly familiar with the indications for magnetic resonance imaging, EEG, brain mapping, evoked potential studies, and other technologies useful in assessing the CNS. In the research arena, these tools have the potential to further elucidate the role of VSC in brain and spinal cord dysfunction. This type of research is one of the holy grails of chiropractic science. If VSC can disturb CNS function, all other functions are in jeopardy. If the chiropractic adjustment can improve CNS function, improved general wellness would be the expected result.

Terrett[55] recently broke new theoretical ground in this area. Reviewing an extensive body of research, he suggests a possible mechanism for chiropractic resolution of such complaints as visual problems, paresis, dizziness, depression, anxiety, and memory loss. Terrett cites previous research indicating that depressed circulation can cause electric silence in neurons without causing cell death. This level of circulation is called the "ischemic penumbra." With restored circulation, normal function often returns to the involved neural structures. On the basis of this information, Terrett theorizes that cervical VSC can disrupt blood flow to the brain to a degree less than a stroke, plunging portions of the brain into the ischemic penumbra, essentially a state of hibernation. He further theorizes that restoration of blood flow by VSC correction can reactivate these brain centers.

IMMUNE SYSTEM

Controlled Experimental and Clinical Studies

Brennan's research team is the most widely published group in chiropractic neuroimmunology. In a 1991 study, they injected a nontoxic sealant into the posterior facet joints of four dogs at various thoracic and lumbar levels, in an attempt to mimic VSC through surgical joint fixation.[56] Four other dogs underwent sham surgery. White blood cell (WBC) functional activity was measured in both groups during postsurgical recovery.

Although functional activity levels of both lymphocytes and polymorphonuclear neutrophils were depressed in both groups, the dogs that underwent sham surgery recovered normal WBC function more rapidly than did the dogs with spinal joint fixation.

In another study by Brennan et al.,[57] using human volunteers, thoracic manipulation (Diversified maneuvers at levels indicated by motion palpation), sham manipulation (light-force thrust with no audible or palpable joint release), and soft tissue manipulation (light massage at the gluteal area) groups were compared. Blood was drawn both before and after these interventions. Both polymorphonuclear neutrophils and monocytes demonstrated increased functional activity following thoracic manipulation, but not following sham or soft tissue manipulation. The difference between groups was statistically significant. A second component of this study explored the role of a particular neurotransmitter (substance P) in spine-to-WBC communication. The results were inconclusive.

A small but potentially ground-breaking clinical study was offered in 1994 by Selano et al.[58] Ten human immunodeficiency virus (HIV)-positive patients were randomly assigned to two groups. The experimental group received upper cervical adjustments according to Grostic protocols, while the control group received sham adjustments (the Grostic instrument trigger was depressed, but no impulse was delivered to the atlas vertebra). The duration of the study was 6 months, with visit frequency not noted.

The most interesting outcome measure in this study was the CD4 count at the beginning and end of the study, since a decline in the level of this particular WBC is an important measure of acquired immunodeficiency syndrome (AIDS)-related immunodeficiency. In the control group, CD4 count declined by a mean of 7.96 percent. In the experimental group, CD4 count increased by a mean of 48 percent. Despite the small number of subjects in this study, the results approached statistical significance.

Major Descriptive Research

In a review of uncontrolled pilot investigations, Allen[59] covered studies indicating increased serum immunoglobulin levels and increased lymphocyte counts following chiropractic adjustments. Allen's review also offers an instructive summary of Brennan's work.

Van Breda and Van Breda[60] surveyed parents, who were either medical doctors or doctors of chiropractic, regarding various aspects of their children's health histories. The "chiropractic" children were typically adjusted once per week or more, while "medical" children were not adjusted at all. At least one bout of otitis media was reported among 80 percent of the medical children versus 31 percent of the chiropractic children. At least one bout of tonsillitis was reported among 42 percent of the medical children versus 27 percent of the chiropractic children. The difference between groups was statistically significant for both conditions.

Rose-Aymon et al.[61] presented a survey involving pediatric patients of chiropractors. Although a small sample size precludes assessment of statistical significance, the pilot data suggest an inverse relationship between the frequency of chiropractic care and the incidence of chickenpox, mumps, measles, and German measles.

Thomas and Wilkinson[62] published a case study of an adult woman with frank spina bifida from T11 to L2. Among other problems, she suffered from long-standing recurrent bladder infections despite a daily regimen of antibiotics. With chiropractic care (a variety of techniques over 5 years), her infections became less frequent, and at the time of the report the patient had been infection free for more than 1 year without antibiotics.

Araghi[63] presented the case of a 2-year-old girl with myasthenia gravis (MG). After 5 months of steady deterioration despite medical attention, the patient began to respond after a single Gonstead adjustment at the upper cervical and sacroiliac levels. Myasthenia gravis is now widely seen as an autoimmune condition, in which the acetylcholine receptors at the myoneuronal junction are attacked by the patient's own WBCs.

Implications for Chiropractic Assessment

Because lymphatic tissue is widely distributed throughout the body, measures of immunosuppression do not identify spinal levels likely to be subluxated. Nevertheless, research presented to date strongly suggests that general immunosuppression is a feature of VSC. As such, certain types of blood analysis may provide useful outcome measures, especially in the research arena and in the chiropractic-medical co-management of selected patients.

Brennan's research team is the first chiropractic group to seriously explore molecular communication pathways between the nervous system and the immune system. Before their investigations, receptors for a variety of neurotransmitters had been identified on certain populations of WBCs. Some WBCs apparently also secrete neurotransmitters, establishing a possible molecular infrastructure for two-way communication between neuron and WBC. Fidelibus[64] presents an interesting review of this research. WBCs can act as if they are mobile neurons with defensive capabilities. The theoretical and applied aspects of this research area are attracting increased interest in the chiropractic scientific community.

With the rise of new antibiotic-resistant disease organisms, the importance of alternative strategies for boosting the competence of the immune system cannot be overestimated. For this reason, neuroimmunology seems destined to become another important area in chiropractic research.

PERSPECTIVES ON RECENT SOMATOVISCERAL RESEARCH

Over the years, it has been suggested that the visceral benefits of the chiropractic adjustment are apparent rather than real. Nansel and Szlazak[65] provide a recent example of this viewpoint. Based on their review of the literature, they suggest that referred spinal pain mimics visceral disorders and that the relief of this referred pain creates the impression of a cure for a disorder that never existed. They assert that autonomic reflex disorders generated by VSC are highly localized and thus irrelevant to general health and wellness.

Taken as a whole, the literature reviewed in this chapter is difficult to reconcile with such a view. Improvement in such dysfunctions as disturbed brain wave patterns, immunodeficiency, seizure disorders, learning disorders, tunnel vision and blindness, pyloric stenosis, duodenal ulcer, elevated serum cholesterol, cardiac arrhythmia, essential hypertension, pulmonary hypoventilation, dyspnea, sexual dysfunction, bowel dysfunction, bladder dysfunction, and dysmennorhea is not easily explained by the abolition of "mimics." Unless and until the vast majority of these findings is decisively refuted by future studies, the most logical conclusion is that the visceral significance of VSC goes well beyond mimicry and skin-deep autonomic reflexes.

Apparent organ dysfunction without frank organic abnormality may simply be an early phase of a process that eventuates in true visceral disease. Disease and "dis-ease" are not mutually exclusive; they may simply represent stages along a continuum.

The general framework of D.D. Palmer's science of tone remains valid and useful. VSC disturbs tone, most importantly neurologic tone. This disturbed tone (or "dis-ease") is deleterious to general health and wellness. While this framework certainly includes simple back pain and referred visceral pain, it also encompasses the broad range of findings reviewed above. In the final section of this chapter, we briefly explore the potential of this traditional paradigm in chiropractic's scientific future.

FUTURE RESEARCH HORIZONS

Stephenson[3] maintains that life is the expression of intelligence through matter. Life functions depend on the free and timely flow of information—a measurable aspect of intelligence—and the integrity of matter. Within this framework, all health problems represent disruption in an organism's matter or interference with information flow, or both. All health interventions seek to improve material (structural) integrity and/or informational fidelity.

The various health professions tend to emphasize either the material aspect or the informational aspect of life. While both approaches are valuable, a focus on matter often leads to the diagnostic tunnel vision of reductionistic thinking.

In an often cited anecdote, D.D. Palmer[2] relates the case of J.M., the farmer. J.M. suffered from chronic ankle pain, and had expended considerable time and money having various practitioners examine and treat his ankle. The underlying assumption by J.M. and his previous practitioners was that something was wrong with the matter in his ankle (e.g., torn ligaments, tendons, joint capsules). Palmer made no such assumption. Finding no apparent local problem in the ankle, he used nerve tracing, which led him to a subluxation in the lumbar spine. Correction of this subluxation brought immediate improvement in J.M.'s ankle pain.

Palmer's focus was primarily on the tone of the nervous system—the free and timely flow of information. This focus provides built-in protection against the hazardous assumption that the location of pain is the location of its cause. Palmer's science of tone is explicitly grounded in information-centered, not matter-centered, clinical logic.

We have argued that chiropractic's clinical logic should be applied to the scientific endeavor.[66,67] Seeing an injured back or neck as damaged matter leads conventional health researchers to ask certain questions and to omit others. Seeing the injured back or neck as a site of disturbed information flow would suggest additional questions to chiropractic researchers.

Even in such a well-established field as cost-effectiveness research, the difference between the two approaches could be vast. For example, rather than limiting themselves to the matter-centered question of how quickly injured workers return to work from lower back injuries, information-centered researchers might also ask about the rate of future hip, knee, ankle, and foot pain in workers with low back injuries. Similarly, questions about female workers with lower back injuries might be supplemented with inquiries about future rates of dysmenorrhea or cystitis.

Conventional ergonomics would view a poorly designed computer work station as a source of neck strain and carpal tunnel syndrome. An information-centered chiropractic researcher might also investigate the effect of such a work station on the future incidence of alimentary disorders, cardiac arrhythmia, pulmonary dysfunction, learning disabilities, and disorders of any other organ or system vulnerable to disturbed information flow in the spine.

For conventional researchers in the field of aging, VSC would be perceived as a possible accelerator of degenerative arthritis. For information-centered chiropractic researchers, any biologic marker of aging would be worthy of study, including reaction time, memory, visual acuity, blood pressure, skin hydration, and immune responses. The aging process could be a third important area in chiropractic research.

We conclude with the hope that D.D. Palmer's information-centered science of tone will energize the research community with an orthopedic neurology of the viscera, unique perspectives in neuroimmunology, new insights into brain function, a holistic approach to ergonomics, and nonpharmaceutical options in geriatrics. This might only be the beginning of a fully realized paradigm shift.

Terminology

chiropractic analysis
descriptive study
disease
dis-ease
ischemic penumbra
Meric technique
nerve tracing
paradigm
paradigm shift
outcome measure
somatic dysfunction
somatic dyspnea
tone

Review Questions

1. What methods of autonomic assessment were incorporated into chiropractic analysis during the profession's first three decades?

2. What methods has Browning proposed for assessing the lower sacral nerve roots?

3. Is somatic dyspnea always accompanied by reduced lung volumes?

4. What special measures should be taken in terms of clinical assessment and patient education when a patient is on antihypertensive medication?

5. What procedures are useful in monitoring central nervous system function? (Include physical examination, diagnostic imaging, and electrodiagnostic procedures.)

6. In what sense do white blood cells resemble neurons?

7. What evidence can be cited from the scientific literature to support the contention that spinal pain is not the only rationale for chiropractic adjustment?

Concept Questions

1. How can the whole-person benefits of chiropractic be explained to the general public, while avoiding unwarranted claims that the adjustment is a cure-all?

2. What might be the full implications of Terrett's theory of brain hibernation for society as a whole? (Address this question broadly. Consider traffic safety, learning disorders, domestic violence, creativity, and so forth.) What testable hypotheses are suggested by these implications?

3. Clinical ethics have been profoundly influenced by Hippocrates, who urged practitioners to exercise utmost caution in avoiding harm to patients. What are the ethical implications of chiropractic's infor-

mation-centered clinical logic? What testable hypotheses do these suggest? (Consider such problems as the rise of antibiotic-resistant pathogens, abuse and side effects of drugs, surgical mishaps, and the rising cost of health care.)

References

1. Homola S: Thirty years after "bonesetting, chiropractic and cultism": confessions of a chiropractic heretic. Chiropr Hist 15:15, 1995

2. Palmer DD: The Science, Art and Philosophy of Chiropractic. Portland Printing House, Portland, OR, 1910

3. Stephenson RW: Chiropractic Textbook. Palmer School of Chiropractic, Davenport, IA, 1948

4. Kyneur JS, Bolton SP: Chiropractic equipment. p. 262. In Peterson D, Wiese G (eds): Chiropractic: An Illustrated History. CV Mosby, St. Louis, 1995

5. Thomason PR, Fisher BL, Carpenter PA, Fike GL: Effectiveness of spinal manipulative therapy in treatment of primary dysmenorrhea: a pilot study. J Manipulative Physiol Ther 2:140, 1979

6. Kokjohn K, Schmid DM, Triano JJ, Brennan PC: The effect of spinal manipulation on pain and prostaglandin levels in women with primary dysmenorrhea. J Manipulative Physiol Ther 15:279, 1992

7. Leboeuf C, Brown P, Herman A et al: Chiropractic care of children with nocturnal enuresis: a prospective study. J Manipulative Physiol Ther 14:110, 1991

8. Reed WR, Beavers S, Reddy SK, Kern G: Chiropractic management of primary nocturnal enuresis. J Manipulative Physiol Ther 17:156, 1994

9. Liebl NA, Butler LM: A chiropractic approach to the treatment of dysmenorrhea. J Manipulative Physiol Ther 13:101, 1990

10. Gemmell HA, Jacobson BH: Chiropractic management of enuresis: time-series descriptive design. J Manipulative Physiol Ther 12:386, 1989

11. Blomerth PR: Functional nocturnal enuresis. J Manipulative Physiol Ther 17:335, 1994

12. Browning JE: Uncomplicated mechanically induced pelvic pain and organic dysfunction in low back patients. JCCA 35:149, 1991

13. Browning JE: Distractive manipulation protocols in treating the mechanically induced pelvic pain and organic dysfunction patient. Chiropr Tech 7:1, 1995

14. Browning JE: Mechanically induced pelvic pain and organic dysfunction in a patient without low back pain. J Manipulative Physiol Ther 13:406, 1990

15. Miller WD: Treatment of visceral disorders by manipulative therapy. p. 295. In Goldstein M (ed): The Research Status of Spinal Manipulative Therapy. National Institute of Neurological and Communicative Disorders and Stroke, Bethesda, MD, 1975

16. Nielsen NH, Bronfort G, Bendix T et al: Chronic asthma and chiropractic spinal manipulation: a randomized clinical trial. Clin Exp Allergy 25:80, 1995

17. Masarsky CS, Weber M: Chiropractic management of chronic obstructive pulmonary disease. J Manipulative Physiol Ther 11:505, 1988

18. Peet JB, Marko SK, Piekarczyk W: Chiropractic response in the pediatric patient with asthma: a pilot study. Chiropr Pediatr 1:9, 1995

19. Bachman TR, Lantz CA: Management of pediatric asthma and enuresis with probable traumatic etiology. p. 14. In Proceedings of the National Conference on Chiropractic Pediatrics. International Chiropractors Association, Arlington, VA, 1991

20. Nilsson N, Christiansen B: Prognostic factors in bronchial asthma in chiropractic practice. Chiropr J Aust 18:85, 1988

21. Masarsky CS, Weber M: Somatic dyspnea and the orthopedics of respiration. Chiropr Tech 3:26, 1991

22. Yates RG, Lamping CL, Abram NL, Wright C: Effects of chiropractic treatment on blood pressure and anxiety: a randomized, controlled trial. J Manipulative Physiol Ther 11:484, 1988

23. Plaugher G, Bachman TR: Chiropractic management of a hypertensive patient: a case study. J Manipulative Physiol Ther 16:544, 1993

24. Peterson KB: Two cases of spinal manipulation performed while the patient contemplated an associated stress event: the effect of the manipulation/contemplation on serum cholesterol levels in hypercholesterolemic subjects. Chiropr Tech 7:53, 1995

25. Lott GS, Sauer AD, Wahl DR, Kessinger J: ECG improvements following the combination of chiropractic adjustments, diet, and exercise therapy. Chiropr: J Res Chiropr Clin Invest 5:37, 1990

26. Pikalov AA, Kharin VV: Use of spinal manipulative therapy in the treatment of duodenal ulcer. J Manipulative Physiol Ther 17:310, 1994

27. DeBoer KF, Schutz M, McKnight ME: Acute effects of spinal manipulation on gastrointestinal myoelectric activity in conscious rabbits. Manual Med 3:85, 1988

28. Fallon JP, Lok BJ: Assessing the efficacy of chiropractic care in pediatric cases of pyloric stenosis. p. 72. In Proceedings of the National Conference on Chiro-

practic Pediatrics. International Chiropractors Association, Arlington, VA, 1994

29. Pluhar GR, Schobert PD: Vertebral subluxation and colic: a case study. Chiropr: J Chiropr Res Clin Invest 7:75, 1991

30. Hyman CA: Chiropractic adjustments and infantile colic: a case study. p. 65. In Proceedings of the National Conference on Chiropractic Pediatrics. International Chiropractors Association, Arlington, VA, 1994

31. Klougart N, Nilsson N, Jacobsen J: Infantile colic treated by chiropractors: a prospective study of 316 cases. J Manipulative Physiol Ther 12:281, 1989

32. Falk JW: Bowel and bladder dysfunction secondary to lumbar dysfunctional syndrome. Chiropr Tech 2:45, 1990

33. Eriksen K: Effects of upper cervical correction on chronic constipation. Chiropr Res J 3:19, 1994

34. Wagner T, Owen J, Malone E, Mann K: Irritable bowel syndrome and spinal manipulation: a case report. Chiropr Tech 7:139, 1995

35. Nyiendo J, Olsen E: Visit characteristics of 217 children attending a chiropractic college teaching clinic. J Manipulative Physiol Ther 11:78, 1988

36. Briggs L, Boone WR: Effects of a chiropractic adjustment on changes in pupillary diameter: a model for evaluating somatovisceral response. J Manipulative Physiol Ther 11:181, 1988

37. Gilman G, Bergstrand J: Visual recovery following chiropractic intervention. Chiropr: J Res Chiropr Clin Invest 6:61, 1990

38. Gorman RF: Automated static perimetry in chiropractic. J Manipulative Physiol Ther 16:481, 1993

39. Gorman RF: Monocular visual loss after closed head trauma: immediate resolution associated with spinal manipulation: J Manipulative Physiol Ther 16:308, 1993

40. Gorman RF, Anderson RL, Hilton D et al: Case report: spinal strain and visual perception deficit. Chiropr J Aust 24:131, 1994

41. Gorman RF: The treatment of presumptive optic nerve ischemia by spinal manipulation. J Manipulative Physiol Ther 18:172, 1995

42. Giesen JM, Center DB, Leach RA: An evaluation of chiropractic manipulation as a treatment of hyperactivity in children. J Manipulative Physiol Ther 12:353, 1989

43. Phillips CF: Case study: the effect of utilizing spinal manipulation and craniosacral therapy as the treatment approach for attention deficit hyperactivity disorder. p. 57. In Proceedings of the National Conference on Chiropractic and Pediatrics. International Chiropractors Association, Arlington, VA, 1991

44. Thomas MD, Wood J: Upper cervical adjustments may improve mental function. J Manual Med 6:215, 1992

45. Arme J: Effects of biomechanical insult correction on attention deficit disorder. J Chiropr Case Rep 1:6, 1993

46. Araghi HJ: Oral apraxia: a case study in chiropractic management. p. 34. In Proceedings of the National Conference on Chiropractic and Pediatrics. International Chiropractors Association, Arlington, VA, 1994

47. Woo CC: Traumatic spinal myoclonus. J Manipulative Physiol Ther 12:478, 1989

48. Duff BA: Documented chiropractic results on a case diagnosed as myoclonic seizures. J Chiropr Res Clin Invest 8:56, 1992

49. Goodman R: Cessation of seizure disorder: correction of the atlas subluxation complex. p. 46. In Proceedings of the National Conference on Chiropractic and Pediatrics. International Chiropractors Association, Arlington, VA, 1991

50. Hospers LA: EEG and CEEG studies before and after upper cervical or SOT category II adjustment in children after head trauma, in epilepsy, and in "hyperactivity." p. 84. In Proceedings of the National Conference on Chiropractic and Pediatrics. International Chiropractors Association, Arlington, VA, 1992

51. Stude DE, Mick T: Clinical presentation of a patient with multiple sclerosis and response to manual chiropractic adjustive therapies. J Manipulative Physiol Ther 16:595, 1993

52. Kirby SL: A case study: the effects of chiropractic on multiple sclerosis. Chiropr Res J 3:7, 1994

53. Woo CC: Post-traumatic myelopathy following flopping high jump: a pilot case of spinal manipulation. J Manipulative Physiol Ther 16:336, 1993

54. Plaugher G, Rowe DJ, Gohl RA: Chiropractic management of spinal fractures and dislocations with closed reduction methods: a report of nine cases. p. 79. In Wolk S (ed): Proceedings of the 1992 International Conference on Spinal Manipulation. Foundation for Chiropractic Education and Research, Arlington, VA, 1992.

55. Terrett AGJ: Cerebral dysfunction: a theory to explain some of the effects of chiropractic manipulation. Chiropr Tech 5:168, 1993

56. Brennan PC, Kokjohn K, Triano JJ et al: Immunologic correlates of reduced spinal mobility: preliminary

observations in a dog model. p. 118. In Wolk S (ed): Proceedings of the 1991 International Conference on Spinal Manipulation. Foundation for Chiropractic Education and Research, Arlington, VA, 1991

57. Brennan PC, Kokjohn K, Triano JJ et al: Enhanced phagocytic cell respiratory burst induced by spinal manipulation: potential role of substance P. J Manipulative Physiol Ther 14:399, 1991

58. Selano JL, Hightower BC, Pfleger B et al: The effects of specific upper cervical adjustments on the CD4 counts of HIV positive patients. Chiropr Res J 3:32, 1994

59. Allen JM: The effects of chiropractic on the immune system: a review of the literature. Chiropr J Aust 23:132, 1993

60. Van Breda WM, Van Breda JM: A comparative study of the health status of children raised under the health care models of chiropractic and allopathic medicine. J Chiropr Res 5:101, 1993

61. Rose-Aymon S, Aymon M, Prochaska-Moss G, et al.: The relationship between intensity of chiropractic care and incidence of childhood diseases. J Chiropr Res 1:70, 1989

62. Thomas RJ, Wilkinson M: Chiropractic care in adult spina bifida: a case report. Chiropr Tech 2:191, 1990

63. Araghi HJ: Juvenile myesthenia gravis: a case study in chiropractic management. p. 122. In Proceedings of the National Conference on Pediatrics and Chiropractic. International Chiropractors Association, Arlington, VA, 1993

64. Fidelibus JC: An overview of neuroimmunomodulation and a possible correlation with musculoskeletal system function. J Manipulative Physiol Ther 12:289, 1989

65. Nansel D, Szlazak M: Somatic dysfunction and the phenomenon of visceral disease simulation: a probable explanation for the apparent effectiveness of somatic therapy in patients presumed to be suffering from true visceral disease. J Manipulative Physiol Ther 18:379, 1995

66. Masarsky CS, Weber M: Stop paradigm erosion. J Manipulative Physiol Ther 14:323, 1991

67. Masarsky CS, Weber M: Cost-effectiveness research with a wide-angle lens. ICA Rev Chiro Jan/Feb: 9, 1993

68. Rogers AW: Textbook of Anatomy. Churchill Livingstone, Edinburgh, 1992

12

Nociceptors, Pain, and Chiropractic

Geoffrey Bove

*I*t may seem obvious that chiropractic and pain, or its relief, have a great deal to do with each other. Chiropractic doctors and students need a strong background in the basic concepts of the neurophysiology of pain. The purpose of this chapter is to present and clarify key issues in the basic science of pain and to direct the reader to more complete works in each general area. All of the following information is clinically relevant, although it may not seem so upon first reading. If the reader perseveres, the final section will be very rewarding, as the concepts presented will provide a scientific rationale for chiropractic treatment, including repeated and ancillary treatments.

Pain and associated terms are first defined. The nociceptor, a structure capable of transducing an event that can lead to pain, is then defined anatomically and functionally. Changes in the central nervous system (CNS) following noxious stimuli are overviewed. Finally, a clinical example demonstrates how these basic scientific concepts fit with the day-to-day practice of chiropractic, and a new hypothesis on a possible mechanism of action of manipulation will be presented.

DEFINITIONS

Taxonomy is important for any discipline, and discussions of pain are clearest when appropriate terms are used. The following terms were defined by a committee of experts from diverse specialties, in association with the International Association for the Study of Pain (IASP).

Pain An unpleasant sensory and emotional experience associated with actual or potential tissue damage, or described in terms of such damage, is what we call pain. Biologists agree that pain is a sensation, but its unpleasantness carries an emotional component. Thus, the foundation of this definition is that pain is subjective and that it may or may not have an objective component. It is possible to have pain without peripheral noxious stimuli; the definition does not link pain to any particular stimulus. Pain is defined by each person based on individual experiences, usually related to injury. However, a report of pain in the absence of apparent cause cannot be dismissed, since psychological reasons are often sufficient to cause pain.

Nociceptor The nociceptor is a receptor that is preferentially sensitive to a noxious stimulus or to a stimulus that would become noxious if prolonged. The nociceptor is a sensory structure that transduces noxious stimuli, communicating them to the central nervous system. Terms like pain sensor or pain receptor should be avoided. Some nociceptors respond to non-noxious stimuli as well, but their discussion falls outside the scope of this chapter.

205

Nociception Nociception is an activity in a neural structure considered capable of leading or contributing to a sensation of pain. Nociception is objective, as the activity can be measured, at least in the laboratory. Nociception does not necessarily lead to pain, especially in the peripheral nervous system. To cause pain, the activity must be of sufficient intensity or frequency to activate the second or higher-order neurons in the nociceptive pathway.

Noxious Stimulus Noxious is defined as harmful, and a noxious stimulus is defined in the laboratory as a stimulus that damages normal tissue. While there are stimuli that are noxious by this definition, but are not painful (such as radiation injury and cutting the wall of the small intestine), there is no descriptive term for this subset of noxious stimuli.

Nociceptive This adjective is not defined by the IASP but is often misused to modify *stimulus*. A stimulus cannot be nociceptive, but it can be noxious. However, an activated nociceptor is nociceptive.

Allodynia Pain due to a stimulus that does not normally induce pain is termed allodynia. It describes an objective response to clinical stimuli, when the normal stimulus can be tested elsewhere in the body. Allodynia is a loss of specificity of any sensory modality, with the final perception being pain. A simple example of allodynia is the pain following light brushing after a sunburn.

Hyperalgesia Hyperalgesia is an increased response to a stimulus that is normally painful. This term is distinct from allodynia. In allodynia, the modality of stimulus differs from the perceptual modality, whereas in hyperalgesia the modalities are the same.

NOCICEPTORS

The Defensive Function of Pain

There has been much debate over the existence of specific receptors for noxious stimuli, with researchers divided into two camps, proponents of the specificity theory versus the pattern theory of sensation. In brief, the specificity theory states that there are specific receptors for different sensory modalities, nociception leading to pain being one of them. The pattern or intensity theory presumes that primary afferents have similar responsiveness

and that the intensity of the response coupled with CNS integration of patterns of input leads to a particular sensation. Debates between the two groups have spawned much innovative experimentation. Although it is likely that both theories have their truths, the bulk of experimental studies indicate systematic differences in primary afferent unit characteristics and support the conclusion that pain is a sense, like touch or smell. Birder and Perl[2] recently published an excellent review on cutaneous sensory receptors. Combined with the recent reviews by Cervero[3] and Wall,[4] a broad perspective on this topic emerges.

Nociceptors serve a primordial function for an organism, providing information about harmful and potentially harmful events that may cause loss of function or life. Even simple organisms effectively have nociceptors; protochordates display the "coiling reflex," withdrawing from a noxious stimulus.[5] Through evolution, this defense mechanism was conserved and refined, though the basic function of signaling harmful events remained unchanged. Indeed, children born without nociceptors are repeatedly injured and usually die from complications of minor infections or trauma. Rats devoid of nociceptors through neonatal capsaicin treatment also have a short life span and are always bruised and unusually incautious.

On a moment-to-moment basis, nociceptors help us decide when to shift from a position that can cause a leg to "go to sleep" (possible beginnings of sciatic or peroneal neuropathy) and signal that we have a pebble in a shoe or that it is time to go to the dentist. Inflammation causes pain, perceived in part through activity of nociceptors that respond to mediators released by the process. In general, nociceptors exist where it makes sense for them to be, which is anywhere that the organism may be subjected to harmful stimuli.

Anatomy and Physiology of Nociceptors

Nociceptors in the peripheral nervous system are pseudounipolar dorsal root ganglion neurons with unmyelinated or thinly myelinated axons. The unmyelinated axons are referred to as C-fibers, with conduction velocities of 2.5 m/sec, and the thinly myelinated axons are referred to as A-axons, with conduction velocities of 2.5 to 40 m/sec. When innervating deep tissues such as muscle, they are referred to as group IV units (with C-fibers) and group III units (with A-fibers). The two projecting axons from a nociceptor cell body can be of different caliber, and an individual A-fiber can thin to C-fiber caliber as it passes distally.[6,7] Because the C-fiber and A-nociceptors are somewhat overlapping in function, for present purposes these will be considered together under the heading "nociceptor." There are many subcategories of nociceptors, but a thorough discussion of these is beyond the scope of this chapter, and the reader is referred to excellent reviews by Cervero,[3] Kumazawa,[8] Mense,[9] and Schaible and Grubb.[10]

The distal projection of nociceptive neurons terminates in what has classically been called a "free nerve ending." This is an unfortunate term, as it implies a nonspecialized structure; in truth, the specialization of these terminals remains elusive, especially for C-fiber nociceptors. Cutaneous nociceptors usually have one or more very small (less than 1-mm²) receptive points at which they respond most strongly, and these points are usually surrounded by a zone of lesser sensitivity. Nociceptive receptive fields in subcutaneous tissues have similar properties but have been found to branch repeatedly, thereby creating more complex receptive fields.[6]

As mentioned in the preceding definitions, the presence of these structures in itself does not confirm that the structure is a nociceptor; this has to be confirmed by a number of procedures, discussed briefly below. It should be kept in mind that axons belonging to the autonomic nervous system are also unmyelinated (C-fiber), but at this point are not known to have any afferent function. Afferent fibers that are intermingled with autonomic nerves, such as those accompanying splanchnic nerves, are not part of the autonomic nervous system, but are simply following a convenient path to their innervation target. Their cell bodies reside in the dorsal root ganglia, and they are part of the peripheral nervous system. Some of these neurons are probably nociceptors.

The skin is the largest organ in the body and is most subject to external stimuli. It follows that it is heavily innervated by nociceptors, as well as by sensory structures subserving other modalities. The densest nociceptive innervation is in the cornea, pointing to its relative importance and vulnerability.

Muscles, joint capsules, periosteum, and most viscera are also innervated by nociceptors, though less densely. This may be due to the lesser vulnerability of these tissues. Blood vessels are known to have a rich innervation, consisting of somatic afferent as well as autonomic fibers, and indeed these structures are painful when stimulated.[12] Recently, nerve sheaths and their accompanying blood vessels have been shown to have nociceptive nerve fibers.[11] Since blood vessels and nerves travel to virtually every tissue in the body, these units may provide a major source of nociceptive input. The paraspinal tissues, including the muscles, joints, and periosteum,[13–16] are innervated by small-diameter nerve fibers, and even small inclusion bodies of the zygapophyseal joint can become innervated.[17]

Small-caliber nerve fibers can be found microscopically using numerous staining procedures. They can also be stained with antibodies for various peptides, and a knowledge of the peptide functions gives insight into the function of the cell. However, functional testing using specific stimuli is usually necessary to prove that the cell is indeed nociceptive. Although functional information on the innervation of paraspinal tissues is scarce, the few available reports show a substantial nociceptor population, supporting the structures as potential pain sources.[11,13,18]

How Nociceptors Are Studied

Nociceptors can be studied in a variety of ways, in humans and animals. In humans, this can be as simple as applying a stimulus and getting a subjective report from the subject, but since the stimuli that are known to evoke responses from nociceptors also evoke responses from mechanoreceptors, and often thermoreceptors, the results are usually similarly nonspecific.

Capsaicin, the hot ingredient in peppers, has gained popularity because it is fairly specific for nociceptors. Numerous studies have used subdermal injections of capsaicin to study a variety of psychophysical parameters. In animals, this chemical has been used to give strength to the assertion that a receptor being tested is nociceptive. It is also possible to study individual nociceptors in both animals and humans. Typically, a nerve is dissected, and filaments 5–15 um are carefully teased from it and placed over electrodes connected to amplification and recording devices. This approach isolates a small number of axons; the process is repeated until only one unit can be recorded. The receptive field is then searched for and, after it is found, the receptive properties are determined. A similar process, called microneurography, can be done in human volunteers. Here, fine-needle electrodes are placed into nerves and the receptive fields characterized. Another process used in animals uses microelectrodes to record from individual cells in ganglia. A fine electrode is advanced into the ganglion, and the electrical activity of individual cells can be recorded. Much of the information that follows was gathered using methods similar to these.

Nociceptor Function

In normal tissue, nociceptors do not exhibit afferent activity at a level that reaches consciousness. Their activity in the absence of applied or evident stimuli is usually either absent or less than 0.5 Hz.[19] As noted above, nociceptors respond to damaging or potentially damaging stimuli. Experimentally, cells are characterized as nociceptors if they respond to applied noxious mechanical, thermal, and/or chemical stimuli. Noxious chemical stimuli include components found in inflammatory milieu, including bradykinin, histamine, serotonin, and hydrogen ions (protons, from low pH [acid][20] (Table 12-1). These substances have been tested on animal and human nociceptors in a variety of preparations,[21] evoking discharge from individual nociceptors and causing behavioral changes and reports of pain. While individual chemicals elicit responses from varying populations of nociceptors, the combination of mediators, found in vivo, is most effective.[20]

In diseased or damaged tissue, the properties of nociceptors can change. In a phenomenon called *sensitization*, they develop ongoing activity, their thresholds to noxious stimuli are reduced, and their receptive fields often increase in size. The effect can occur with even a brief stimulus, and can last for hours.[22] In skin, this effect is seen even in response to a small burn. The spontaneous pain and increased sensitivity of the damaged area, outlasting the stimulus, is mediated by sensitized nociceptors, though other receptor types may play a role during injury. Sensitization has been shown to occur in nociceptors from cutaneous and deep tissues, but the details of the process remain poorly understood.

Sympathetic stimulation affects nociceptors in certain situations. Under normal conditions, nociceptors do not respond to sympathetic stimulation or application of norepinephrine.[23,24] Sympathetic stimulation is sufficient, but not necessary, for nociceptor sensitization.[25,26] However, during chronic inflammation or following nerve injury, sympathetic stimulation becomes an effective stimulus,[27–31] but only for C-fiber nociceptors.[32] It is well known that pain and psychological stressors increase sympathetic discharge leading to increased levels of norepinephrine.[33–35] This supports our clinical observations that reducing pain and psychological stressors facilitate a more rapid recovery.

At the beginning of this century, it was discovered that electric stimulation of dorsal roots caused cutaneous vasodilation and plasma extravasation when the intensity was high enough to excite unmyelinated fibers.[36] This was termed the axon

Table 12-1. Chemical Sensitivites of Nociceptors

Substance	Source	Effect on Nociceptor
Acid and potassium	Damaged cells	Activation/sensitization
Serotonin	Platelets	Activation
Bradykinin	Plasma kininogen	Activation
Histamine	Mast cells	Activation
Prostaglandins	Arachidonic acid-damaged cells	Sensitization
Leukotrienes	Arachidonic acid-damaged cells	Sensitization
Substance P	Primary afferent neuron	Sensitization

(Modified from Fields,[85] with permission.)

reflex. Later, a population of nerves that mediated the response to injury was described, and termed the nocifensor system, referring to neurons that release initiators and mediators of inflammation into the skin.[37]

More recently, the nerves having axon reflexes were found to be nociceptors,[38] strongly suggesting that nociceptors have both sensory and efferent functions. The most important mediators (neuropeptides) released by these nerves are calcitonin gene-related peptide (CGRP) and substance P, which are co-localized in their terminals[39–41] (Fig. 12-1). Substance P and CGRP are potent vasodilators, and CGRP potentiates the effects of substance P.[42–47] Moreover, substance P contributes to nociceptor sensitization[48] and is thought to participate in the immune response.[49] When electrically stimulated proximally, nociceptor terminals release these peptides and a focal inflammation develops, called neurogenic inflammation.

Neurogenic inflammation has all the components of inflammation evoked by direct injury and has been shown to occur in vivo during experimental arthritis.[50] Nociceptors may be essential for an animal to mount an inflammatory response, through neurogenic inflammation. The development of peripheral experimental arthritis was shown to be at least in part dependent on the presence of afferent innervation.[50] It was also shown that the severity of experimental arthritis is reduced in animals depleted of nociceptors (through neonatal injection of capsaicin).[51] Finally, the increased cerebral blood flow due to meningitis is greatly attenuated by denervation of the primary afferents innervating the intracranial structures.[52] These lines of evidence support a critical role of nociceptors in our response to injury.

Spinal Cord Projections of Nociceptors

Nociceptive dorsal root ganglion neurons project into the spinal cord through Lissaur's tract, where they branch T-wise, sending branches 1 to 5 segments rostral and caudal (1 to 2 for C-fiber nociceptors, 1–5 for A-nociceptors).[53] C-fiber nociceptor branches terminate in laminae I and II outer,[54] and A fibers also project to laminae V and X.[55] Whereas appendicular tissues have unilateral representation,

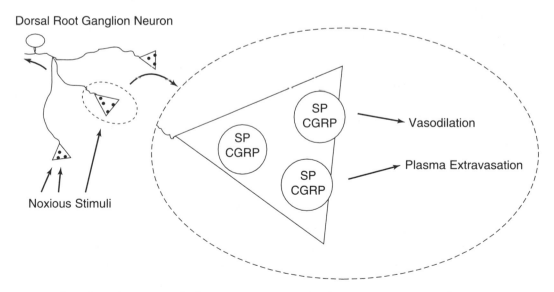

Fig. 12-1. Overview of plasma extravasation leading to neurogenic inflammation. Secretory vesicles containing substance P and calcitonin gene-related peptide release their contents when the mechanical, chemical, or thermal stimuli generates action potentials in the primary afferent branches. These substances act on blood vessels and mast cells to promote inflammation.

dorsal horn neurons have been recorded that respond to bilateral paraspinal tissue stimulation.[56,57] Most dorsal horn neurons are classified as wide dynamic range, meaning that they respond to noxious and innocuous stimuli. A smaller percentage of dorsal horn neurons is specific for nociception.

Central Mechanisms Related to Nociception

Obviously, nociceptors are not the only players in the perception of pain. In a classic study, Adriaensen et al.[58] demonstrated that while sustained skin pinching led to increasing reports of pain with time, the neural discharge from nociceptors supplying the area decreased. Explaining this paradox is difficult, but it is probable that other nociceptors are recruited and that the spinal cord and higher centers are changing their "gain" in response to the input from the nociceptors.

There is substantial evidence that peripheral noxious stimulation leads to changes in the central nervous system, collectively called spinal cord plasticity (for recent reviews, see Coderre et al.[59] and Woolf[60]). These changes lead to sensitization of CNS neurons and may cause hyperalgesia, allodynia, and spontaneous discharge, all of which can be maintained in the absence of afferent input from the original source. The type and intensity of stimulus necessary to produce these changes are unclear. Additionally, because spinal cord neurons have receptive fields that converge from many tissue types, sometimes bilaterally,[56] allodynia and hyperalgesia may occur in tissues remote from the injury. Indeed, these symptoms are observed among the plethora of acute and chronic back pain presentations; CNS plasticity could help explain these variable presentations.

When their peripheral axons are injured, the central projections of dorsal horn neurons can sprout into wider territories in the spinal cord. This occurs with neurons with myelinated or unmyelinated axons.[61,62] The sprouting of presumably nociceptive terminals in the superficial dorsal horn could explain hyperalgesia, since the discharge of an individual neuron would be transmitted to more second-order neurons, and their sum may lead to an increased perception of pain. Sprouting of larger fibers, usually non-nociceptive, into the laminae of the spinal cord usually reserved for nociceptor input may explain allodynia, since their discharge is now projecting to nociceptive neurons. Indeed, it is likely that the allodynia during causalgia is mediated by myelinated fibers.[63,64]

The principal concepts of spinal cord plasticity include windup, long-term potentiation (LTP), and long-term depression (LTD). A brief presentation of these processes follows; further details can be found in a review by Pockett.[65] *Windup* was coined for the phenomenon of increasing response of a spinal cord cell to repeated stimuli.[66] When depolarized by the primary afferent, dorsal horn neurons do not fully recover their resting potential before another volley from the primary afferent neuron arrives, and is thus more susceptible to firing (*facilitation*). This process typically lasts seconds to minutes. It is possible that repeated episodes of windup may induce LTP or LTD, but this has not been studied. LTP is similar to windup but lasts much longer, sometimes months. It requires a high-frequency conditioning discharge by the primary afferent neuron[67] and results in increased synaptic efficiency. It differs from windup in that the increased synaptic efficiency is not related to a change in the tonic membrane potential of the postsynaptic cells and involves changes in postsynaptic receptor properties, and perhaps increases in the number of receptors.[68]

Once established, nothing is known to reverse LTP except induction of LTD. LTD can be established by both high- and low-frequency conditioning stimuli and involves a long-lasting decrease in synaptic efficacy. It is hypothesized that LTP is responsible for chronic pain and, if so, LTD induction by stimulating an appropriate nerve may relieve it.[65] This may be the mechanism behind the anecdotal effectiveness of various forms of clinical electrical stimulation, but this remains to be demonstrated.

Molecular Changes Related to Nociception

When primary afferent neurons are stimulated, their central terminals release SP, CGRP, and glutamate onto central neurons. Besides transmitting information to higher-order neurons, genes in second- and higher-order neurons increase their expression of some proteins. Even a brief stimulus can induce some genes to increase their activity, a process called upregulation. The c-*fos* and c-*jun* genes have been intensely studied, and their protein products can be visualized indirectly using immunohisto-chemical techniques. Studies using these techniques have confirmed the projection of the nociceptive primary afferents, though the stimuli used are usually not specific for nociceptors.[69–72]

These protein products of c-*fos* and c-*jun* initiate a cascade resulting in the production of enkephalins and dynorphin by higher centers.[73] Enkephalin is an inhibitor of dorsal horn cells, but dynorphin has varied effects on spinal cord neurons, inhibiting one-third of them, sensitizing another one-third, and increasing their receptive field size.[74] This effect could also contribute to primary and secondary hyperalgesia and to chronic pain. The details of this process are being intensely studied.

CLINICAL APPLICATIONS

Nociception and Facet Syndrome

The preceding sections have presented information relevant to the initiation and maintenance of nociception and pain. How are these principles relevant to a patient's condition? Let us apply these mechanisms to a clinical condition—acute facet syndrome—and then explore a new hypothesis on the mechanism of injury leading to chronic pain.

Facet syndrome is described as a sprain of the zygapophyseal joints; it can either be acute or chronic. The acute form can follow an excessive movement in any plane or combination of planes of motion, and most likely involves pinching the articular capsule. This structure is relatively small—why can the pain be hard to localize and difficult to manage?

For our purposes, we will assume that the injury was restricted to the left L5-S1 joint and involved pinching of the joint capsule or an inclusion body. The joint capsules are innervated by nociceptors,[18,57] which would respond to the vigorous and harmful mechanical stimulation with a high-frequency discharge. It would also lead to mast cell degranulation, releasing histamine that heightens the response. The proximal terminals of the primary afferent neurons would release substance P and CGRP into the surrounding tissue, which could diffuse into the joint space. This, in turn, would lead to the development of inflammation in the joint and capsule. Inflammation is characterized by the increased concentrations of bradykinin, serotonin, histamine, prostaglandins and by a lowered pH, all

of which are effective stimuli for nociceptors. Inflammation is also characterized by hyperemia, which raises the local temperature. Although the temperatures reached during inflammation may not be sufficient to stimulate nociceptors, it is likely that the increased temperature would facilitate the effect of the other stimuli. A vicious cycle is created, and surrounding nociceptors may be recruited. Also, we must remember that the nociceptors that have been damaged or sensitized may be responding to products of increased sympathetic stimulation.

Reasons for Extension of Symptoms

So far we have a patient who should have only focal back pain. So, why do these patients usually present with poorly defined symptoms that seem to extend to other areas? Besides the local effect, the nociceptors would stimulate neurons in the CNS (otherwise there would be no perception at all). The innervation of the facet joint in question is through the posterior ramus of the spinal nerve from L4 to S1, and these nerves likely synapse with neurons in cord levels L2 to S2; it should be emphasized here that the projection from paraspinal tissues is bilateral.[56,57] This has two possible effects: first, the neurons are receiving input from many structures, and therefore the localization of the symptom will be poor; second, this may cause axon reflexes in any tissue innervated by these levels, causing release of substance P and CGRP by antidromic mechanisms and the development of neurogenic inflammation to some degree. In presumed facet joint syndrome cases, paraspinal, gluteal, and even leg pain are common and could be explained by this mechanism.

The initial incident was probably severe for the tissue, but patients usually present with symptoms that can be elicited by maneuvers that do not usually cause pain. This allodynia, which gives us positive orthopedic and neurologic tests, is probably mediated by changes in the peripheral and central nervous systems as outlined above. The initial barrages sensitized the primary afferent neuron and led to windup and LTP in the spinal cord and possibly higher centers. This left the patient with hypersensitive tissues, so that any movements could reinitiate or aggravate the processes, including any processes in other remote sites. (This is not to say that all movements are bad; there is substantial evidence that stimulating mechanoreceptors inhibits nociceptor activity, at least in the acute situation, and may be beneficial. Also, it is known that movements direct proper orientation of collagenous tissue.) Also, the neurogenic inflammation could lead to allodynia and hyperalgesia in the referred symptom areas.

The above sequence of events describes the pain-dysfunction cycles often used to illustrate musculoskeletal disease processes. It is thought that clinical efforts directed at breaking these cycles will aid the patient's recovery. However, most musculoskeletal injuries do get better on their own, probably through the gradual subsiding of the processes described. One major problem with the theory is that it does not explain a major population of musculoskeletal pain sufferers—those with chronic pain in the absence of detectable pathology. In many cases, these patients are thought to have suffered permanent plastic changes in the CNS, leading to the perception of spontaneous pain thought to be originating from a peripheral site. However, it seems likely that a persistent peripheral pathology has remained undetected and maintains the peripheral noxious input and associated pain.

Role of Nervi Nervorum

Nerves that innervate the nerve sheaths were described as early as 1884[75] and were described more recently by Hromada.[76] Although their existence has been hypothesized as contributory in neuropathic and nerve trunk pain[77,78] this anatomic feature has received little subsequent attention. Recently, nociceptors were characterized that innervate the sheaths of nerves and the connective tissue surrounding the neurovascular bundles.[11,79] Appropriately termed nervi nervorum, these nociceptors were found to have substantial branching both within the neurovascular bundle and to other tissue types, such as muscle and tendon sheath. They were found to be located preferentially at fascial foramina, and to respond to traction and direct pressure.[11]

Mechanisms of Axon Injury

These nervi nervorum axons are at particularly high risk of injury from traction and friction when they pierce a connective tissue plane or bony foramen, such as the thoracolumbar fascia or intervertebral foramen. In the facet syndrome example, the branches of the spinal nerve must pierce the inter-transverse ligament to reach its target innervation.[80] There is ample opportunity for nociceptive axons innervating this nerve sheath to become injured during a facet syndrome.

First, they can be injured simply by the traction placed on them during excessive movements. Second, they can be damaged by chronic friction due to any scar tissue formed during the repair of the initial injury. (Patients in general limit their movements to reduce pain, and tissue healing in the absence of motion is undirected and leads to irregular collagen formation, and therefore improper tissue biomechanics.) The scar tissue formation is nonspecific and can involve the nerve bed, in which the nerve is supposed to move freely. Any adhesion between a nerve and its bed will focus shear forces on the interface, the nerve sheath. Shear forces are also an effective noxious stimulus for nociceptive nervi nervorum. Facet joints that are biomechanically deranged as a result of injury often hypertrophy, causing friction injuries and contributing to entrapment neuropathies of the spinal nerve. It is reasonable to apply this accepted etiology to much smaller nerves.

Innervation of Scar Tissue

Perhaps most importantly, damaged axons will regrow, and partial nerve injury leads to what has been termed a "neuroma in continuity."[81] This regrowth is thought to innervate scar tissue preferentially. Since all tissues have nerves passing through them, and because it is likely that they all are innervated, this effect could occur at some level during many types of injury. It is this combination, the innervation of scar tissue in a nerve bed by sprouts of damaged nervi nervorum, that may explain patients who have "healed," yet have a persistent, movement-related source of nociceptive input adequate to maintain allodynia and hyperalgesia through local and central mechanisms. These patients will likely exhibit few objective findings using standard orthopedic tests and are unlikely to recover without active treatment. Figure 12-2 presents a summary of this proposed mechanism.

Manual Therapy: Theorized Effects on Adhesions

What can be done for this condition? Many manual therapy techniques use forces adequate to break up

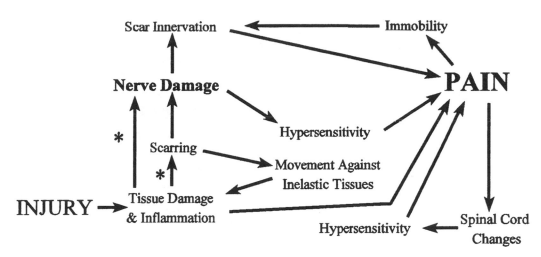

Fig. 12-2. Hypothesized cascade of events leading to chronic pain from injury of nervi nervorum. Manipulation is thought to interrupt the process (asterisks).

adhesions. Some even hypothesize that this is the mechanism behind their efficacy. Indeed, if there is an adhesion or an innervated scar, it makes sense that removing it could lead to a resolution of symptoms. However, surgical intervention intrinsically leads to further scar tissue formation, though surgical excision of scar tissue in the intervertebral foramen has been shown to reduce leg pain and positive straight-leg raises.[82–84] It is reasonable to believe that manual therapies, including joint manipulation, do break similar adhesions, removing the source of nociceptive input by breaking the axons transmitting the impulses. Of course, this is an injury in itself; therefore, repeated motion of the area, possibly through further manipulation, is probably necessary to prevent re-formation of the problem. Directed movements of the injured parts by the patient may also be necessary to promote proper orientation of the repairing tissue, and more importantly to prevent the sprouting nociceptor from extending beyond the nerve sheath.

PAIN AND NOCICEPTION: KEY CONCEPTS IN REVIEW

Pain and nociception are related but different events. Neural events leading to pain usually involve activation of nociceptors innervating a threatened or damaged tissue. Once activated, nociceptors transmit information to the spinal cord for process-

ing and may initiate and mediate inflammation. The response properties of nociceptors are plastic; typically, they become more sensitive with further stimulation. This sensitization also occurs in the CNS, with the development of windup and long-term potentiation. The projection of nociceptors in the spinal cord supports the observation of referred pain, and neurogenic inflammation that can actually cause these sites to have inflammation through axon reflexes in the absence of pathology.

An example of the possible roles played by these processes was presented, along with the hypothesis that damage to the nervi nervorum may lead to a persistent source of nociceptive input in the absence of detectable pathology. It is possible that methods directed at breaking up adhesions, such as spinal manipulation, work through these mechanisms to break the pain-dysfunction cycles of chronic pain.

Terminology

afferent
allodynia
axon reflex
conduction velocity
efferent
group III nociceptor
group IV nociceptor
hyperalgesia
nerve sheath

nervi nervorum
neurogenic inflammation
neuroma
nociception
nociceptive
nociceptor
noxious stimulus
ongoing activity
pain
plasma extravasation
receptive field
sensitization

Review Questions

1. What is the difference between pain and nociception?

2. What is the conduction velocity of the neurons that subserve nociception?

3. What is an axon reflex, and how is it related to neurogenic inflammation?

4. Where are nociceptors located?

5. Damage to nociceptor axons leads to what anatomic changes?

6. To what levels in the spinal cord can a C-fiber nociceptor projecting through the L4 dorsal root project?

7. What is a possible clinical effect of long-term potentiation?

8. Describe the nervi nervorum.

9. What nociceptors are likely to be activated during a positive straight-leg raise?

10. How can light brushing cause pain?

Concept Questions

1. A runner presents with diffuse back and buttock pain, worse on the left, and left posterior calf pain. Onset followed an increase in training intensity. Examination demonstrates excessive left talar eversion with taut and tender left external hip rotators. You correctly make a descriptive diagnosis of piriformis syndrome, secondary to internal rotation of the leg. Explain the development of symptoms using the concepts presented in this chapter.

2. A local herbalist gives you a poultice that he claims reduces the pain of sprains. You use it on the next patient that you see, and not only does the patient report less pain within 30 minutes, but you observe that local redness and swelling are reduced. Being familiar with nociceptor physiology, you think that it may be affecting them directly. How would you investigate your hypothesis?

3. A patient presents with bilateral foot pain. The symptoms started on the right; after an exacerbation 2 weeks ago, the left side also started hurting. Your examination indicates a biomechanical lesion on the right, but a normal left foot, though it is somewhat tender to palpation. You make a diagnosis of right plantar fasciitis. Why does the patient have symptoms on the left? Do you treat the left foot?

REFERENCES

1. Merskey H, Bogduk N: Classification of Chronic Pain. IASP Press, Seattle, 1994

2. Birder LA, Perl ER: Cutaneous sensory receptors. J Clin Neurophysiol 11:534, 1994

3. Cervero F: Sensory innervation of the viscera: peripheral basis of visceral pain. Physiol Rev 74:95, 1994

4. Wall PD: Comments after 30 years of the gate control theory. Pain Forum 5:12, 1996

5. Carew TJ, Walters ET, Kandel ER: Classical conditioning in a simple withdrawal reflex in Aplysia californica. J Neurosci 1:1426, 1981

6. Duclaux R, Mei N, Ranieri F: Conduction velocity along the afferent vagal dendrites: a new type of fiber. J Physiol (Lond) 260:487, 1976

7. Morrison JFB: Splanchnic slowly adapting mechanoreceptors with punctate receptive fields in the mesentery and gastrointestinal tract of the cat. J Physiol (Lond) 233:349, 1973

8. Kumazawa T: Functions of the nociceptive primary neurons. Jpn J Physiol 40:1, 1990

9. Mense S: Nociception from skeletal muscle in relation to clinical pain. Pain 54:241, 1993

10. Schaible HG, Grubb BD: Afferent and spinal mechanisms of joint pain. Pain 55:5, 1993

11. Bove GM, Light AR: Unmyelinated nociceptors of rat paraspinal tissues. J Neurophysiol 73:1752, 1995

12. Bazett HC, McGlone B: Note on the pain sensations which accompany deep punctures. Brain 51:18, 1928

13. Cavanaugh JM, El-Bohy A, Hardy WN et al: Sensory innervation of the soft tissues of the lumbar spine of the rat. J Orthop Res 7:378, 1989

14. El-Bohy A, Cavanaugh JM, Getchell ML et al: Localization of substance P and neurofilament immunoreactive fibers in the lumbar facet joint capsule and supraspinous ligament of the rabbit. Brain Res 460:379, 1988

15. Giles LGF, Harvey AR: Immunohistological demonstration of nociceptors in the capsule and synovial folds of human zygapophyseal joints. Br J Rheumatol 26:362, 1987

16. Giles LGF, Taylor JR, Cockson A: Human zygapophyseal joint synovial folds. Acta Anat (Basel) 126:110, 1986

17. Giles LGF, Taylor JR: Intra-articular synovial protrusions in the lower lumbar apophyseal joints. Bull Hosp J Dis Orthop Inst 42:248, 1982

18. Yamashita T, Cavanaugh JM, El-Bohy AA et al: Mechanosensitive afferent units in the lumbar facet joint. J Bone Joint Surg 72A:865, 1990

19. Lundberg LE, Jorum E, Holm E, Torebjörk HE: Intraneural electrical stimulation of cutaneous nociceptive fibres in humans: effects of different pulse patterns on magnitude of pain. Acta Physiol Scand 146:41, 1992

20. Reeh P: Chemical excitation and sensitization of nociceptors. p. 119. In Urban L (ed): Cellular Mechanisms of Sensory Processing. Springer-Verlag, Berlin, 1994

21. Handwerker HO, Reeh PW: Nociceptors in animals. p. 1. In Besson JM, Guilbaud G, Ollat H (eds): Peripheral Neurons in Nociception: Physiopharmacological Aspects. John Libbey Eurotext, Paris, 1994

22. Perl ER, Kumazawa T, Lynn B, Kenins P: Sensitization of high threshold receptors with unmyelinated (C) afferent fibers. Prog Brain Res 43:263, 1976

23. Shea VK, Perl ER: Failure of sympathetic stimulation to affect responsiveness of rabbit polymodal nociceptors. J Neurophysiol 54:513, 1985

24. Barasi S, Lynn B: Effects of sympathetic stimulation on mechanoreceptive and nociceptive afferent units from the rabbit pinna. Brain Res 378:21, 1986

25. Sanjue H, Jun Z: Sympathetic facilitation of sustained discharge of polymodal nociceptors. Pain 38:85, 1989

26. Koltzenburg M, Kress M, Reeh PW: The nociceptor sensitization by bradykinin does not depend on sympathetic neurons. Neuroscience 46:465, 1992

27. Devor M, Jänig W: Activation of myelinated afferents ending in a neuroma by stimulation of the sympathetic supply in the rat. Neurosci Lett 24:43, 1981

28. Sato J, Perl ER: Adrenergic excitation of cutaneous pain receptors induced by peripheral nerve injury. Science 251:1608, 1991

29. Koltzenburg M, Budweiser S, Kees S et al: Receptive properties of nociceptors in a peripheral neuropathy. Soc Neurosci Abs 19:325, 1993

30. Selig DK, Meyer RA, Campbell JN: Noradrenergic excitation of cutaneous nociceptors two weeks after ligation of spinal nerve L7 in monkey. Soc Neurosci Abs 19:326, 1993

31. Sato J, Suzuki S, Iseki T, Kumazawa T: Adrenergic excitation of cutaneous nociceptors in chronically inflamed rats. Neurosci Lett 164:225, 1993

32. Bossut DF, Perl ER: Effects of nerve injury on sympathetic excitation of a delta mechanical nociceptors. J Neurophysiol 73:1721, 1995

33. Cannon WB: Bodily Changes in Pain, Hunger, Fear, and Rage. New York, D. Appleton and Co., 1929

34. Selye H: The general adaptation syndrome and diseases of adaptation. Yearbook Pathol Clin Pathol 7, 1950

35. Ecker A: Norepinephrine in reflex sympathetic dystrophy: an hypothesis. Clin J Pain 5:313, 1989

36. Bayliss WM: On the origin from the spinal cord of the vasodilator fibres of the hind-limb, and on the nature of these fibres. J Physiol (Lond) 26:173, 1900

37. Lewis T: The nocifensor system of nerves and its reactions. BMJ 1:431, 1937

38. Kenins P: Identification of the unmyelinated sensory nerves which evoke plasma extravasation in response to antidromic stimulation. Neurosci Lett 25:137, 1981

39. Alvarez FJ, Cervantes C, Blasco I et al: Presence of calcitonin gene-related peptide (CGRP) and substance P (SP) immunoreactivity in intraepidermal free nerve endings of cat skin. Brain Res 442:391, 1988

40. Gulbenkian S, Merighi A, Wharton J et al: Ultrastructural evidence for the coexistence of calcitonin gene-related peptide and substance P in secretory vesicles of peripheral nerves in the guinea pig. J Neurocytol 15:535, 1986

41. Gibbins IL, Furness JB, Costa M et al: Co-localization of calcitonin gene-related peptide-like immunoreactivity with substance P in cutaneous, vascular and visceral sensory neurons of guinea pigs. Neurosci Lett 57:125, 1985

42. Brain SD, Tippins JR, Morris HR et al: Potent vasodilator activity of calcitonin gene-related peptide in human skin. J Invest Dermatol 87:533, 1986

43. Holzer P: Peptidergic sensory neurons in the control of vascular functions: mechanisms and significance in the cutaneous and splanchnic beds. Rev Physiol Biochem Pharmacol 121:49, 1992

44. Kenins P, Hurley JV, Bell C: The role of substance P in the axon reflex in the rat. Br J Dermatol 111:551, 1984

45. LeGreves P, Nyberg F, Terenius L, Hökfelt T: Calcitonin gene-related peptide is a potent inhibitor of substance P degradation. Eur J Pharmacol 115:309, 1985

46. Uddman R, Edvinsson L, Ekblad E, Hakanson R, Sundler F: Calcitonin gene-related peptide (CGRP): perivascular distribution and vasodilatory effects. Regul Pept 15:1, 1986

47. Ishida-Yamamoto A, Tohyama M: Calcitonin gene-related peptide in the nervous tissue. Prog Neurobiol 33:335, 1989

48. Cohen RH, Perl ER: Contributions of arachidonic acid derivatives and substance P to the sensitization of cutaneous nociceptors. J Neurophysiol 64:457, 1990

49. Mantyh PW: Substance P and the inflammatory and immune response. Ann NYork Acad Sci 632:263, 1991

50. Rees H, Sluka KA, Westlund KN, Willis WD: Do dorsal root reflexes augment peripheral inflammation? Neuroreport 5:821, 1994

51. Levine JD, Dardick SJ, Roizen MF, Helms C, Basbaum AI: Contribution of sensory afferents and sympathetic efferents to joint injury in experimental arthritis. J Neurosci 6:3423, 1986

52. Weber JR, Angstwurm K, Bove GM et al: The trigeminal nerve augments regional cerebral blood flow during experimental bacterial meningitis. J Cereb Blood Flow Metab 16:1319–1324, 1996

53. Light AR: Normal anatomy and physiology of the spinal cord dorsal horn. Appl Neurophysiol 51:78, 1988

54. Sugiura Y, Lee CL, Perl ER: Central projections of identified, unmyelinated (C) afferent fibers innervating mammalian skin. Science 234:358, 1986

55. Light AR, Perl ER: Spinal termination of functionally identified primary afferent neurons with slowly conducting myelinated fibers. J Comp Neurol 186:133, 1979

56. Gillette RG, Kramis RC, Roberts WJ: Characterization of spinal somatosensory neurons having receptive fields in lumbar tissues of cats. Pain 54:85, 1993

57. Gillette RG, Kramis RC, Roberts WJ: Spinal projections of cat primary afferent fibers innervating lumbar facet joints and multifidus muscle. Neurosci Lett 157:67, 1993

58. Adriaensen H, Gybels J, Handwerker HO, Van Hees J: Nociceptor discharges and sensations due to noxious mechanical stimulation—a paradox. Hum Neurobiol 3:53, 1984

59. Coderre TJ, Katz J, Vaccarino AL, Melzack R: Contribution of central neuroplasticity to pathological pain: review of clinical and experimental evidence. Pain 52:259, 1993

60. Woolf CJ: Recent advances in the pathophysiology of acute pain. Br J Anaesth 63:139, 1989

61. Cameron AA, Pover CM, Willis WD, Coggeshall RE: Evidence that fine primary afferent axons innervate a wider territory in the superficial dorsal horn following peripheral axotomy. Brain Res 575:151, 1992

62. Woolf CJ, Shortland P, Coggeshall RE: Peripheral nerve injury triggers central sprouting of myelinated afferents. Nature 355:75, 1992

63. Campbell JN, Raja SN, Meyer RA, Mackinnon SE: Myelinated afferents signal the hyperalgesia associated with nerve injury. Pain 32:89, 1988

64. Price DD, Bennett GJ, Rafii A: Psychophysiological observations on patients with neuropathic pain relieved by a sympathetic block. Pain 36:273, 1989

65. Pockett S: Spinal cord synaptic plasticity and chronic pain, review. Anesth Analg 80:173, 1995

66. Mendell LM: Physiological properties of unmyelinated fiber projection to the spinal cord. Exp Neurol 16:316, 1966

67. Randic M, Jiang MC, Cerne R: Long-term potentiation and long-term depression of primary afferent neurotransmission in the rat spinal cord. J Neurosci 13:5228, 1993

68. Bliss TVP, Collingridge GL: A synaptic model of memory: long-term potentiation in the hippocampus. Nature 361:31, 1993

69. Bullitt E: Induction of c-fos-like protein within the lumbar spinal cord and thalamus of the rat following peripheral stimulation. Brain Res 493:391, 1989

70. Bullitt E: Somatotopy of spinal nociceptive processing. J Comp Neurol 312:279, 1991

71. Menétrey D, Gannon A, Levine JD, Basbaum AI: Expression of c-fos protein in interneurons and projection neurons of the rat spinal cord in response to noxious somatic, articular, and visceral stimulation. J Comp Neurol 285:177, 1989

72. Swett JE, Woolf CJ: The somatotopic organization of primary afferent terminals in the superficial laminae of the dorsal horn of the rat spinal cord. J Comp Neurol 231:66, 1985

73. Iadorola MJ, Brady LS, Draisci G, Dubner R: Enhancement of dynorphin gene expression in spinal cord following experimental inflammation: stimulus specificity, behavioral parameters and opioid receptor binding. Pain 35:313, 1988

74. Hylden JLK, Nahin RL, Traub RJ, Dubner R: Effects of spinal kappa-opioid receptor agonists on the responsiveness of nociceptive superficial dorsal horn neurons. Pain 44:187, 1991

75. Horsley V: On the existence of sensory nerves and nerve endings in nerve trunks. Proc R Med Chir Soc 196, 1884

76. Hromada J: On the nerve supply of the connective tissue of some peripheral nervous tissue system components. Acta Anat (Basel) 55:343, 1963

77. Asbury AK, Fields HL: Pain due to peripheral nerve damage: an hypothesis. Neurology 34:1587, 1984

78. Zochodne DW: Epineurial peptides: a role in neuropathic pain? Can J Neurol Sci 20:69, 1993

79. Bove GM, Light AR: Calcitonin gene-related peptide and peripherin immunoreactivity in nerve sheaths. Somatosens Mot Res 12:49, 1995

80. Bogduk N, Twomey LT: Clinical Anatomy of the Lumbar Spine. Churchill Livingstone, Melbourne, 1987

81. Bennett GJ: An animal model of neuropathic pain: a review. Muscle Nerve 16:1040, 1993

82. Epstein JA, Epstein BS, Rosenthal AD et al: Sciatica caused by nerve root entrapment in the lateral recess: the superior facet syndrome. J Neurosurg 36:584, 1972

83. Epstein JA, Epstein BS, Lavine LS et al: Lumbar nerve root compression at the intevertebral foramina caused by arthritis of the posterior facets. J Neurosurg 39:362, 1973

84. Lerman VI, Drasnin HV: Adhesive lesions of the nerve root in the dural orifice as a cause of sciatica. Surg Neurol 4:229, 1975

85. Fields HL: Pain McGraw-Hill, New York, 1985

13

Appropriate Care, Ethics, and Practice Guidelines

J.F. McAndrews

A profession's maturity is defined by the knowledge and behavior of its members. True professionalism in health care requires that interest in economics be subordinated to the best interest of the patient, that guidelines based on objective information be developed and respected, that members of the profession be knowledgeable about the scientific literature relating to their practice, that research be encouraged so that the new knowledge it reveals can accrue to the benefit of present and future patients, and that those who aspire to professional stature interact with each other in a professional rather than political manner. By these measures, the chiropractic profession is now far more mature than a generation ago, but still falls well short of its potential.

Chiropractic has made tremendous strides in the past quarter-century with regard to educational standards (see Ch. 2) and the development of a solid scientific research base (see Chs. 10 and 11). As a result, chiropractic has been recognized increasingly as a valid form of health care by government agencies, private insurers, and the health care community as a whole. Full integration into the mainstream health care system, however, still appears to be a generation or two away.

Why? Aftereffects of the decades-long antichiropractic boycott by organized medicine (for which the U.S. Supreme Court in 1990 affirmed liable the American Medical Association [AMA]) still cast a pall over chiropractors' relations with other health professions and the general public. But it is too easy to blame others. Chiropractors must also look within.

Substantial improvement is required in two critical areas: respect for reasonable, objectively based practice guidelines, and development of a profession-wide ethic of financial fairness.

PRACTICE GUIDELINES: WHAT THEY ARE AND WHY THEY ARE NEEDED

The Political Imperative

By the early 1990s, chiropractic leaders understood that a significantly more fact-based era had begun, in which political muscle and agility could not be relied upon to take the place of objectively agreed upon measures of clinical efficacy. The profession faced an urgent need to design and develop its own practice guidelines. Failure to do so would have allowed the resultant vacuum to be filled by default, with guidelines prepared by medical directors, nurses, MBAs, attorneys, managed care organizations, insurers, and third-party payers.

Guidelines for Chiropractic Quality Assurance and Practice Parameters,[1] which grew out of the 1992 Mercy Center Consensus Conference, placed the chiropractic profession at the cutting edge of the guidelines movement. In contrast to professions that attempted to delay the inevitable or, like the orthopedic surgeons, that allowed their guidelines to be prepared by a single individual, chiropractors convened a consensus conference representing an appropriate balance of opinions in the profession and then debated the issues until consensus was reached. Minority opinions were included in the published report, which is specifically intended to be a living document, open to ongoing revision as new information emerges.

Because chiropractic proactively moved forward with this project, the specter of chiropractic guidelines prepared by outsiders was averted. The consensus conference, by bringing together so diverse a profession, set a positive tone for chiropractic's future.

The Need for Objectivity

Science seeks to counter the well-known inclination of the human mind to fool itself. That a particular patient, or group of patients, recovers from back pain or any other ailment after receiving chiropractic adjustments does not necessarily indicate a cause-and-effect relationship between the adjustments and the recovery. The placebo effect and the natural course of the illness must be factored into the equation.

To clarify these crucial issues, practice guidelines identify and organize available hard data in the peer-reviewed literature. Where such data are lacking or inconclusive, a consensus process is used to determine which procedures are safe and appropriate. One of the great virtues of the guidelines development process is that identifying areas in which insufficient objective information exists encourages outcome studies and other research in these weak areas.

Most of chiropractic history has been marked by a freewheeling empiricism in which individual practitioners developed new techniques, applied them immediately in patient care, and then taught them to as many colleagues as possible. This in some ways

has served the profession well—many current chiropractic techniques originated in this manner. But anecdotal evidence, no matter how powerful, does not qualify as proof. All chiropractic methods, and those of other health care disciplines, must eventually be subjected to rigorous scientific investigation, facing what Thomas Huxley called "the great tragedy of science: the destruction of a beautiful hypothesis by an ugly fact." Such scrutiny can cause intense uncertainty as the process unfolds. It is possible that some widely used chiropractic methods may fail to pass muster. In the current era, however, there is no good alternative to this system. If chiropractors wish to become full participants in the health care mainstream, they must abide by the emerging rules of the level playing field.

Because the Mercy conferees required that all claims either be documented in the scientific literature or acquire a measurable and significant level of consensus, the report they produced has stood up exceedingly well when presented to agencies that require high standards of documentation, such as the Agency for Health Care Policy and Research (AHCPR) panel on acute low back problems in adults. Professions that appeared before the AHCPR panel lacking such documentation were markedly less successful than chiropractic. In the long run, such documentation spells the difference between integration and isolation. No responsible professional wishes to permanently relegate his profession to the fringe.

Key Areas in the Mercy Guidelines

The Mercy Guidelines address all key areas of chiropractic practice in a manner consistent with AHCPR procedures for guideline development. They cover a wide range of diagnostic and therapeutic procedures employed by contemporary chiropractors, determining in each case whether such procedures are supported by scientific data, evaluating and rating the quality of that data, and, in the absence of conclusive data, seeking a consensus of clinical opinion.

The Mercy Guidelines include the following areas:

1. History and physical examination
2. Diagnostic imaging
3. Instrumentation

4. Clinical laboratory
5. Record keeping and patient consents
6. Clinical impression
7. Modes of care
8. Frequency and duration of care
9. Reassessment
10. Outcome assessment
11. Collaborative care
12. Contraindications and complications
13. Preventive maintenance and public health
14. Professional development

Addressing all these topics in detail is beyond the scope of this chapter. However, practicing chiropractors and chiropractic students have a responsibility to read the Guidelines and to consider the appropriateness of bringing their practices into accord with the consensus recommendations.

Critiques of the Mercy Guidelines

Probably the most common criticism of the Guidelines is that the document is difficult to read. Unfortunately, documents prepared by committees are seldom hailed for their high literary quality. Most other critiques of the Guidelines identify certain perceived failings, which on deeper analysis turn out to be failures of the profession, not of the Guidelines. These include concerns about inadequate research, inadequate objective thinking, and inadequate organization of results and outcomes. All these need improvement, but guidelines can only reflect the current state of professional development. Furthermore, while imperfections are certainly present, *Guidelines for Chiropractic Quality Assurance and Practice Parameters* compares quite favorably with guidelines prepared by other professions and specialties.

Other criticisms of the Mercy Guidelines relate to recommendations on duration of care, the appropriate number of visits for various conditions, and the suggestion that cases not demonstrating clear improvement within a 1-month period be referred out. In particular, strong concerns have been raised about insurance companies using the Guidelines as a basis for cutting off reimbursement for chiropractic care sooner than is warranted.

Instances undoubtedly exist where the Guidelines have been misused, whether from malice or igno-

rance. The flaw, however, lies not in the Guidelines themselves, but in their misuse. The Mercy document specifically states that the purpose of such recommendations is "to assist the clinician in decision making based on the expectation of outcome for the *uncomplicated case* [emphasis in original]. They are *not* designed as a prescriptive or cookbook procedure for determining the absolute frequency and duration of treatment/care for any specific case."[1] Furthermore, guidelines should not be confused with standards. Guidelines are voluntary, standards are mandatory.

DURATION OF CARE

Duration of care is a major unresolved issue in chiropractic. Depending on which chiropractor a patient sees, the recommended course of care for the same condition may vary drastically, from several visits with one doctor to several dozen—sometimes hundreds—with another. Such variations appear in all regions, among graduates of all chiropractic colleges, and in urban, suburban, and rural settings.[2,3] Reducing these variations is crucial to the further advancement of the chiropractic profession.

Abuses of the System

The question of why a patient needs to return to a chiropractor for a series of visits is legitimate and controversial. Like it or not, chiropractors have a reputation for lengthy courses of care. In the absence of a rational, patient-centered explanation, the unfortunate corollary assumption is that such extended care is primarily for the financial benefit of the chiropractor. Sadly, in some instances this is indeed the case. Let us confront such abuses of the system first, and then explore how duration of care can be addressed within a patient-centered framework.

During the early 1990s, I participated in a retrospective review of a year's already-paid chiropractic claims, in which I saw page after page of outrageous overtreatment by chiropractors. In one case there were 278 visits for a diagnosis of mitral valve disorder; in another, 155 visits for a uterine infection. *Such doctors are a danger to society.* In another case, a chiropractor had taken 70 radiographs of a 12-year-old girl. In my opinion, this person should be behind bars.

Honest chiropractors pay a terrible price for the fraud merchants among us. One particularly disturbing example of overutilization and its consequences involves a highly respected health maintenance organization (HMO), John Deere, which initially included chiropractic benefits in its health plan. During the first year of Deere's HMO operation, two doctors of chiropractic, involved in the highly dubious practice of "forgiving" deductibles and copayments, so that their patients had no out-of-pocket expenses, billed the HMO $1 million each! Almost immediately, chiropractic benefits were removed from the plan. The damage caused by unscrupulous practitioners such as these is incalculable. Many thousands of people with a genuine need for chiropractic care will not receive it as a result of these practitioners' unmitigated greed.

Unethical practices like these have created a situation where all chiropractors are tarred with the same brush. The title "doctor of chiropractic" is too often associated with "scam artist" or "trumped-up" fraudulent insurance claims. In addition, when these cases of abuse are subjected to the glare of media attention, chiropractic care becomes associated with the 1½ to 3-minute office visits common in such assembly line operations. It is a sad state of affairs. Chiropractors cannot reform the entire health care system, but the profession can certainly clean up its own backyard. Unless honest chiropractors speak out against this behavior, the entire profession will continue to be judged guilty by association.

Guidelines for Duration of Care

Consensus recommendations on "reasonable and customary" care

What constitutes an appropriate course of care? How many visits are necessary? The North American Spine Society (NASS), the RAND consensus panel, and the Mercy Consensus Conference have attempted to define a reasonable and customary number of visits with relation to particular conditions, correctly distinguishing acute cases from chronic, and complicated from uncomplicated.

The NASS, for example, suggests two to five chiropractic treatments per week for the first 2 weeks in acute low back cases, decreasing to one to two treatments per week with an optimum treatment dura-

tion of one month and maximum treatment of 2 to 4 months.[4]

The RAND Consensus Panel and the Mercy Guidelines recommend two weeks of initial care for the uncomplicated acute case. If no positive result is evident within this time frame, 2 weeks of an alternative chiropractic method may be appropriately employed. But if no demonstrable improvement is noted at the end of this second 2-week period, the patient should be referred. Profession-wide attention to this guideline would dramatically rein in overutilization.

Of course, if subjective and objective improvement is noted, treatment may continue, though with a decreasing frequency of visits. The following conclusions from a study by Haldeman and Nyiendo, cited in the Mercy Guidelines,[1] are helpful in evaluating a reasonable course of care:

1. Patients with chronic disorders may require more treatment/care to resolve symptomatic episodes.
2. Lordotic areas of the spine, on average, required twice the care of complaints involving the thoracic and transitional regions.
3. Most cases studied resolved well within 6 weeks of intervention consistent with the expectations from natural history.
4. Patients for whom care is necessary beyond 6 weeks may require up to 11 (mean 3.8) additional sessions before reaching resolution.

Why So Many Visits?

Determining a reasonable and customary number of visits for a particular condition is an important endeavor, but it does not confront the deeper issue of *why* such visits are necessary. What exactly does the doctor of chiropractic do—and why—during such time periods and visits?

Individuals and groups within the profession offer a wide variety of answers, whose diversity adds to the confusion already felt by the public as well as small and large purchasers of health care, particularly employers. Even utilization review companies often display uncertainty when it comes to this subject. Although certain elements, including many medical physicians and some insurers, may not want to understand, others are diligently seeking a rational and objective explanation. It is the responsibility of chiropractors to provide one.

The following discussion is offered as a rational basis for chiropractors to explain to patients, insurers, and other health professionals what chiropractors do, as well as why multiple visits are often required for them to accomplish it.

A FACT-BASED RATIONALE FOR CHIROPRACTIC CARE

The correction of malfunctioning musculoskeletal joints or articulations (subluxations) is a central goal of the chiropractor.[5] But correction of joint dysfunction does not occur in a vacuum. Attending a dysfunctional joint may be (1) a neurologic component; (2) muscular, ligamentous, disc, or other soft tissue damage or derangements; and (3) extensive and complex compensation to the original dysfunction, affecting the function of various other joints and tissues of the musculoskeleton.[6,7]

The neurologic component, which constitutes an important part of the chiropractic hypothesis, centers on the fact that nerve supply to the tissues surrounding the joint may exert either adverse or beneficial effects on the healing process. Time is required for healing to occur, even after joint dysfunction has been partly or completely corrected by the chiropractor. Since soft tissue injury may result in adhesions, deformation of certain tissues, tearing, or rupture,[8] the chiropractor seeks to make joint function corrections, in many cases, over a period of time that allows maximum restoration of normal joint mobility. This approach is intended to avoid fixating the joint either in an abnormal position or within an abnormal range of motion. Because certain soft tissues have a minimal blood or nerve supply,[9] proper healing and normal repositioning or mobilization of the injured joint requires more time than, for example, a cut on the skin. Furthermore, the weight-bearing function of the musculoskeleton also tends to interfere with this process of healing and normalization.[10]

During this healing process, periodic visits with the chiropractor are required in order to evaluate changes in structural balance and in the dynamic relationships among bones, discs, muscles, and ligaments. When necessary, the chiropractor shepherds the healing process by adjusting, manipulating, or otherwise intervening to aid these structures on their road to recovery.

Compensation

Compensations are more complex phenomena, but they follow a logical pattern. For example, a secretary is talking on the telephone, holding it by the force of her neck muscles against her shoulder while taking notes. The sustained contraction of the neck musculature creates waste products in the muscles; the muscles quickly become fatigued and enter a phase of spasm. This may involve the large muscles of the neck, or the small muscles which control, in part, relationships between the vertebrae.

When the secretary puts her phone down and straightens her neck to its normal position, one or more of the muscles remains in a contracted state. The joint at this site cannot move normally now; it is dysfunctional. At this time, there may or may not be a state of pain and stiffness. All 24 movable segments of the spine function as a whole—somewhat like a shaft of wheat in the wind—with each segment contributing its share of movement to the movement of the entire structure.[11] Thus, one dysfunctional joint will alter, to some degree, the full and normal movement of the entire spine.[12] The normal part of the spine must compensate.

Certain segments will rotate in directions opposite that of the "fixed" or dysfunctional neck joint. Others will rotate in the other direction. A mild compensatory S curve will develop.[13] To accomplish this, certain muscles throughout the spine must contract on one side, while their counterparts on the opposite side relax. The spine is now in a state of substantial compensatory distortion, placing abnormal loading on many of the tissues and joints, downward to the lower back or even the ankle, and upward to the skull. In time this compensation may create other symptoms, such as lower back pain and headaches. In some cases, symptoms will emerge in the arms and legs, or in the rib cage.

If the original neck problem and its compensation are left untreated for a long period, other structures that articulate with the now abnormally curved spine (e.g., the rib cage) may alter their configuration.

This might take the form of a bulge on one side of the back and on the opposite side in the front of the body. One shoulder may be carried higher than the other, or the pelvis may no longer move in symmetric motion when walking or running.

The longer this situation exists, the more established it becomes. So a fairly innocent, acute beginning—a small neck muscle spasm—has led to a chronic, extensive compensatory distortion that may, at any time and in many possible locations, result in pain or disability. If the condition began in the neck, it could ultimately result in lower back pain; if it began in an ankle, it could result in hip or knee pain; if it began in the lower back, it could manifest in the upper back, or perhaps the upper neck.

The entire musculoskeleton may be affected. Balance between the right and left sides of the body may be substantially disrupted. If the secretary in our example is a jogger, she may find that her otherwise very healthy attempt to exercise creates new problems arising from compensatory imbalances.

Chronicity

To carry this example of the secretary's neck muscle spasm further, let us now suppose that she comes to the doctor of chiropractic, 5 years after the initial incident, for pain in her back and shoulder. The chiropractor must rule out a range of potential causes with a broad screening diagnostic examination. He or she must ascertain that there are no contraindications to spinal corrective procedures (adjustments) and confirm that there are no parallel problems necessitating referral to a medical physician for additional evaluation.

Assuming that the problem originated as detailed above, the chiropractor must evaluate the entire compensatory distortion, differentiating between the compensation and the original joint dysfunction in the neck. After locating the offending spinal segment, the chiropractor works to restore it to its normal function and mobility. He must then evaluate and treat the rest of the spine to reduce the compensatory distortions. Failure to do so may cause the original problem to return repeatedly. The spine, in effect, splints itself against further distortion, but also against an unaided return to normal. The chronicity of the problem adds to the chiropractor's challenge.

Logically, a long-term distortion that alters the loading or foundational aspects of the human frame and spine may result in degenerative joint dysfunction, bulging discs, ligaments that have exceeded their coefficients of elasticity, and other changes that are not correctable.[14] These must be included in the chiropractor's professional evaluation of the patient.

With this background, we now have the answers to our original questions: Why doesn't the chiropractor simply correct the neck problem in one or two visits and then dismiss the patient? And, why does the patient need to return to the chiropractor for repeated visits? A well-reasoned explanation of compensation and chronicity is central to making the answers understandable not only to chiropractic patients, but also to employers, insurance companies, health consultants, and government officials. In the current political and economic environment of retrenchment in health care, the fact that a certain number of visits is usual and customary attains maximum viability when presented within a context of solid, patient-centered reasons that explain *why* it is usual and customary.

Chiropractors must evaluate each case on its own merits, so that for those cases requiring extended care, a coherent, fact-based explanation can be provided. Practitioners who take advantage of patients' vulnerability by having them return to the office for an unnecessary number of times, or who recommend the same large number of visits for virtually every patient, have abandoned professionalism and bring disrepute on the entire profession. In addition to its inherent immorality, such unethical behavior makes it extremely difficult to collect meaningful data from the field to arrive at evidence-based mean values of visits required for a particular condition.

ETHICAL CHALLENGES

Confronting the Charge of "Unscientific Cultism"

As part of its former campaign to contain and eliminate chiropractic, the AMA once charged that chiropractic is an "unscientific cult."[15,16] It is worthwhile to confront the questions raised by such charges directly. Appropriate responses include not only self-defense but self-analysis and self-criticism.

The allegation that chiropractic is unscientific has been answered since the 1970s with an ongoing commitment to research and rigorous educational standards. As stated earlier, when the validity of chiropractic research has been subjected to rigorous scrutiny by independent bodies such as the AHCPR, it has stood up extremely well. Similarly, chiropractic educational institutions have demonstrated sufficient rigor to achieve and maintain accreditation by both the Council on Chiropractic Education and various nonchiropractic regional accrediting agencies.

Charges of cultism are less easily resolved. Let us first define the qualities of cultism:

• Unquestioning loyalty to the principles of a founder or leader

• Unwillingness to analyze objectively information that conflicts with the received precepts of the founder or leader

• Unwillingness to change one's beliefs even when a preponderance of new evidence contradicts them

• The belief that one possesses the sole and singular truth

• Elevation of slogans to the status of ultimate truths

In my opinion, examples of jingoistic chiropractic slogans include "innate rules," "subluxation kills," and "above down, inside out." These clarify nothing about chiropractic science and create an aura of strangeness that continues to hover over the profession.

Chiropractors are not unique in the healing arts in sometimes demonstrating cultist qualities, but the uncomfortable truth is that the persistence of such behaviors among a vocal minority of chiropractors leaves a continuing stain on the reputation of the profession. In my years as a chiropractic college president, and as a representative of the chiropractic profession in Washington, D.C., with the International Chiropractors Association and later with the American Chiropractic Association, the greatest obstacle I saw to the advancement of the profession was the persistence of stridently vocal chiropractors with irrational, cult-like opinions. They are a minority, but they can and do cause the profession great harm.

Appropriate Terminology

During the first few decades of the twentieth century, development of a vocabulary unique to chiropractic was an astute survival tactic. Charged with, and in some cases jailed for, practicing medicine without a license, chiropractic leaders maneuvered brilliantly, denying the charges by asserting that:

1. Medicine is the diagnosis and treatment of disease.
2. Chiropractors do not diagnose or treat disease.
3. Therefore, chiropractors are not guilty of practicing medicine.

This rationale required significant semantic contortions. Normal use of the English language includes as diagnosis all methods used by a doctor to determine the nature of the patient's condition, and defines as treatment all measures used by the doctor to influence that condition. Thus, the average intelligent English speaker would recognize analysis of spinal subluxations as diagnosis, and application of chiropractic adjustments as treatment.

In the process of circumventing attempts to control chiropractic with medical practice laws, many chiropractors enshrined their tactic as something close to holy writ. At the more traditionalist schools, generations of chiropractic students were taught (and in a few cases still are taught) that chiropractors do not diagnose or treat disease. Instead of diagnosing, they *analyze.* Instead of treating, they *adjust.*

In my opinion, such cultish language has become highly counterproductive. Chiropractic is now mature enough to converse with other health professions in a common lexicon. This does not mean that chiropractors must reject their natural healing roots and endorse allopathic principles, nor does it mean that all terminology developed by the chiropractic profession should be jettisoned. It does mean that members of all professions, and their patients, benefit from professionals speaking the same language.

Cooperation need not imply co-optation. Chiropractic terms such as *subluxation* and *adjustment* to a considerable degree have entered the common domain of scientific language. But to vigorously assert, at the dawn of the 21st century, that the chiropractic adjustment is not a form of treatment borders on the absurd and is properly perceived as such by impartial listeners.

STEPS TOWARD INTEGRATION INTO MAINSTREAM HEALTH CARE

At a 1995 conference on alternative medicine sponsored by Harvard University's School of Graduate Education, it was noted that one of the most significant achievements for any group wishing to join the health care mainstream is the creation of an infrastructure.[17] Chiropractic stood out among the many groups represented because it already has a substantial portion of such a structure in place: licensure laws, a national association, state associations, an accrediting agency, established and accredited colleges, and ongoing scientific research efforts. These elements constitute substantive movement toward full professional status.

What further steps are necessary to solidify mainstream status? At a minimum, the following are urgently required:

1. Assertive, ongoing efforts by chiropractors to foster collegial relations with medical professionals.
2. Establishment of a proper ethic of interprofessional referral, in which medical physicians know which cases chiropractors should refer to them, and which cases they should refer to chiropractors. In both cases, such referrals require that the patient be returned to the original referring doctor, as is the case when MDs refer to other MDs. For many years, referrals from chiropractors to medical physicians constituted a transfer of the patient, rather than a true referral, and remnants of this pattern still exist. Lack of an explicit ethic on DC–MD referral remains a barrier to better interprofessional communication, and therefore to improved patient evaluation and care.
3. An organized effort by licensing boards to acquire peer-review authority immunized from antitrust laws, followed by the assertive use of this authority to change the behavior of practitioners who violate laws and ethical standards.
4. The active discouragement of "practice-building" programs that celebrate and glorify practitioners on the basis of elevated income. One significant step in this direction would be for all chiropractic publications to refuse all advertising promising to increase the doctor's income.

These efforts will work best if pursued simultaneously. They include individual action (reaching out to MDs), group action (mutual agreement with the medical profession on interprofessional referral), legal action (securing immunized peer review, and applying it in a rigorous effort to raise standards), and moral action (rejection of programs that identify income as the prime measure of success). Though the desired changes will not happen overnight, the actions required to secure their eventual accomplishment must be undertaken without delay. The future of chiropractic depends on it.

Terminology

boycott
chronicity
compensation
cultism
duration of care
empiricism
joint dysfunction
level playing field
Mercy Guidelines
utilization review (UR)

Review Questions

1. What are three characteristics of a mature profession?

2. Why did the chiropractic profession develop practice guidelines?

3. How did the Mercy Consensus Conference deal with minority opinions?

4. What were some criticisms of the Mercy Guidelines?

5. What is the longest period of time that a chiropractor should wait before referring a patient who is not showing clinical progress?

6. According to Haldeman and Nyiendo, which areas of the spine generally require longer periods of treatment?

7. What is musculoskeletal compensation?

8. Name two unethical practices, and describe why they are unethical.

9. What are the characteristics of cultism?

10. What are the key components of a health profession's infrastructure?

Concept Questions

1. Why does chiropractic care sometimes require an extended period of treatment?

2. How should the chiropractic profession deal with practitioners who violate the profession's ethics?

3. How should the chiropractic profession distinguish between cooperation and co-optation in relations with the medical profession? What are some examples of each?

References

1. Haldeman S, Chapman-Smith D, Peterson DM: Guidelines for Chiropractic Quality Assurance and Practice Parameters: Proceedings of the Mercy Center Consensus Conference. Aspen, Gaithersburg, MD, 1993

2. Shekelle PG, Markovich M, Louie R: Comparing the costs between provider types of episodes of back care. Spine 20:221, 1995

3. Hurwitz EL, Coulter ID, Adams AH et al: Utilization of chiropractic services in the United States and Canada. Am J Pub Health (submitted for publication), 1997

4. North American Spine Society: Common diagnostic and therapeutic procedures of the lumbosacral spine. Spine 16:1161, 1991

5. Gatterman MI: Foundations of Chiropractic: Subluxation. Mosby–Year Book, St. Louis, 1995

6. Jirout J: Studies in the dynamics of the spine. Acta Radiol 46:55, 1965

7. Lantz CA: The vertebral subluxation complex. p. 149. In Gatterman MI (ed): Foundations of Chiropractic: Subluxation. Mosby–Year Book, St. Louis, 1995

8. Frank W, Woo SL-Y, Amiel D et al: Medial collateral ligament healing: a multidisciplinary assessment in rabbits. Am J Sports Med 11:379, 1983

9. Hell JE: Vascular distensibility and functions of the arterial and venous systems. p. 171. In Guyton A (ed): Textbook of Medical Physiology, 9th Ed. WB Saunders, Philadelphia, 1996

10. Bullough PG, Vigorita JJ: Atlas of Orthopedic Pathology With Clinical and Radiological Correlations. Gower Medical, New York, 1984

11. Blunt EL, Gatterman MI, Bereznick DE: Kinesiology: an essential approach toward understanding the chiropractic subluxation. p. 170. In Gatterman MI (ed): Foundations of Chiropractic: Subluxation. Mosby–Year Book, St. Louis, 1995

12. Goel VK, Clark CR, McGowan D, Goyal S: An in-vitro study of the kinematics of the normal, injured and stabilized cervical spine. J Biomech 17:363, 1984

13. Hviid H: Functional radiography of the cervical spine. Ann Swiss Chiro Assoc 3:37, 1965

14. Lantz CA: Immobilization degeneration and the fixation hypothesis of chiropractic subluxation. Chiro Res J 1:21, 1988

15. Wardwell WI: Chiropractic: History and Evolution of a New Profession. Mosby–Year Book, St. Louis, 1992

16. *Wilk v. AMA*, 895 F2D 352 Cert den, 112.2 Ed 2D 524, 1990

17. Mason M: Centering on alternatives. Washington Post, April 3, 1995

14

The Comparative Safety of Chiropractic

William J. Lauretti

I will follow that system of regimen which, according to my ability and judgment, I consider for the benefit of my patients, and abstain from whatever is deleterious and mischievous.

Hippocratic oath[1]

The ancient Hippocratic appeal to physicians to "first, do no harm" has a powerful attraction among members of the health care professions and in the popular imagination. After all, if a doctor's job is to heal, shouldn't patients receive benefit from a doctor's ministrations, and not further injury? Unfortunately, the doctor—as a professional, as a healer, and as a human being—must occasionally face the specter of inadvertently doing harm to a patient.

Chiropractic has come under increased scrutiny as a result of its widespread use and entry into the health care mainstream. Despite considerable progress in interprofessional relations between chiropractors and medical physicians in recent years, the adversarial climate of the past has not entirely disappeared. Within this context, the possibility of adverse reactions to chiropractic treatment is a politically and emotionally charged issue. In certain cases, the popular media and some biomedical journals have inflamed the issue by emphasizing negative reactions to spinal manipulation, evaluating it in isolation, rather than comparing it with common medical treatments for similar problems.

Most chiropractors perform thousands of manipulations annually without any serious complications and observe that many patients benefit greatly from manipulation. Many of these therapeutic successes occur after more aggressive therapies, medications, and/or surgery have failed. Such personal experience with the safety and efficacy of spinal manipulation can lead individual chiropractors to devalue reports of adverse reactions. The incongruity between the positive personal experience of chiropractors using manipulation and recurring negative stories about manipulation's dangers sets the stage for a "chiropractic paradox":

- According to conventional medical wisdom, chiropractic spinal manipulation has a very limited role to play in conventional health care, if any.[2] In some cases, particularly involving the cervical spine, some medical authorities see manipulation as being "too risky to perform."[2-4]

- Yet, millions of people receive chiropractic spinal manipulation each year, without apparent harm and with apparent benefit.
- Furthermore, by far, most chiropractors and other practitioners of manual medicine have never personally experienced a serious complication during treatment. Most chiropractors view manipulation as safe and noninvasive, and frequently perform the procedure on family members and loved ones and receive it themselves with hardly a thought of hazardous complications.

It is crucial to avoid evaluating the risks of chiropractic manipulation in a clinical vacuum, with inappropriate emphasis on the perceived risks of manipulation and corresponding underemphasis on the considerable scientific evidence favoring its safety and efficacy. The solution to the "chiropractic paradox" lies in the answer to two key questions: how risky is spinal manipulation, and how do its risks and benefits compare with other conventional treatments for similar conditions?

CERVICAL ADJUSTMENTS: CONSERVATIVE CARE OR A RISKY GAMBLE?

"Every neurologist in this room has seen two or three people who have suffered this [cerebrovascular accident] after chiropractic manipulation"

William Powers, Washington University, St. Louis. The Washington Post, February 20, 1994[5]

Manipulation of the cervical spine has been questioned more frequently than any other commonly applied chiropractic procedure. Reports of serious complications from neck manipulation have appeared intermittently in the medical literature since at least 1934.[6] The issue reached a peak in the popular media in early 1994, when the Associated Press ran an article describing a survey performed by several Stanford University faculty members. This survey asked members of the American Academy of Neurology practicing in California whether they had encountered patients who apparently suffered a stroke from "chiropractic manipulation." Of 486 neurologists polled, only 177 (36 percent) responded to the survey, with 37 reporting that they

recalled treating a total of 55 strokes appearing to stem from chiropractic manipulation.[7] To place these numbers in some perspective, in the two years covered by this survey (1990–1991) approximately 9,000 licensed chiropractors were practicing in California. According to national averages, these chiropractors saw 100 million patient visits and likely performed 35 to 50 million cervical manipulations during those two years.[8]

This survey had significant methodologic problems, including a low response rate, possible bias, and/or possible poor recall by participants.[9] Yet, hundreds of newspapers across North America carried the story, some with sensational headlines, such as "Warning! Chiropractors Can Kill You!"[10] Many respected newspapers included Dr. Powers's statement that "every neurologist in this room has seen two or three people" who had suffered a stroke at the hands of a chiropractor.[5] Even accepting the methodologic limitations of the Stanford study, Powers's statement is highly inaccurate. Of the neurologists responding to the survey, only *20 percent* reported seeing one or more strokes that appeared to stem from chiropractic manipulation.

A positive effect of this story is that it highlighted the need for chiropractors to inform themselves fully about the potential risks of neck manipulation. With accurate, up-to-date information, chiropractors can institute preventive measures to decrease risk to patients as well as provide reasoned responses to journalists, patients, and medical colleagues concerned that chiropractic treatment is unacceptably hazardous.

MECHANISMS OF STROKE FROM CERVICAL MANIPULATION

The most likely mechanism of stroke from cervical manipulation involves injury to the vertebral artery as it courses through the transverse foramina of the upper cervical vertebrae into the base of the skull (Fig. 14-1). Between the first two cervical vertebrae, the vertebral artery makes a sharp bend upward and laterally to enter the transverse process of the atlas vertebra. The artery is relatively fixed to the transverse processes by fibrous tissue at this point and is less freely movable.

The vertebral artery emerges from the transverse process of atlas and winds posteriorly and laterally

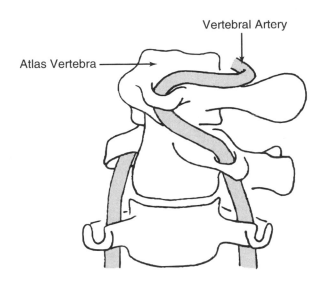

Vertebral Artery

Atlas Vertebra

Figure 14-1. The stretch applied to the vertebral artery with cervical rotation is a possible mechanism for vertebrobasilar stroke from manipulation. (From Terrett and Kleynhans,[72] with permission.)

around the posterior arch of atlas. Then it ascends into the foramen magnum and joins with its counterpart to form the basilar artery. This vertebrobasilar system comprises the main blood supply of the brainstem.

Vigorous rotation of the neck may traumatize the vertebral artery along its course, most likely between atlas and axis or atlas and occiput. This may cause dissection or tearing of the artery wall, or the trauma may lead to formation of a blood clot, which can break free and lodge in one of the other ascending blood vessels. Either event can result in ischemia to the brain stem—a cerebrovascular accident (CVA). Alternately, the force of rotation may cause vasospasm in one vertebral artery. If pre-existing arteriosclerosis or a developmental anomaly has compromised flow in the contralateral artery, this may also result in brain stem ischemia.

Cervical manipulation is not the only mechanism to initiate this type of injury. The literature contains numerous reports of similar vascular accidents resulting from common medical procedures such as administering anesthesia during surgery[11,12] or during neck extension for radiography.[13] Cases of vertebrobasilar stroke have been reported that apparently occurred during normal activities, such as swimming, yoga, star gazing, overhead work,[14] and

even during sleep.[15] "Beauty Parlor Stroke," caused by cervical hyperextension over a sink while washing the hair, is also well documented.[16] Cases of spontaneous vertebrobasilar stroke, with no apparent precipitating event, have been reported as well.[17,18]

Strokes of the vertebrobasilar circulation usually present with brain stem signs, such as severe nausea and vomiting, visual problems, or vertigo. Strokes of the posterior circulation can also result in Wallenberg syndrome, characterized by loss of the ability to sense pain and temperature of the face on the ipsilateral side of the lesion, and of the body on the contralateral side. Extreme cases can demonstrate "locked-in syndrome," wherein the patient is completely paralyzed except for eye movements.

It is important to note that only a minority of vertebrobasilar strokes are fatal or result in such severe disability. In Terrett's summary of 183 cases of vertebrobasilar stroke following manipulation reported in the worldwide medical literature,[19] about one-fourth of the cases resolved completely or almost completely. Death occurred in 33 cases (18 percent), while 6 cases (3 percent) resulted in the locked-in syndrome with tetraplegia.

It has been argued that the rate of strokes following manipulation may be significantly underreported in the literature.[2] But it may also be likely that the cases that resulted in death or major neurologic deficits are proportionally overreported in the literature. Serious and impressive cases seem more likely to warrant description in a published case report.

Occasionally, a report implicates manipulation in nonvertebrobasilar strokes, usually strokes of the internal or external carotid circulation.[20] However, nothing in the literature provides a plausible anatomic or pathophysiologic mechanism for such an event. The association between manipulation and carotid stroke is speculative.

INCIDENCE OF STROKE FROM MANIPULATION: SUMMARY OF STUDIES

Every published study estimating the incidence of stroke from chiropractic cervical manipulation agrees that the risk is one to three incidents per million treatments (Table 14-1). Several studies have documented large numbers of cervical manipulations without any reports of stroke or major neurological complication. One report[21] documents approximately 5 million cervical manipulations performed at the National College of Chiropractic Clinic from 1965 to 1980, without a single case of vertebral artery stroke or serious injury. Henderson and Cassidy[22] reported a survey done at the Canadian Memorial Chiropractic College outpatient clinic, where more than a half-million treatments were given over a 9-year period, again without serious incident. Eder and Tilscher[23] offered a report of 168,000 cervical manipulations over a 28-year period, without a single significant complication.

A survey of 203 members of the Swiss Society for Manual Medicine[24] noted a practitioner-reported rate of 1 serious complication per 400,000 cervical manipulations, without any reported deaths, among approximately 1.5 million cervical manipulations.

Notably, these practitioners were nonchiropractors who received an average of about 38 days of training in manipulation. This survey represents the highest incidence rate of complications from cervical manipulation reported in the literature.

In another survey, based on a computerized registration system in Holland, Patjin[25] found an overall rate of 1 complication in 518,886 manipulations. The Stanford survey of California neurologists[6] described earlier also suggests a rate of about 1 stroke per 500,000 manipulations. Other experts on manipulation[26] have published opinions that the risk of stroke from cervical manipulation is "two or three more-or-less serious incidents" per million treatments. This figure has also been accepted in court testimony.[27]

Table 14.1. Studies That Have Estimated the Probability of Stroke Following Cervical Manipulation

Source	Methods	Findings
Jaskoviak[21]	Report based on clinical files of the National College of Chiropractic Clinic	No cases of vertebral artery injury or stroke in 5 million cervical manipulations in a 15-year period
Henderson and Cassidy[22]	Survey done at Canadian Memorial Chiropractic College Clinic	No cases of vertebral artery injury or stroke in more than 500,000 treatments over a 9-year period
Dvorak and Orelli[24]	Survey of 203 members of the Swiss Society of Manual Medicine (all nonchiropractors)	One serious complication per 400,000 cervical manipulations; no reported deaths
Patjin[25]	Review of computerized registration system in Holland	Overall rate of complication of 1 in 518,000 manipulations
Haldeman et al.[28]	Extensive literature review to formulate practice guidelines	1–2 incidences of stroke per million manipulations
Carey[29]	Claims reviewed from Canada's largest chiropractic malpractice company	13 CVA incidents reported throughout Canada in a 5-year period, and no deaths among an estimated 50 million neck manipulations; estimated rate of 1 CVA per 3 million neck manipulations
National Chiropractic Mutual Insurance Company (NCMIC) Data	According to unpublished case records, NCMIC paid an average of 20 claims per year, 1991–1993 for stroke following manipulation; Based on national averages, we calculate that NCMIC's 24,000 insured DCs perform about 43 million cervical manipulations per year	20 strokes per year in approximately 43 million cervical manipulations yields a rate of 1 stroke per 2 million cervical manipulations
Klougart et al.[32]	Survey of Danish chiropractors over a 10-year period, cross-referenced with official complaints and insurance records	An overall rate of 1 "irreversable CVA after chiropractic treatment" per 1,320,000 cervical spine treatment sessions

After an extensive literature review performed to formulate practice guidelines, Haldeman et al.[28] concurred that "the risk of serious neurological complications [from cervical manipulation] is extremely low, and is approximately one or two per million cervical manipulations."

Carey,[29] the president of Canada's largest chiropractic malpractice insurance carrier, reviewed claims of CVA from chiropractic manipulation in Canada between 1986 and 1991. He estimated that about 50 million neck manipulations were performed in Canada during that period, 13 of which resulted in significant CVA, without any reported deaths. This article suggests that the incidence of CVA from neck manipulation is about 1 incident per 3 million neck manipulations.

In addition to these published studies, data from the National Chiropractic Mutual Insurance Company (NCMIC), which insures more than 50 percent of chiropractors in the United States, is also useful in determining the frequency of these incidents. According to NCMIC's president (personal communication with L. Sportelli, Dec. 21, 1994), during 1991 to 1993, NCMIC closed a total of 96 claims for CVA. Of these, 61 were closed with payment and 35 without payment. Assuming that claims closed without payment were without merit, this would represent an average of 20 legitimate CVA claims per year. If NCMIC chiropractors are similar to the national average, they see approximately 120 patients visit per week.[30] Curtis and Bove[31] report that rotary adjustments of the cervical spine comprise about 30 percent of the visits made to chiropractors. Therefore, the 24,000 chiropractors insured by NCMIC each performed 1,800 cervical manipulations in each of those three years, for a total of 43 million cervical manipulations per year. The 20 strokes represent a rate of less than one stroke per 2 million cervical manipulations.

Finally, in what might be the best documented study to date, Klougart et al.[32] sought to identify the total number of CVAs related to chiropractic manipulation that occurred in Denmark over a 10-year period. They surveyed all members of the Danish Chiropractors' Association, and cross-referenced the members' reports of CVA occurrences with published cases, official complaints, and insurance data. Then they estimated the total number of neck manipulations performed by chiropractors over the same time period from the survey responses cross-referenced with insurance reimbursement data. They found five cases of "irreversible CVA after chiropractic treatment" occurred in Denmark between 1978 and 1988, in the course of 6,600,000 cervical spine treatment sessions. They estimated a risk of 1 CVA per 1,320,000 cervical spine treatment sessions, and 1 CVA per 414,000 cervical spine sessions using rotation techniques in the upper cervical spine.

Taken together, the various studies form a remarkably consistent pattern regarding the frequency of stroke from cervical manipulation. In summary, a reasonable estimate of the risk of stroke from cervical manipulation is one-half to two incidents per million manipulations performed, and the risk of death from manipulation-induced CVA is about 1 in 4 million manipulations.

Researching this issue more thoroughly presents many difficulties. Ideally, a randomized controlled trial should be used to explore the relation between neck manipulation and stroke. However, a reliable randomized controlled trial requires the researcher to follow 3 times as many patients as the reciprocal of the expected reaction rate in order to be 95 percent confident that a single reaction will occur.[33] Thus, based on the best estimates currently available, a randomized controlled trial would require observing 1.5 to 6 million neck adjustments in order to be valid. The time, money, and personnel required for such a prospective study would appear prohibitive.

Retrospective case studies may be the only feasible way to study this phenomenon. Unfortunately, many published case reports have serious drawbacks. Some are poorly documented and fraught with serious questions regarding the cause-and-effect relationship between the manipulation and the stroke.[33] Others have misrepresented the profession of the practitioner, using the term "chiropractic" despite the fact that the involved practitioner was not a chiropractor.[34]

REDUCING THE RISKS

Although it is clear from all the available evidence that stroke after manipulation is quite rare, this is no reason for complacency on the part of chiropractors. Strokes from manipulation appear to fall into three patterns: manipulating the high-risk patient, inappropriate manipulative technique, and strokes occurring in patients who apparently could not have been previously identified as being high risk.

Identifying the High-Risk Patient

Certain patients have an identifiable pre-existing abnormality that can be exacerbated into a completed stroke by neck manipulation. The problem in some cases can be identified by risk factors in the health history, by "red flags" in the presenting complaint, or by a reaction to a provocative test that makes their pre-existing condition apparent.

Occasionally, investigators identify smoking and use of birth control pills as risk factors for stroke from manipulation.[35] These are established risk factors for most strokes; however, it is doubtful they are significant risk factors for manipulative iatrogenesis.[36,37] Characteristics such as age, gender, and the presence of cervical osteoarthritis also do not appear to be significant risk factors for stroke from manipulation.

Perhaps the most significant risk factors are found in the nature of the patient's presenting complaints. Case reports suggest that some patients may have shown signs and symptoms of vertebrobasilar insufficiency prior to the manipulation that went unrecognized until it was too late. In these cases, the manipulation probably exacerbated the pre-existing condition. In other cases, the condition may have inevitably worsened as part of its natural course, though manipulation was blamed for causing the stroke.

It is vital for chiropractors and other practitioners of manual therapies to recognize the signs and symptoms of vertebrobasilar ischemia, which Terrett[19] refers to as the *5 Ds And 2 Ns:*

1. Dizziness, vertigo, or light-headedness
2. Drop attacks
3. Diplopia or other visual problems
4. Dysarthria (speech difficulty)
5. Dysphagia (difficulty in swallowing)
6. Ataxia of gait or hemiparesis
7. Nausea or vomiting
8. Numbness or hemianesthesia

If a patient presents with any of these signs or symptoms, the practitioner should carefully consider the possibility of vertebrobasilar insufficiency. A patient complaining of dizziness presents a particular diagnostic challenge. The dizziness or vertigo may have its origin in a musculoskeletal lesion of the cervical spine, in which case cervical manipulation may be the treatment of choice.[38,39] However, the dizziness or vertigo might be an early sign of vertebrobasilar insufficiency, in which case a neck adjustment might precipitate a stroke. There is no simple and reliable method to differentiate these entities. The practitioner should determine if neck rotation and extension aggravate the dizziness (which suggests a vascular etiology), if any other of the "5Ds And 3Ns" are present, and whether cervical manipulations have aggravated the symptoms in the past. *When in doubt, a prudent course is to treat the neck with other nonmanipulative conservative methods such as soft tissue massage, physiologic therapeutics, or nonforce chiropractic techniques.* If the dizziness improves under this course of care, it suggests a musculoskeletal, nonvascular etiology.

Screening Tests

Various authorities recommend premanipulative screening maneuvers to identify high-risk patients.[35,40] These tests attempt to stress the cervical spine in rotation and extension, while the practitioner watches for adverse effects suggesting vertebrobasilar insufficiency. However, the literature offers little evidence supporting the efficacy of these tests.[41] Their use may only serve to give the practitioner a false sense of security. Nonetheless, this type of premanipulative maneuver has become the de facto legal standard of care in many areas. The use of premanipulation screening tests should not be discouraged, since they are generally safe and may reveal patients with gross cerebrovascular pathology. However, their value in predicting the safety of a neck adjustment in any particular patient is questionable.

Advanced Imaging Methods

Doppler Ultrasonography

In recent years, there has been discussion about the possibility that high-technology imaging methods may present us with a reliable means of screening patients who are at risk of developing vertebrobasilar ischemia from manipulation. Two of the most advanced imaging modalities considered in this regard are Doppler ultrasonography and duplex ultrasound scanning.

In ultrasonography, a high-frequency sound wave is emitted from a source and passes through a medium (tissue) until it reaches a barrier. A portion of this pulsed sound wave is then reflected back toward the source where it can be imaged or measured. Doppler ultrasonography is based on analyzing frequency shifts in the reflected echoes. When a sound wave is reflected by a moving particle, the frequency of the reflected wave is shifted depending on whether the particle is moving toward or away from the sound source. The degree of the frequency shift depends on the speed of the moving particle. Doppler ultrasonography can detect blood flow within arteries by measuring the frequency shifts of sound waves reflected off moving blood cells.

Duplex Ultrasound Scanning

Duplex ultrasound scanning combines Doppler flow analysis with a complementary modality called real-time B-mode ultrasonography. This allows an image composed of dots to be created from the reflected sound wave; the brightness of each dot is dependent on the amplitude of the returning echo. The image is updated rapidly enough to allow the examiner to see physiologic changes in real-time, such as the motion of blood vessel walls.[42]

In theory, Doppler ultrasonography, particularly with duplex ultrasound scanning, should allow blood flow in the vertebral arteries to be imaged and assessed in a noninvasive manner. One study[43] showed that duplex sonography could be used to record Doppler signals in the vertebral arteries in 89 percent of healthy volunteers. However, the clinical utility of these tools for screening high-risk patients before cervical manipulation is far from established. For example, Thiel et al.[44] used duplex scanning to study the vertebral arteries (VAs) in 42 subjects. Thirty of these subjects were controls with no signs or symptoms of vertebrobasilar insufficiency, and 12 subjects had previously had a positive functional VA vascular test (e.g., clinical symptoms of arterial insufficiency on sustained neck rotation and extension). Duplex scanning detected no differences in VA diameter between the right and left

sides in any of the subjects (whether experimental or control), and the investigators found no difference in VA blood flow when any of the subjects held the various head positions that simulated the functional VA vascular tests. The results of this study cast serious doubt on the value of duplex scanning to correlate clinical findings from VA vascular tests with true VA insufficiency.

If the value of duplex ultrasonography is uncertain for assessing reduced VA blood flow with neck rotation, its value is even more questionable in predicting whether or not cervical manipulation will injure the artery by causing a dissection or vasospasm. At this time, Doppler and duplex ultrasonography have not been established as reliable or specific screening tools to determine the safety of neck manipulation in a particular patient.

Using Appropriate Manipulative Technique

In reviewing case reports of CVA following neck manipulation, two points are apparent. First, where the reports describe the technique used, it appears that the vast majority occurred with rotary cervical adjustments, particularly in the upper neck. Second, inexperienced, poorly trained, or untrained personnel seem to have performed the manipulation in a disproportionate number of cases where a serious injury occurred. Only properly trained, experienced, and qualified persons should perform neck manipulation.

Neck manipulations that use a strong rotary motion seem to be the most risky. One authority suggests discontinuing rotary neck adjustments entirely.[36] Other investigators have suggested that family physicians not refer to practitioners who use rotary cervical manipulation.[45] Given the good clinical results many practitioners report with this technique and the infrequent incidence of adverse effects, these suggestions seem extreme. However, it underscores the importance of good technique. If a rotary manipulation is used, it is important to de-emphasize excessive neck rotation, and emphasize lateral flexion to bring the joints to their physiologic end range before thrusting.

Although there is no empiric evidence that more forceful manipulations are riskier, given what we know about the pathophysiology of vertebral artery dissections, the practitioner should apply only the amount of thrust necessary to bring the joint just beyond the elastic barrier and barely into the paraphysiologic range (Fig. 14-2). This technique generally yields adjustments where only a single audible "pop" is heard, rather than multiple cavitations. It is important to avoid "following-through" in neck adjustments—the practitioner should release the force immediately after feeling the joint cavitate. Cervical rotation should not be continued to the anatomic end range of the joint.

Another group of patients who experienced strokes, apparently resulting from improper care, are those who experienced a mild or possibly uncompleted stroke from an initial manipulation, but whose condition was then greatly exacerbated by another manipulation from a practitioner who ignored the early signs of a lesser stroke. If a patient exhibits any of the key warning signs or symptoms or any other neurologic complication after a neck manipulation, *do not re-manipulate the patient*. The literature contains reports in which a practitioner re-manipulated a patient hoping to correct what appeared to be a mild "bad reaction."[46,47] In some cases, the second manipulation appears to have changed what could have been a mild and tempo-rary case of reversible ischemia into a completed and irreversible stroke.

If a patient shows any of the signs or symptoms described above (e.g., dizziness, ataxia, dysphagia), allow the patient to rest quietly. Observe closely. If the symptoms do not resolve, or if they worsen, the patient needs to be hospitalized immediately. Describe what happened to the emergency department physician, so that the patient can receive proper care as soon as possible.

Unpredictable Strokes

In some cases, a stroke occurs in the absence of identifiable risk factors, and despite a skillfully applied manipulation. For practitioners, the existence of such cases is a humbling, even frightening, prospect because it means that even responsible and highly skilled doctors are capable of initiating strokes through manipulation.

This sort of unpredictable adverse reaction is comparable to a severe idiosyncratic allergic reaction (e.g., anaphylactic shock) to an analgesic or an unpredictable severe complication from a routine surgery. The possibility of being injured by an unforeseen event is a fact of modern life, whether

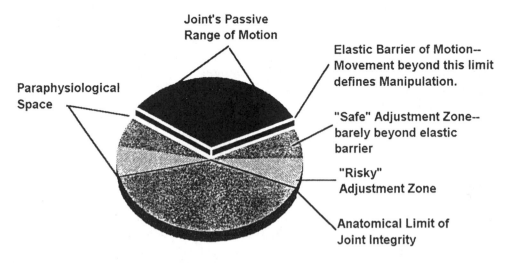

Figure 14-2. A manual adjustment applied with minimal force uses only the amount of thrust necessary to bring the joint past its passive range of motion, beyond the elastic barrier, and barely into the "paraphysiologic space." An adjustment that uses more force brings the joint closer to its anatomic limit of integrity, thereby risking trauma to the joint or nearby vascular and neurologic structures.

that event is an unavoidable auto accident, an unexpected adverse reaction to medication, or an unpredictable stroke from manipulation.

OTHER MANIPULATION RISKS

Although the possibility of stroke from cervical manipulation is the most publicized and serious complication from manipulation, other cases of adverse effects from manipulation have been reported. Terrett and Kleynhans[48] classified complications of manipulation into four categories:

- *Accidents:* Serious impairments, permanent or fatal (include stroke from cervical manipulation, cauda equina syndrome from lumbar manipulation, and serious neurologic syndromes caused by disc herniation or fracture)
- *Incidents:* Consequences of manipulation noticeable by their seriousness or their long duration (includes milder cases of disc pathology or injury, most fractures, and temporary cases of neurologic injury)
- *Reactions:* Consequences of manipulation that are slight and short-lived (include increased pain after manipulation, mild to moderate sprains and strains, and other mild or transient responses)
- *Indirect complications:* Consequences of using manipulation in cases in which it cannot benefit the condition and delays diagnosis and rational treatment (include cases of missed diagnosis, use of manipulation as a treatment for an inappropriate condition, and excessive treatment)

Cauda Equina Syndrome

Cauda equina syndrome is usually described as the most serious accident that can result from lumbar spine manipulation. This condition results from compression to the cauda equina as the nerves pass through the lower part of the lumbar spinal canal, usually resulting from a large posteromedial disc herniation. The immediate effect can be a dramatic loss of bowel and bladder function. This appears to be an exceedingly rare complication from lumbar manipulation.

In a detailed literature review of spinal manipulation for low back pain, Shekelle et al.[49] estimated the occurrence of cauda equina syndrome from lumbar manipulation to be less than one case per 100 million manipulations. Terrett and Kleynhans[48] analyzed other disc-related complications from low back manipulation and found only 65 cases reported in the worldwide literature in the 80 years of 1911 to 1991. They also noted that manipulative iatrogenesis is more common with manipulation under anesthesia, accounting for more than 44 percent of reported cases.

Additional Major Complications

Other major complications from manipulation are attributable to missed diagnosis and inappropriate use of manipulation. A variety of conditions are relative or absolute contraindications for manipulation. These include metastatic tumors, unstable fractures, osteopenia, free disc fragments, and space-occupying lesions. Other investigators have described these contraindications in detail.[50,51] All clinicians should also be familiar with the diagnostic "red flags" indicating that a patient with back pain might have a potentially serious condition[52] (Table 14-2). The presence of any of these "red flags" in a patient presenting with back pain should alert the clinician to the possibility that the pain is nonmechanical in origin and should suggest the need for further diagnostic procedures.

Less Serious Complications

Other less serious complications of manipulation include sprains or strains, rib fractures, post-treatment soreness, and exacerbation of symptoms. While these adverse reactions are probably far more common than the major complications of manipulation, their self-limiting and relatively benign nature makes them a less pressing issue among chiropractors, patients, and chiropractic critics.

Good communication between doctor and patient can often help prevent a minor reaction from developing into a major issue. For example, it is prudent to advise patients that they may experience some increased soreness after an initial adjustment. If these reactions occur, they are usually mild and transitory, but they can be alarming to a new patient who is unaware that they may occur. New patients should be told to contact the doctor if there is a significant reaction. This allows the doctor to assess the

Table 14-2. Red Flags for Potentially Serious Conditions

Possible Fracture	Possible Tumor or Infection	Possible Cauda Equina Syndrome
From medical history		
Major trauma, such as vehicle accident or fall from height	Age over 50 or under 20 History of cancer	Saddle anesthesia Recent onset of bladder dysfunction, such as urinary retention, increased frequency, or overflow incontinence
Minor trauma or even strenuous lifting (in older or potentially osteoporotic patient)	Constitutional symptoms, such as recent fever or chills or unexplained weight loss Risk factors for spinal infection: recent bacterial infection (e.g., urinary tract infection); IV drug abuse; or immune suppression (from steroids, transplant, or HIV) Pain that worsens when supine; severe nighttime pain	Severe or progressive neurologic deficit in the lower extremity
From physical examination		
		Unexpected laxity of the anal sphincter Perianal/perineal sensory loss Major motor weakness: quadriceps (knee extension weakness); ankle plantar flexors, evertors, and dorsiflexors (foot drop)

(Courtesy of Bigos S et al.[52])

RISKS OF "CONVENTIONAL" TREATMENT FOR NECK AND BACK DISORDERS

Need for a Balanced Perspective

When looking at possible complications of chiropractic treatment, certain critics[4] imply that nearly any degree of risk is unacceptable. The musculoskeletal conditions for which manipulation is usually used are perceived to be self-limiting or unimportant. According to this logic, any complication encountered from treating such relatively benign conditions is objectionable.

An example of this viewpoint is found in a 1993 *Neurosurgery* article,[3] which concluded that "the risk/benefit ratio for patients with midline neck pain is unacceptably high, and cervical spinal manipulation therapy should be discouraged as treatment. Moreover, it is unlikely that a sufficiently high benefit for spinal manipulation therapy in

patients with benign disease processes will be achieved to justify the risk of severe complications, no matter how infrequent the occurrence."

The *Neurosurgery* article clearly implies that spinal manipulation therapy is riskier than other options but provides no comparative analysis to justify this conclusion. To properly assess the risks of chiropractic treatment, it must be compared against the risks of other treatments for similar conditions. For example, even the most conservative conventional treatment for neck and back pain—prescription nonsteroidal anti-inflammatory drugs (NSAIDs)—may carry significantly greater risk than manipulation. Less conservative treatments, such as neck surgery, are also used for some conditions similar to those chiropractors treat with spinal manipulation. There is a 3 to 4 percent rate of complication for cervical spine surgery and 4,000 to 10,000 deaths per million.[53] These risk rates are several orders of magnitude greater than the most extreme estimates of manipulation risks.

Even bed rest, a mainstay of conservative treatment for back and neck pain in the past, carries substantial risks. These risks include muscle atrophy (1.0 to 1.5 percent of muscle mass lost per day); cardiopulmonary deconditioning (15 percent loss in aerobic capacity in 10 days); bone mineral loss with hypercalcemia and hypercalciuria; and the risk of thromboembolism.[52] The social and psychological side effects of prolonged bed rest are also considerable. Current evidence suggests that more than two to four days of bed rest does more harm than good.

Moreover, "doing nothing," that is, not treating patients with neck and back pain, carries risks as well. These may include increased rates of disability, abuse of analgesics or illegal drugs for pain relief, and disruption of work and social activities.

Effectiveness of Chiropractic Manipulation Versus Other Treatments

Numerous recent studies have found that spinal manipulation provides superior clinical outcomes compared to other common treatments for neck and back complaints. These studies are described in detail in Chapter 10.

Ironically, despite their widespread use, the evidence supporting the effectiveness of NSAIDs for neck and back pain is limited. The AHCPR Guideline for Treatment of Acute Low Back Pain[52] found only four randomized controlled trials for NSAIDs that met their criteria for adequate evidence of efficacy. Three of the 4 studies found NSAIDs superior to placebo for low back pain relief in the short term. For comparison, the AHCPR found 12 randomized controlled trials for manipulation which met the criteria for review. The evidence for NSAIDs in the treatment of neck pain is even slimmer. A recent MEDLINE search (1966–1996), failed to identify even a single randomized controlled trial examining the use of NSAIDs specifically for neck pain.[54]

In reviewing the evidence supporting common treatments for neck pain, Bogduk[55] concluded that recommendations to use NSAIDs, exercise, and cervical collars were not valid. He noted, "Of all the various therapies for neck pain, only early manual therapy for whiplash has been vindicated in the literature." Another review article[56] noted that, "although NSAIDs are good analgesics in many clinical settings, there are limited data supporting their use over pure analgesics or physical modalities in non-inflammatory musculoskeletal disorders." In a

recent review of medications used for neck pain, Dillin and Uppal[57] noted that the current standard of accepted practice "may rest on a quagmire of possibly valid, but unproven, treatments." To date, there has been only one large-scale randomized trial comparing manipulative therapy to general practitioner management (including NSAIDs) in the treatment of back and neck pain.[58] This trial found manipulative treatment significantly superior, with the advantages for the group treated with manipulation persisting at the 12-month follow-up.

NSAIDs: IS THERE SAFETY IN NUMBERS?

The most common conventional first-line treatment for most musculoskeletal pain syndromes is NSAIDs.[57] This broad class of prescription and over-the-counter drugs includes common aspirin, ibuprofen, naprosyn, Voltaren, and similar drugs. NSAIDs are generally considered safe. They are among the most prescribed drugs in the United States and represent about 5 percent of all prescriptions filled in this country,[62] or some 90 million prescriptions annually.[63] NSAIDs also account for millions of dollars in annual sales of over-the-counter formulations.

In spite of their widespread use and perceived safety, NSAIDs have a significant risk of serious complications. Uncommon side effects include renal dysfunction, hypersensitivity reactions, liver damage, and central nervous system damage.[64,65]

The most common and most serious adverse effects associated with NSAIDs are gastrointestinal ulcers and hemorrhage. These complications of NSAIDs are likely an integral consequence of their pharmacology. NSAIDs probably provide their analgesic and anti-inflammatory properties by inhibiting the synthesis of prostaglandins. However, prostaglandins are essential for promoting the health of the gastrointestinal mucosa by acting to reduce gastric acid secretion, increasing the production of gastric mucosal blood volume and increasing the production of duodenal bicarbonate.[66] Unlike other common gastric ulcers, ulcers from the use of NSAIDs do not appear to be related to *H. pylori* infection and are not responsive to antibiotic therapy.

Gastrointestinal ulcers can present serious problems and occasionally lead to fatal complications such as hemorrhage and perforation. At any given time, the chance of a patient on NSAID therapy having a gastric ulcer is 10 to 20 percent, a rate 5 to 10 times greater than that in nonusers.[63] One retrospective study[67] reported that nearly 80 percent of all ulcer-related deaths occurred in patients using an NSAID.

NSAIDs are often used for the long-term treatment of chronic conditions such as rheumatoid arthritis. However, these drugs are also commonly used for symptomatic relief of musculoskeletal conditions. A diagnosis of "osteoarthritis" accounts for more than one-half of NSAID prescriptions.[68] Many patients with symptoms of musculoskeletal pain, particularly chronic pain, receive a clinical diagnosis of "osteoarthritis"or "spondylosis."[55,57] These are exactly the type of patients chiropractors often treat effectively with manipulation.

Fries[61] estimated 13 million regular users of NSAIDs in the United States. Eight million of these patients have osteoarthritis or "miscellaneous conditions." He used data from the Arthritis, Rheumatism and Aging Medical Information System (ARAMIS), a chronic disease database of 46,000 individuals in the US and Canada. He found the rate of hospitalization from gastrointestinal bleeding to be 0.4 percent per year higher than the expected rate among patients receiving NSAIDs for "osteoarthritis." He estimated the death rate for NSAID-associated gastrointestinal problems to be 0.04 percent per year among osteoarthritis patients receiving NSAIDs, or 3,200 deaths in the United States per year.

Complications from NSAID use are not only the result of chronic, long-term use. One meta-analysis[69] actually found short-term use of NSAIDs to be associated with a higher risk of gastrointestinal complications than with chronic use. The odds ratio for adverse gastrointestinal events associated with NSAID use was 1.92 for more than three months of NSAID exposure, but 8.00 for less than one month of NSAID exposure.

Most studies of NSAID complications have dealt only with the prescription version of these medications. In recent years, an increasing number and variety of NSAIDs have become available in nonprescription strength. Widespread use of these over-the-counter NSAIDs may represent an increasing and underrecognized cause of peptic ulcer disease and ulcer-related hemorrhage.[70]

Recent studies also raise serious questions regarding the appropriateness of using NSAIDs in cases of osteoarthritis. Brandt[71] noted a lack of evidence that NSAIDs favorably influence the progression of joint breakdown in osteoarthritis. He also noted that several animal studies and human clinical studies have actually implicated NSAIDs in the *acceleration* of joint destruction.

Need for Consistent Standards

There is a long history of pointed, and often acrimonious, criticism of spinal manipulation in mainstream medical literature. The most common criticisms focus on the lack of definitive studies that clearly demonstrate the effectiveness of manipulation and on anecdotes illustrating the supposed dangers of the procedure. Much of the criticism appears to be sincere but misguided—motivated more by misunderstanding than by malice.

Of necessity, the healing arts have always been practiced based both on pragmatism and pure science. Even today, only a minority of mainstream medical methods have been exposed to careful scientific scrutiny.[59] On the level playing field of the contemporary health care system, each method

Table 14-3. Estimated Risks of Common Chiropractic Treatments, Common Medical Treatments, and Accidents

Procedure or Activity	Estimated Risk	Reference
Risk of developing cauda equina syndrome from lumbar manipulation	1 in 100,000,000	49
Risk of death from neurologic complications from cervical manipulation	1 in 4,000,000	54
Risk of death in fatal air crash, flying 425 miles (e.g., Boston to Washington, DC) on a scheduled commercial airline	1 in 4,000,000	60
Risk of death in motor vehicle accident, driving 14.5 miles	1 in 4,000,000	60
Risk of stroke or serious neurologic complication from cervical manipulation	1 in 1,000,000	54
Risk of being disabled in motor vehicle accident, driving 1.1 miles	1 in 1,000,000	60
Risk of death, per year, from GI bleeding due to NSAID use for osteoarthritis and related conditions	400 in 1,000,000	61
Overall mortality rate for spinal surgery	7 in 10,000	52
Death rate from cervical spine surgery	4–10 in 10,000	53
Rate of serious or life-threatening complications from spinal stenosis surgery	5 in 100	52

must be fairly judged according to consistent standards. Spinal manipulation should not be held to standards different than those required of other methods.

Terminology

ataxia
cauda equina syndrome
cerebrovascular accident (CVA)
contraindication
absolute contraindication
relative contraindication
Doppler ultrasonography
hemianesthesia
iatrogenic disorder
ischemia
locked-in syndrome
MEDLINE
manipulation
nonsteroidal anti-inflammatory drugs (NSAIDs)
osteoarthritis
randomized controlled trial
red flag
vertebrobasilar insufficiency
Wallenberg syndrome

Review Questions

1. Which artery is most likely to be injured from cervical manipulation? Other than cervical manipulation, what are some other ways that this artery might be injured?

2. What is a reasonable estimate of the risks for a stroke following cervical manipulation?

3. What are the eight signs and symptoms of vertebrobasilar ischemia? Why is it important for chiropractors to be aware of and recognize the presence of these signs and symptoms?

4. Why does a patient with complaints of dizziness or vertigo present a dilemma to a practitioner of cervical manipulation? What is a prudent course of action to take in treating these patients?

5. What specific type of neck adjustment seems to be most associated with an increased risk of vertebrobasilar stroke? How can technique be modified to decrease the risks?

6. What signs and symptoms might a patient experience following a neck adjustment that could indicate that a potentially serious complication has occurred? What is a prudent course of action to follow if a patient presents with these signs and symptoms? What actions are imprudent?

7. Name five major contraindications for manipulation in general.

8. What are the "red flags" for possible fracture in a patient with back pain? What are the red flags for possible tumor or infection? What are the red flags for possible cauda equina syndrome?

9. What are some possible adverse effects from the use of NSAIDs for treatment of musculoskeletal pain? What is the most common and serious adverse effect?

Concept Questions

1. What factors should go into performing a risk-benefit analysis of a particular treatment? How do you determine whether the risks are acceptable? Who should determine this?

2. For what types of conditions are the risks of spinal manipulation acceptable, and why? For what types of conditions are the risks unacceptable? Why? For these conditions, what are some alternative treatments a chiropractor could use with risks that are more acceptable?

3. How would you design a scientific study to better determine the risks of various chiropractic treatments? What strengths and weaknesses would your study have? How practical would it be to actually perform this study? How costly would it be to perform the study, and where could you obtain funding?

References

1. Thomas CL (ed): Taber's Cyclopedic Medical Dictionary. FA Davis, Philadelphia, 1985
2. Anonymous: Chiropractors: Consumer Reports 59: 383, 1994
3. Powell FC, Hanigan WC, Olivero WC: A risk/benefit analysis of spinal manipulation therapy for relief of lumbar or cervical pain. Neurosurgery 33:73, 1993
4. Wiesel SW, Feffer HL, Rothman RH: Neck Pain. The Michie Company, Charlottesville, VA, 1986,
5. Anonymous. Doctors say twist in neck can trigger a stroke. The Washington Post, 14 (col 1), Feb 20, 1994
6. *Foster v. Thornton: Malpractice.* death resulting from chiropractic treatment for headache. JAMA 103:1260, 1934
7. Lee KP, Carlini WG, McCormick GF, Albers GW: Neurologic complications following chiropractic manipulation: a survey of California neurologists. Neurology 45:1213, 1995
8. Lauretti WJ: Chiropractic complications, letter. Neurology 46:884, 1996
9. Haldeman S: Chiropractic complications, letter. Neurology 46:884, 1996
10. Anonymous: Warning! Chiropractors Can Kill You! The Examiner, p. 15(col 3), March 22: 1994
11. Tettenborn B, Caplan LR, Sloan MA et al: Postoperative brainstem and cerebellar infarcts. Neurology 43:471, 1993
12. Fisher M: Basilar artery embolism after surgery under general anesthesia: a case report. Neurology 43:1856, 1993
13. Fogelholm R, Karli P: Iatrogenic brainstem infarction. Eur Neurol 13:6, 1975
14. Okawara S, Nibblelink D: Vertebral artery occlusion following hyperextension and rotation of the head. Stroke 5:640, 1974
15. Hope EE, Bodensteineer JB, Barnes P: Cerebral infarction related to neck position in an adolescent. Pediatrics 72:335, 1983
16. Weintraub MI: Beauty parlor stroke syndrome: report of five cases. JAMA 269:2085, 1993
17. Swenson RS: Spontaneous vertebral artery dissection: a case report. J Neuro Sys 1:10, 1993
18. Mas J, Goeau C, Bousser MG et al: Spontaneous dissection aneurysms of the internal carotid and vertebral arteries: two case reports. Stroke 16:125, 1985
19. Terrett AGJ: Vertebrobasilar Stroke Following Manipulation. National Chiropractic Mutual Insurance Company, West Des Moines, IA, 1996
20. Beatty RA: Dissecting hematoma of the internal carotid artery following chiropractic cervical manipulation. J Trauma 17:248, 1977

21. Jaskoviak P: Complications arising from manipulation of the cervical spine. J Manipul Physiol Ther 3:213, 1980

22. Henderson DJ, Cassidy JD: Vertebral artery syndrome. p. 194. In Vernon H (ed): Upper Cervical Syndrome: Chiropractic Diagnosis and Treatment. Williams & Wilkins, Baltimore, 1988

23. Eder M, Tilscher H: Chiropractic Therapy: Diagnosis and Treatment. [English transl.] Aspen, Gaithersburg, MD, 1990

24. Dvorak J, Orelli F: How dangerous is manipulation to the cervical spine? Manual Med 2:1, 1985

25. Patijn J: Complications in manual medicine: a review of the literature. Manual Med 6:89, 1991

26. Guttman G: Injuries to the vertebral artery caused by manual therapy. [English abs.] Manuelle Med 21:2, 1983

27. *Mason v Forgie, S/C/1569/82*, Court of Queen's Bench, New Brunswick, Canada, decision dated December 27, 1984, accepting expert evidence of Scott Haldeman DC MD PhD: 19, 27

28. Haldeman S, Chapman-Smith D, Petersen DM: Guidelines for Chiropractic Quality Assurance and Practice Parameters. Aspen, Gaithersburg, MD, 1993

29. Carey PF: A report on the occurrence of cerebral vascular accidents in chiropractic practice. JCCA 37:104, 1993

30. Plamandon RL: Summary of 1992 ACA annual statistical survey. ACA J Chiro 30:36, 1993

31. Curtis P, Bove G: Family physicians, chiropractors, and back pain. J Fam Pract 35:551, 1992

32. Klougart N, Leboeuf-Yde C, Rasmussen LR: Safety in chiropractic practice. Part I. The occurrence of cerebrovascular accidents after manipulation to the neck in Denmark from 1978–1988. J Manipul Physiol Ther 19:371, 1996

33. McGregor M, Haldeman S, Kohlbeck FJ: Vertebrobasilar compromise associated with cervical manipulation. Top Clin Chiro 2:63, 1995

34. Terrett AGJ: Misuse of the literature by medical authors in discussing spinal manipulative therapy injury. J Manipul Physiol Ther 18:203, 1995

35. Carver G, Willits J: Comparative study and risk factors of a CVA. J Am Chiropr Assoc 32:65, 1995

36. Terrett AGJ: Vascular accidents from cervical spine manipulation: the mechanisms. Chiro J Aust 17:131, 1987

37. Haldeman S, Kohlbeck FJ, McGregor M: Cerebrovascular complications following cervical spine manipulation therapy: a review of 53 cases. In Conference Proceedings of the Chiropractic Centennial Foundation, Washington, DC, July 6–8, 1995

38. Chapman-Smith D: Vertigo. Chiropr Report 5(5):1, 1991

39. Fitz-Ritson D: Assessment of cervicogenic vertigo. J Manipul Physiol Ther 14:193, 1991

40. George PE, Silverstein HT, Wallace H, Marshall M: Identification of the high-risk pre-stroke patient. J Chiro 15:S26, 1981

41. Côté P, Kreitz BG, Cassidy JD, Thiel H: The validity of the extension-rotation test as a clinical screening procedure before neck manipulation: a secondary analysis. J Manipul Physiol Ther 19:159, 1996

42. Steinmetz OK, Cole CW: Noninvasive blood flow tests in vascular disease. Can Fam Physician 39:2404, 1993

43. Schoning M, Walter J: Evaluation of the vertebrobasilar-posterior system by transcranial color duplex sonography in adults. Stroke 23:1280, 1992

44. Thiel H, Wallace K, Donat J, Yong-Hing K: Effect of various head and neck positions on vertebral artery blood flow. Clin Biomech 16:105, 1994

45. Assendelft WJJ, Bouter LM, Knipschild PG: Complications of spinal manipulation: a comprehensive review of the literature. J Fam Pract 42:475, 1996

46. *Blakewell v Kahle:* Medicolegal abstracts. Chiropractors: rupture of brain tumor following adjustment. JAMA 148:699, 1952

47. *York v Daniels:* Medicolegal abstracts. Chiropractors: injury to spinal meninges during adjustments. JAMA 159:809, 1955

48. Terrett AGJ, Kleynhans AM: Complications from manipulation of the low back. Chiro J Aust 22:129, 1992

49. Shekelle PG, Adams AH, Chassin MR et al: Spinal manipulation for low-back pain. Ann Intern Med 117:590, 1992

50. Dvorak J, Kränzlin P, Mühlemann D, Wälchi B: Musculoskeletal Complications. p. 549. In Haldeman S (ed): Principles and Practice of Chiropractic. 2nd Ed. Appleton & Lange, Norwalk, CT, 1992

51. Gatterman MI: Chiropractic Management of Spine Related Disorders. Williams & Wilkins, Baltimore, 1990

52. Bigos S, Bowyer O, Braen G et al: Acute Low Back Problems in Adults. Clinical Practice Guideline No. 14. AHCPR Publ. Nos. 95-0642-3. U.S. Department of Health and Human Services, Public Health Service, Agency for Health Care Policy and Research, Rockville, MD, 1994

53. Cervical Spine Research Society Editorial Committee: The Cervical Spine. 2nd Ed. JB Lippincott, Philadelphia, 1989

54. Dabbs V, Lauretti WJ: A risk assessment of cervical manipulation vs. NSAIDs for the treatment of neck pain. J Manipul Physiol Ther 18:530, 1995

55. Bogduk N: Neck pain: how to treat. Aust Dr Wkly (August 21): I–VII, 1992

56. Saag KG, Cowdery JS: Nonsteroidal anti-inflammatory drugs: balancing benefits and risks. Spine 19:1530, 1994

57. Dillin W, Uppal GS: Analysis of medications used in the treatment of cervical disc degeneration. Orthop Clin North Am 23:421, 1992

58. Koes BW, Bouter LM, van Mameren H et al: Randomized clinical trial of manipulative therapy and physical therapy for persistent back and neck complaints. BMJ 304:601, 1992

59. Smith R: Where is the wisdom? The poverty of medical evidence, editorial. BMJ 303:798, 1991

60. National Safety Council: Accident Facts 1995 Ed. National Safety Council, Itasca, IL, 1995

61. Fries JF: Assessing and understanding patient risk. Scand J Rheumatol, suppl. 92:21, 1992

62. Burke LB, Baum C, Jolson HM et al: Drug Utilization in the United States: 1989. Eleventh Annual Review. Department of Health and Human Services, Office of Epidemiology and Biostatistics, Center for Drug Evaluation and Research, Food and Drug Administration, Rockville, MD, 1991

63. Babb R: Gastrointestinal complications of nonsteroidal anti-inflammatory drugs. West J Med 157: 444, 1992

64. Carson JL, Willett LR: Toxicity of nonsteroidal anti-inflammatory drugs: An overview of the epidemiological evidence. Drugs, suppl. 1. 46:243, 1993

65. Saag KG, Cowdery JS: Nonsteroidal anti-inflammatory drugs: balancing benefits and risks. Spine 9:1530, 1994

66. Bach GL: Introduction. Scand J Rheumatol, suppl. 96:5, 1992

67. Armstrong CP, Blower AL: Nonsteroidal anti-inflammatory drugs and life threatening complications of peptic ulceration. Gut 28:527, 1987

68. Savvas P, Brooks PM: Nonsteroidal anti-inflammatory drugs: risk factors versus benefits. Aust Fam Physician 20:1726, 1991

69. Gabriel SE, Jaakkimainen L, Bombardier C: Risk for serious gastrointestinal complications related to use of nonsteroidal anti-inflammatory drugs: a meta-analysis. Ann Intern Med 115:787, 1991

70. Wilcox CM, Shalek KA, Cotsonis G: Striking prevalence of over-the-counter nonsteroidal anti-inflammatory drug use in patients with upper gastrointestinal hemorrhage. Arch Intern Med 154:42, 1994

71. Brandt KD: Should osteoarthritis be treated with nonsteroidal anti-inflammatory drugs? Rheum Dis Clin North Am 19:697, 1993

72. Terrett AGJ, Kleynhans AM: Cerebrospinal complications of manipulation. p. 579. In Haldeman S (ed): Principles and Practice of Chiropractic. 2nd Ed. Appleton & Lange, Norwalk, CT, 1992

15
Chiropractic and the Law

Alan Dumoff

I am not an advocate for frequent changes in laws and constitutions, but laws and institutions must go hand and hand with the process of the human mind. As that becomes more developed, more enlightened, as new discoveries are made, new truths discovered and manners and opinions change, with the change of circumstances, institutions must advance also to keep pace with the times. We might as well require a man to wear still the coat which fitted him when a boy as civilized society to remain under the regimen of their barbarous ancestors.

Thomas Jefferson,
in a letter to Samuel Kercheval, 1816

Several generations after these words were written, the art and science of chiropractic began. This development brought new ways of understanding and treating disease and challenged state and private institutions that were developing to regulate, and in some cases, monopolize, the business of health care. Chiropractors have had many successes crafting a role in the health care system and continue to face numerous challenges in an increasingly regulated and managed care system.

Chiropractic has always reflected a somewhat idiosyncratic professional community. Many chiropractors are understandably uneasy with the unprecedented oversight and complexity in utilization reviews, quality assurance concerns, and the overarching control over medical care exercised by managed care and governmental programs. The increasingly bureaucratic nature of the health care delivery system has been counterbalanced to some extent by a resurgence of interest in natural healing systems, which has created additional opportunities for the chiropractic profession.

Chiropractic is sufficiently established that there is question as to whether it should be referred to as an "alternative" healing system. However, it clearly does offer an alternative to allopathic healing. As alternative and complementary care take an increasingly larger role in the health care system, chiropractic plays a unique role in this progression. Chiropractic has the mixed blessing of being the best established of the alternative modalities, not only as a method of patient care but also as a target of mainstream medical concern. Chiropractic is advancing on many fronts. Legal actions against noncompetitive institutional practices and inappropriate denials by insurance companies, state laws banning discrimination against chiropractic in health insurance policies, reimbursement for a wider range of services by Medicare and worker's compensation programs, continuing development of professional standards of care, and expanded interpretation of scope of practice are areas of continuing struggle as the profession seeks to expand its legal purview to fit the range of competence it can offer its patients.

HISTORICAL DEVELOPMENT

When D.D. Palmer delivered his first adjustment in 1895, the professional landscape comprised a lively competition between physicians and surgeons, osteopaths, homeopaths, eclectic herbalists, and a variety of other healers. At the turn of the century, what is now known as scientific medicine was at its very inception. Ether and antiseptics had only been on the medical scene for a generation,[1] and the use of the "heroic" efforts of blistering, bleeding, and cathartics were in decline. Medical schools began to grow in earnest at this juncture, a growth that bloomed into a more professional education following the Flexner Report's recommendations. By 1895, one-half of the states had passed medical practice acts limiting the practice of medicine to those educated at allopathic medical schools.[2]

As medical schools elevated their educational quality in the early part of the century, other professional and economic factors converged to accelerate the development of the medical profession. The founding of third-party payors, including Blue Cross–Blue Shield and indemnity insurance policies, steered access to care sharply in the direction of medically trained providers. The growth of medical hospitals and investment in the pharmaceuticals industry also consolidated medical economic strength. These events established medical care as an industry and planted seeds for the struggle between chiropractic and conventional medicine.

Limited license statutes began shortly after the passage of the medical practice acts, as states recognized that practitioners such as dentists were required to focus on particular areas not within the training of medical physicians. Chiropractic played an important role in this process. By the 1920s, chiropractic was flourishing, with approximately 36,000 practitioners, a figure that has slowly grown to approximately 52,000 in the United States today.[3] Chiropractic was widely recognized at the beginning of the century and was tolerated to the extent that many of the states without chiropractic licensing allowed large numbers of chiropractors to practice.[1] The Federation of Chiropractic Licensing Boards was established in 1933 to promote unified standards in licensing and to provide assistance to individual state licensing boards. By 1974, chiropractic was licensed in all 50 states and in the District of Columbia.

Central to the advancement of any health occupation as a licensed profession is the creation of a standardized and accepted competency examination. The National Board of Chiropractic Examiners has been administering the National Board examinations since 1965. Most states also require that chiropractors continue their training by imposing continuing education requirements for license renewal. The only exceptions are Arizona, Connecticut, New Jersey, New York, Utah, Vermont, and Virginia.

Current Efforts to Advance Chiropractic

State and national chiropractic associations are working to further the legal framework under which patients have access to quality chiropractic care. The development of standardized practice guidelines, for example, has been a focus throughout the health care industry. The Congress of Chiropractic State Associations has supported the development of such voluntary standards since 1992, referred to as the "Mercy Guidelines." The American Chiropractic Association (ACA) was recently granted representation on the American Medical Association (AMA) committee which authors the current procedural terminology (CPT) insurance reimbursement codes. Another significant advance in the acceptance of chiropractic is the creation in 1995 of a "Chiropractic Health Care" section of the American Public Health Association (APHA). The APHA maintained an antichiropractic posture until 1982, when it modified its stance in response to efforts of the chiropractic community, including the historic lawsuit *Wilk v. AMA*, highlighted later in this chapter.

Recent Growth in Alternative Practices

The past decade has seen phenomenal growth in public and professional recognition of alternative and complementary health care approaches as a critical ingredient in health and wellness. The role of nutrition and lifestyle; the contributions of alternative approaches, such as acupuncture, herbal medicine, and homeopathy; and the role of attitude and patient responsibility have all gained consumer and scientific acknowledgement. This growing interest is due to the successes of alternative approaches and recognition of the limitations of conventional medicine as a complete approach to health needs. While still termed "alternative," these approaches are a significant aspect of our health care system. Americans make more visits to alternative practitioners than to primary care medical doctors and pay more out of pocket to see these providers than for outpatient medical treatment.[4]

The National Institutes of Health (NIH), through the Office of Alternative Medicine, has a small budget to issue grants as part of a new commitment to research the effectiveness of alternative treatments. More than 40 medical schools are beginning to teach alternative medical practices, and a government panel recently recommended that this practice be extended to all medical school curricula. These changes portend a growing integration of mainstream and alternative modalities, a shift that will create challenges and opportunities for chiropractors.

SCOPE OF PRACTICE ISSUES

In the United States, healing arts practice is regulated predominantly at the state level. While the federal government regulates some aspects of health care through food and drug law, and has a significant impact through its regulation of third-party payment in the form of Medicare (for the elderly and disabled), Medicaid (for the poor), and CHAMPUS (for military dependents), the vast majority of health care regulation is left to the states. This includes licensing or certification of health care providers. Each state decides which types of providers it will authorize, the educational and other requirements for licensure, and the rules to which practitioners must conform their practice. Of particular importance, each state sets the nature and extent of practice allowable for each health profession.

There is significant variation among the 50 states in the scope of practice granted by the state, and chiropractors setting up practice must take special care to learn the nuances of these requirements. Some states have narrow definitions restricting chiropractors to manipulation of the spine, while others allow chiropractors a broad range of treatment modalities to address a broad range of health care complaints. The fact that a procedure is taught in

chiropractic training institutions does not mean that the practice will be within the chiropractor's scope in a particular state.[5] However, the lack of training in a procedure at a chiropractic college can be held to bar the practice.[6]

The grant given chiropractors to practice is considered a *limited* scope of practice. Every health care provider other than medical physicians (MDs and DOs) is given such a limited license. While only medical physicians have a general grant to diagnose and treat any disease or illness and to do so using virtually any modality, limited license practitioners must be sure that they remain within the bounds of their licensed activities and do not infringe upon the practice of medicine. Although courts may not always recognize the requirement, a disciplinary action against a chiropractor for exceeding the scope of practice must demonstrate not only that the statute did not authorize the practice in question but that the activity infringes upon the practice of medicine.[7]

Some chiropractors have attempted to avoid licensure by claiming that they are practicing naturopathy. Some states allow the practice of naturopathy based simply on registration, facilitating entry and ensuring less oversight. Since naturopaths include manipulation in their practice, these chiropractors have reasoned that they should be allowed to practice in this manner. The courts have disagreed, holding that the practice of chiropractic falls under the defined scope of chiropractic and therefore requires such a license.[8]

Legal Status of Chiropractors

Notwithstanding the limited scope of their license, chiropractors are considered independent practitioners. Independent practitioners are able to practice without a supervisory or collaborative relationship with a medical physician or other provider. By contrast, many health care occupations are dependent on some form of supervision or collaboration with a medical physician, including nurses (except for advanced nurse practitioners) and physician assistants. Others, such as acupuncturists, nutritionists, and physical therapists, are either independent or dependent, depending on state law.

The independent status of chiropractors allows them to play the role of gatekeeper in various health care settings. Despite their independent status, some states bar chiropractors from using the term "chiropractic physician."[9]

Statutes also address the ability of chiropractors to include a variety of particular modalities in their practice, such as acupuncture, acupressure, or meridian therapies; nutritional counseling; ancillary procedures, such as electric muscle stimulators, hot and cold packs, diathermy, ultrasound, and massage; laboratory diagnostic procedures; or even whether a chiropractor can perform a physical examination or radiography that extends to parts of the body other than the spine.[7] Chiropractors risk disciplinary proceedings for practicing activities not clearly within their scope of practice. Not surprisingly, these differences among the states reflect the political and legal struggle between the "straight" and "mixer" schools of chiropractic,[10,11] as well as the concerns of those who have sought to limit the reach of chiropractic.

Acupuncture

Acupuncture is generally considered a medical practice because it is offered for the treatment of disease and because it involves penetration of the skin. The practice of acupuncture by chiropractors has been addressed differently among the states. Some states allow chiropractors to practice as part of their standard scope of practice, others allow practice upon completion of some postgraduate training, and most states prohibit such practice under chiropractic licensure. Chiropractors can currently practice acupuncture as part of their scope of practice in Illinois, Iowa, Kansas, New Mexico, and Oklahoma and can do so with some additional training in Alabama, Arizona, Colorado, Florida, Maine, Minnesota, Missouri, North Dakota, South Dakota, Texas, Virginia, and West Virginia.[12] Some chiropractors practice a form of meridian therapy that does not involve the puncture of the skin. This technique is more likely to be acceptable, since it is not an invasive procedure, although results of disciplinary actions have been mixed.[13–15]

Diagnostic Testing

Another issue of contention is the extent to which chiropractors may perform or order diagnostic testing. Some chiropractors perform complete physical examinations, including drawing blood for diagnostic testing or obtaining Papanicolaou smears. Like most questions on scope of practice, the answers arrived at by chiropractic boards and state courts have varied from state to state. The intent of the practitioner may govern the result; the procedure itself may be seen as within the competency of the practitioner, but in some states an intent to diagnose human ailments "unrelated" to chiropractic practice can lead to liability.[16]

Nutritional Counseling

The right of a chiropractor to give nutritional advice has been the subject of much contention and confusion. Allowable conduct under chiropractic practice acts is not always self-evident. Some courts have held, for example, that chiropractors cannot prescribe or otherwise suggest to their patients that they take a supplement available over the counter even where the state practice act allows for giving "dietary advice."[14,17] Nutritional advice has been problematic throughout the alternative health care community, and chiropractors have been a primary target despite the irony that many chiropractors are better trained in nutrition than most medical physicians. These disciplinary actions occur because of a concern that the chiropractor is "prescribing" for a particular ailment in a manner that appears to run counter to the established legal history of chiropractic as a "drugless art."[14,15,18] Courts are particularly concerned when specific remedies are suggested for particular ailments,[19] when the provider does not explain his or her educational background or limited scope of practice,[19] when blood tests are used as a basis for nutritional guidance,[17] or when the provider has otherwise exceeded his or her scope of practice.[14]

Convictions are often based on statements that can be interpreted as a prescription for a specific disease. But practitioners should note that many of these cases contain additional facts that may have added to the court's willingness to find the providers culpable of practicing medicine without a license. A chiropractor, for example, found guilty of medical practice act violations for giving nutritional advice was selling a line of nutritional products at his office. While the language of the court suggests it may have upheld his conviction in any event, these sales may have undercut the argument that the statements were informational, rather than prescriptive.[14]

While scope of practice arises expressly only from the language of the state law, standards of care established by the profession can influence a court in its interpretation where the scope is ambiguous. The ACA holds that "it is appropriate for doctors of chiropractic to recommend the use of vitamins, minerals, and food supplements for their patients, to the extent that this is not in conflict with state statutes and regulations."[20] When weight loss is at issue, an assessment should be made, and the recommendations should not include experimental products. The ACA recommends that the chiropractor's suggestions be supported by independent laboratory data.[20]

The provision of information, as opposed to prescription for a particular disease, may provide protection for chiropractors operating without a clear scope of practice allowing for nutritional consultation. While this is a gray area of law, the provision of information and education, rather than prescription for a particular disease, is on legally safer ground. Providing information is arguably protected by the First Amendment's guarantees of free speech. When one tells a client, "If I had these symptoms, I would suspect a liver deficiency and would try to assist the liver using milk thistle," or, "There is a significant body of evidence that daily use of feverfew can prevent migraines," this is the provision of information and is arguably protected speech. While historically, the protection of free speech is deeply honored and respected by our courts, the hoped-for protection in these statements could be rejected by a disciplinary body or the courts as merely an artifice meant to allow the practice of medicine.

The legal distinction that turns a substance into a drug is the purpose for which it is suggested. Strictly speaking, any material intended for use to mitigate or cure a disease can be considered a drug.[17,21] Most cases disciplining chiropractors for nutritional advice therefore involve prescribing a supplement for a particular disease condition.[18] When garlic is suggested because of its wonderful taste, it is a food; when garlic is suggested because it can mitigate arteriosclerosis by lowering cholesterol, it becomes a drug in the eyes of the law. Simply educating someone that there is evidence that garlic lowers cholesterol, however, without mentioning artery disease, references the nutritional impact on the structure and process of the body without going so far as to prescribe for disease.

Such an approach may provide some protection, as it follows the approach taken by a compromise Congress adopted in 1994 in its regulation of health claims on supplements and other natural products in the Dietary Supplement Health Education Act (DSHEA).[22] This law addresses the issue of health claims that may be made by supplement manufacturers, allowing claims regarding the impact on processes of the body, but not with regard to disease or illness.[23] A supplement manufacturer could claim that calcium supplements improve the strength of bones, for example, but could not claim that calcium mitigates or cures osteoporosis. This distinction does not offer clear protection; it is important to recognize that federal food and drug law holds that "articles (other than food) intended to affect the structure of any function of the body of man..." are drugs.[24]

Nevertheless, discussing structure, rather than disease, when the substance is at least arguably a food, as is the case for many supplements, serves to make the conversation more clearly educational and lessens, if not removes, the intent to prescribe a drug for a particular illness. Since state medical boards largely follow federal food and drug law in interpreting the scope of medical practice acts, framing advice in the same manner Congress allows manufacturers to label supplements under the DSHEA should have some weight in disciplinary matters.

MALPRACTICE AND DISCIPLINARY ISSUES

Ethical Concerns

While ethics are not strictly legal in nature, violations of ethical principles can have legal consequences. State laws generally make the violation of an ethical code a basis for discipline by the state chiropractic board or comparable regulatory body. Ethical codes can also be considered standards of care, making their violation a basis for a malpractice action. Substance abuse is a frequent basis for discipline. If a chiropractor engages in sexual contact with a patient, this ethical breach could be the basis for a malpractice action in addition to an action involving battery (unlawful touching) and informed consent, since a patient is often considered swayed by the authority of the health care provider and thus unable to grant informed consent for sexual activity. There is risk even when it appears that the patient is a willing participant. If the relationship turns sour, apparent consent can be held to have been manipulated under the influence of the doctor–patient relationship.

Certain practice building efforts also raise ethical issues. Many chiropractic colleges and marketing companies teach a variety of practice building techniques. Many of these methods are ethical and uncontroversial. Others raise concerns of professionalism or even health and safety. Advertising free radiographic examinations, for example, may subject patients to unnecessary radiation without documented clinical need.[25] Efforts to incorporate controversial or poorly documented mind/body approaches into practice can also create exposure; informing patients that scoliosis is caused by emotional and psychological problems, for example, has been a basis for discipline.[6]

Malpractice Issues

A health care provider becomes liable in malpractice when the provider (1) Harms a patient, (2) To whom he or she owed a duty of due care, (3) Resulting from a negligent act, (4) That violated the standards of care for the profession.

The issues of harm and duty are usually clear in cases reaching the court. The issue on which litigation generally turns is whether the provider's negligence breached a standard of care and actually harmed the patient. Negligence can arise from *commission*, such as an adjustment that causes injury to a patient, or *omission*, such as failing to diagnose a disease or contraindication or to make a referral to a medical physician or other professional when appropriate.

Malpractice actions against chiropractors are frequently based on allegations that the patient was injured by an adjustment, that the chiropractor should have recognized the treatment was contraindicated, or that the patient was misdiagnosed. One frequent basis for litigation is a claim that the

chiropractor failed to take necessary radiographs or perform other diagnostic tests.[26] Liability can also occur as a result of false representations of the reach of chiropractic care,[27] a claim in which the patient asserts that he or she was fraudulently induced into seeking a treatment for a medical condition not responsive to chiropractic for which medical treatment would have been appropriate. The prescription of herbs for a serious infection or other medical condition is an area of clear malpractice risk.[28] The creation of some pain during a procedure is by itself generally insufficient to create malpractice liability.[29]

Necessity of Referral

One critical area for chiropractors is the duty to refer to a medical doctor or other provider for diagnosis or treatment if the chiropractor has reason to suspect a condition requiring such attention. Chiropractors are particularly vulnerable to such suits, given their limited scope of practice, particularly in states whose statute and judicial environment is not friendly to chiropractors. This obligation can even extend to a requirement that the chiropractor follow up with an ongoing patient to ensure that the patient follows through on the referral.[30]

Given the increasing interest in integrated practices (see Ch. 19), chiropractors should be aware that collaborative practice has risks that, although manageable, are nonetheless real. A provider can be liable for the negligence of another due to association or to joint work with the patient. An attorney can assist in limiting this liability by attention to the scope of practice governing the various providers, representations made to the patients, the legal structure of the practice, quality assurance efforts in choice of colleagues, and other such avenues.

Informed Consent

Like other health care professionals, chiropractors are subject to liability for violating a patient's right to informed consent. This is an action in battery and is a modification of the long-established principle that people have a right to only be touched when they consent to that touch. Given the complexities of the professional health care relationship, the law has imputed a responsibility on the part of health care practitioners to educate their patients on the

VARIATIONS IN INTERPRETATION

The law can be frustrating in the variable way it responds to issues of liability. In New York, a patient fell off an examining table. This accident was ruled to be ordinary negligence, rather than professional malpractice, thus removing the matter from the hearing panel created for malpractice claims.[31] The exact opposite occurred in Louisiana, when a patient fell off an x-ray table. This accident was held to be malpractice, resulting in the dismissal of the suit, brought as ordinary negligence, for failure to bring the matter before the malpractice hearing panel.[32] Such distinctions, and their procedural results, can often drive the outcomes in malpractice litigation.

nature of procedures, including their risks and benefits, before touching patients. When such informed consent is not obtained, the touching can legally convert a healing act to a battery.[33] A practice of adjusting patients unaware of the impending manipulation in order to minimize resistance makes the chiropractor vulnerable to such a suit, as does attempting to treat a presenting symptom from a part of the body distal to the spine without explanation or consent. A finding that the chiropractor misrepresented the treatment can lead to liability for failing to acquire informed consent.[33]

Informed consent forms can also provide some protection for alternative practices that fall outside the standard of care. Chiropractors who incorporate unusual approaches can inform their patients of the risks and benefits of, as well as alternatives to, their techniques. Should an adverse reaction anticipated in the consent form occur, a court might find that the patient assumed the risk of the harm and find that the chiropractor is not liable. A recent medical case that accepted this argument involved the unconventional cancer treatment of Emanuel Revici, a New York medical physician, whose finding of liability was overturned by an appeals court, based on this defense.[34]

Standard of Care

A primary concern for chiropractic has been what standard of care the profession would be held to in malpractice cases; earlier in the century, medical physicians would frequently testify against chiropractors despite their lack of education in and disdain for chiropractic care. Most courts now recognize that the standard of care to be applied for nonmedical health care modalities is the standard of care for that profession; the question is not what a physician should have done, but what a competent chiropractor (or acupuncturist, naturopath, or other relevant provider) would have done. While the practices of chiropractic may seem "nonstandard" to a medical doctor, the legal posture for chiropractic is that the chiropractic body of knowledge provides customary and standard practices for chiropractic.[35,36] Similarly, allegations that a chiropractor failed to diagnose an ailment accurately or recognize a contraindication would generally be tested not by whether a physician would have made the diagnosis, but by whether a similarly trained provider would have. Testimony against a chiropractor, therefore, generally cannot come from a physician but must come from one licensed in chiropractic.[27,33,36]

An important exception to this rule is when chiropractors are found by the court to have exceeded their scope of practice and to have made what would be considered a medical determination. In that event, they will be held to a medical standard of care.[29,37] Chiropractors are limited in their legal ability to diagnose and treat disease; they face malpractice exposure when it can be shown that they exceeded their statutory scope of practice.

Malpractice insurance is an important aspect of protection against claims. It is important to know one's policy and its exclusions. Intentional acts, such as sexual malpractice, are generally not covered. This is also true of needle acupuncture or other modalities outside of the chiropractor's scope of practice.

Malpractice in Practice

An awkward dilemma faced by chiropractors in some jurisdictions is that their liability in malpractice can arguably extend into areas for which it is difficult to protect themselves due to limitations in scope of practice. Chiropractors may be barred, for example, from performing a full physical examination, taking or ordering radiographs of the body other than of the spine, or ordering laboratory tests. Yet chiropractors may be liable in malpractice for failing to determine if a referral is necessary or if a procedure is indicated or contraindicated based on information that would be yielded by these tests.[7,38]

One of the fronts along which the battle is being fought for full recognition of chiropractic is inclusion as "primary care" physicians, a determination that has malpractice implications. A threshold matter in this struggle is the extent to which the state law recognizes the chiropractor as a gatekeeper or independent physician with a broad scope of practice allowing for inclusion in managed care and insurance systems. When a chiropractor achieves some gatekeeper status, there is an increased obligation to make proper referrals when he or she finds signs or symptoms that may reflect a medical condition, particularly if that condition is outside of that chiropractor's scope of treatment.

Even when the condition treated is within the chiropractor's scope of practice, conservative practice still suggests that a referral be contemplated and discussed with the patient in such cases. Whatever the state scheme, there is a risk that a court may find even a back problem to be medical, rather than chiropractic, resulting in a malpractice finding against the chiropractor.[39] The issues of referrals and missed medical diagnoses are less troublesome within managed care networks, since patients generally will have been referred to chiropractors by medical physicians. Thus, the inclusion of chiropractors in managed care networks significantly lessens this primary area of exposure. As chiropractors become gatekeepers in managed care settings, their liability will increase, and the issue of scope of practice limitations may hinder full participation.

THE WILK CASE

The relationship between chiropractic and allopathic medicine is uneasy at best; historically, these two professions have been at war. In a remarkable and significant case, Chester A. Wilk and four other chiropractors successfully sued the AMA for violations of federal antitrust laws.[40] This suit alleged that

the AMA "violated § 1 of the Sherman Antitrust Act[41] by conducting an illegal boycott in restraint of trade directed at chiropractors generally. ..." The court found that the AMA had set out with clear intent to eliminate chiropractic and that the motive for this effort was not protection of patients, but the economic self-interest of its membership. At the heart of this suit was the now infamous "Principle 3" of the AMA, which stated that: "A physician should practice a method of healing founded on a scientific basis; and he should not voluntarily associate with anyone who violates these principles."

The evidence presented at the trial made it clear that the AMA branded chiropractic an "unscientific cult" and intended by Principle 3 to pressure medical physicians into boycotting chiropractors and anyone who associated with them. This boycott was managed by the AMA Committee on Quackery, which moved to limit referral both to and from medical physicians, to deny hospital privileges to chiropractors, and to bar medical and chiropractic physicians from teaching in each other's schools.

Midway through the trial, the *Wilk* plaintiffs dropped their monetary demand in an effort to focus on winning a declaration that the AMA had

PRE-*WILK* MEDICAL STANDARDS

One of the many practices of the AMA that came out at trial was the effort of AMA member physicians to subvert the customary handling of referrals made by chiropractors. The protocol for a referral between health professionals is ordinarily one in which the patient is sent to a specialist who sees the patient, suggests appropriate diagnosis and treatment, and then sends the patient back to the referring physician. AMA physicians were encouraged to give patients referred to them by chiropractors a "quack pack," which was used to discourage the patient from returning to the chiropractor. These clearly anticompetitive activities successfully denied patients both chiropractic services and the advantages of a team containing both medical and chiropractic physicians.

been conducting an illegal boycott. The plaintiffs had lost a jury verdict in a first trial but had that verdict vacated because of improper jury instructions.[40] During the first trial, the AMA had presented the jury with numerous practice building manuals in an effort to show that chiropractors are governed by greed, rather than by patient care. By removing the monetary demand, this evidence was no longer considered relevant, and the second trial focused on the issue of the AMA conduct.

The AMA argued at trial that their motive for the boycott was a genuine and reasonable concern for patient care. One of the core successes of the *Wilk* legal team was that they presented enough evidence of the efficacy of chiropractic that the court found the "patient care defense" objectively unreasonable.[40] The court required the AMA to rescind its position with respect to chiropractic and to widely disseminate a new policy that did not discourage association with chiropractors by its members.

Current Implications of the *Wilk* Decision

The court found that the conspiracy formally ended in 1980, but that the "lingering effects still threatened plaintiffs with current injury.[40] This is as true today as it was when the opinion was written in 1990. While an overt conspiracy may not be in evidence, these lingering effects are felt in the policies of third-party payors, individual decisions of hospitals and other health care institutions to exclude chiropractors, and efforts by some physicians and organizations still dedicated to eliminating chiropractic along with other complementary and alternative forms of health care.

One of the limitations of *Wilk* was that the court did not grant relief against the AMA's co-defendants. In addition to the AMA, the *Wilk* plaintiffs also pursued their action against the Joint Commission on the Accreditation of Hospitals (JCAH) and the American College of Physicians (ACP), as well as several other medical societies. The JCAH and the ACP were dismissed from the suit, and the plaintiffs settled with the American Hospital Association (AHA) and other co-defendants.

As a result of the suit, however, the JCAH and AHA have taken the position that whether a hospital extends privileges to chiropractors is up to each individual hospital. The organizations no longer use the threat of loss of accreditation or professional censure to force hospitals to exclude chiropractors. Whether this brought an end to the conspiracy, or merely decentralized it to local communities, is open to debate and future litigation. Nothing in the *Wilk* opinion expressly prevents individual hospitals from choosing not to grant privileges to chiropractors. Progress in this regard has been definite but very slow; while some hospitals began extending privileges during the early 1980s when the *Wilk* case was first decided, according to the ACA approximately 200 of the 6,500 hospitals in the United States have some form of chiropractic participation, and of these, only about 50 extend staff privileges to chiropractic physicians.[42]

Staffing privileges allow chiropractors access to patients, their medical records, and some support services while they are in the hospital. Some hospitals have taken the extra step of granting chiropractors co-admitting privileges under which they can admit a patient along with a medical physician. These privileges are generally granted either to individual chiropractors or to a group that contracts with the hospital to provide chiropractic services. Some hospitals have even set up chiropractic departments within the hospital. (See Ch. 19 for further details).

Current Litigation: *Wilk* Revisited in the Managed Care Setting

The dominant role played by managed care organizations (MCOs) in the American health care marketplace makes MCO policies toward chiropractic critical to the future of the profession. MCOs have been slow to accept the inclusion of chiropractic, or where services are covered, to accept the full range of chiropractic services. MCOs rarely afford chiropractors status as primary care providers with gatekeeping responsibility. While chiropractors were well entrenched throughout the United States before the inception of the first health maintenance organization (HMOs) in the 1930s, as of 1993 only 16 percent of MCOs covered chiropractic services.[43]

While the battleground over unlawful boycotts by medical doctors against chiropractors during the 1980s was centered in large part on hospital privileges, a key struggle as we approach the next century is full participation of chiropractors in managed care. Antitrust suits are currently being brought alleging a continuing conspiracy on the part of medical societies, hospitals, and MCOs to boycott chiropractic services unlawfully.[44] The AMA, along with various MCOs, is once again being called to defend against allegations of conspiring to restrain the delivery of health care services by chiropractors. At issue in these actions are the exclusion of chiropractors from participation in health plans as gatekeepers or providers, or, when included, restrictions on the scope of benefits that effectively curtail the value offered by chiropractic. These limitations include restrictions on the conditions the plan will cover, limitation of treatment to spinal manipulation, and denial of access to laboratories, radiography facilities, and professional consultation and referral arrangements. Also at issue are internal decision-making arrangements in which only MDs are enfranchised as decision makers. Scientific studies demonstrating the superior efficacy of chiropractic for some conditions are arbitrarily dismissed, and excessive and improper utilization reviews targeting chiropractors are alleged to have occurred.

A primary concern that MCOs must address in choosing providers is the obligation to ensure professional quality. Clearly, the chiropractic profession, with its authorized scope of practice, well-established professional associations, credentialing bodies, peer-review bodies, and established standards of care and ethical conduct is sufficiently developed to meet these quality assurance requirements. One difficulty that health care institutions have faced in bringing chiropractors into their settings has been a perceived variability in chiropractic training. Some hospitals that have experience with chiropractors have found considerable variation in the strength of the curriculum in the sciences and in the ability of chiropractors to provide effective relief for back injuries. Although the skills of medical doctors are also variable, a system based on medical peer review is more comfortable dealing with such variation in their peers. Efforts are being made to incorporate chiropractors into the internal processes at health care institutions, which may eventually make these professional concerns more manageable.

REIMBURSEMENT ISSUES

Insurance Coverage

Coverage for chiropractic care has been increasingly incorporated in insurance contracts. Forty-one states require insurers to reimburse for chiropractic services.[44] This coverage varies considerably by the type and extent of covered services and the diagnoses for which services will be covered.[45] Even when a contract covers chiropractic services, chiropractors sometimes find that their claims are denied because the insurer finds that the treatments are not "reasonable and necessary" or that payment amounts are capped or otherwise reduced. These disagreements have been the subject of considerable litigation, based on varying theories and with mixed success.[47]

Some state laws require that insurers grant parity or otherwise not discriminate against chiropractors in their payment of benefits. These laws are either specific to chiropractors or include "any willing provider," requiring that if a procedure is covered by the insurance policy, a chiropractor or any provider licensed to perform that procedure within his or her scope of practice must be covered under the contract. But even these laws have not achieved their purpose in some cases. A state has the power, for example, to impose limitations on chiropractic care that indirectly affect insurance reimbursement, since states face reduced antitrust limitations. In Louisiana, chiropractors are barred by statute from working in hospitals. An insurance policy allowing 100 percent reimbursement for manipulations performed in a hospital (e.g., by osteopaths), but only 80 percent for outpatient work (e.g., primarily by chiropractors), was upheld as nondiscriminatory despite the disparate impact this had on reimbursement.[47] The court reasoned that the state could rationally limit chiropractors' access to hospitals and that procedures performed in hospitals could be billed differently than those done on an outpatient basis.

The state of Washington recently enacted a controversial requirement that insurance policies allow "every category of health care provider to provide health services or care for conditions included in the Basic Health Plan.[48] This law requires that every health care plan sold in the state, including fee-for-service and managed care plans, must cover all services within the scope of practice of any licensed provider. As with an "any willing provider" law, if a "health plan covers rehabilitation therapy, that service must be covered whether treatment is rendered by an osteopathic physician, a chiropractor, a registered physical therapist, or a licensed massage therapist, so long as the practitioner is operating within his or her scope of practice.[49] What makes this law unique is that it is based on covered conditions, rather than on covered services. "Any willing provider" legislation generally requires that if a service, such as spinal manipulation, is covered, the policy cannot cover osteopaths and exclude chiropractors. The Washington law is much broader, requiring that if a policy covers treatment by any type of provider for a particular condition (e.g., back pain), it must cover treatment of that condition by all licensed providers within their scope of practice.

A coalition of managed care and indemnity health insurance plans have filed suit against the Washington State Insurance Commissioner, alleging that he misinterpreted that statute to require much broader mandatory coverage of alternative providers than the legislature intended.[50] This issue remains unresolved.

Any willing provider laws have also been the subject of a great deal of litigation.[51] The legislative agenda may turn instead to "direct access" laws, which allow managed care plan members to access specialty care without having to access such care through a referral from a primary care gatekeeper. This would allow patients to refer themselves directly to chiropractors and reduce the impacts of medical gatekeepers biased against the treatments chiropractic has to offer.

Federal Programs: Medicare and Worker's Compensation

Insurance coverage for chiropractic has slowly and steadily grown. While many third-party payors cover the range of services within the chiropractor's scope of practice, there are important limitations. Many contracts still specifically exclude chiropractors or limit payment to the diagnosis and manipulation of spinal subluxations. These limitations are due in part to the tendency of insurance policies to follow the lead of the federal government, a key player in

the health care financing system, in determining compensable benefits.

Medicare limits payment to manual spinal manipulation for demonstrated subluxations of the spine. Federal worker's compensation similarly limits reimbursement. This requirement has limited chiropractic to the status of a "manipulation only" profession, as federal programs and some insurance polices will only reimburse for Current Procedural Terminology (CPT) codes for spinal manipulations, despite the range of services offered by chiropractors. Medicare will only pay for chiropractic services if a radiograph demonstrates the presence of a subluxation and the chiropractor reasonably finds that the subluxation has resulted in a neuromusculoskeletal condition for which manipulation is the appropriate treatment. Yet Medicare will not reimburse for these radiographs, nor will it cover other diagnostic efforts in the patient's interest. The ACA is actively working to change this situation, seeking both payment for a wider range of diagnostic categories and services and relief from the requirement that patients be exposed to radiographs, regardless of clinical need. As a part of this effort, the ACA was granted an unprecedented seat on the AMA committee developing recommendations to the Medicare system on reimbursement criteria and reasonable payment levels.

While the courts allow the standard of care for chiropractic to be set by chiropractors in malpractice cases as noted above, there are still barriers to such professional self-direction in the field of worker's compensation. Unlike malpractice, the issue of worker's compensation is statutory, and the language of some state statutes raises questions about whether a physician from one modality of practice can opine that care being given pursuant to a worker's compensation claim is reasonable and necessary.[52]

A central issue in worker's compensation is whether chiropractors can serve as the primary physician in treating worker's compensation clients. While chiropractors can generally serve in this capacity, certain mechanisms can work to exclude chiropractors. In some states, for example, employers are required to list a specified number of physicians available to a claimant, but there is nothing to require the list to include chiropractic physicians.

Personal injury cases are an important source of income for many chiropractors, and the testimony of the chiropractor regarding the nature and extent of the injury is an important aspect of these cases. A primary issue here is the standard to be applied to the testimony. The trend is to recognize that chiropractic issues are to be judged by chiropractic, not medical, standards.[53]

Reimbursement Mechanics

Utilization review (UR) committees are key centers of decision making in virtually all reimbursement systems. The function of UR is to review submitted claims to determine whether the services provided are reasonable and necessary. Chiropractors often have particular difficulty with such reviews, in part because many UR committees still do not have chiropractors conducting the review of their work. Even when chiropractors sit on the UR committee, the pressure to contain costs can result in determinations that do not follow the minimal standards of the profession. A chiropractic reviewer might, for example, deny payment for radiography, with the conclusion that medical radiographs were available, even though the medical radiographs were recumbent, rather than weight bearing, and thus not acceptable for certain chiropractic purposes. Such decisions are difficult to reverse—UR committees and private companies performing UR functions enjoy limited immunity from civil action.[54]

Insurers and UR companies frequently refer patients for independent medical examinations (IME), which can include referral to a chiropractor for a second opinion. IMEs raise numerous legal issues. When coverage for chiropractic is denied, one of the first places to seek information is the records of the examining physician. This can be difficult to accomplish, as the records are not generally available to the claimant. Another issue is whether a chiropractor takes on malpractice liability by providing such an opinion. Courts generally conclude that no doctor–patient relationship is formed by such an examination, and there is thus no malpractice liability.[55,56] This same reasoning has also barred actions for simple negligence in the performance of the duties for an examining physician, with courts reasoning that the only action in negligence that can be brought is one for profes-

sional negligence (i.e., malpractice), which requires a doctor–patient relationship.[56]

Careful record keeping is an important aspect of billing. One common pitfall is to record dates of services inaccurately. Such inaccuracy can lead to allegations of billing fraud. A surprising number of physicians alter charts in an effort to respond to litigation, an action that can severely damage the doctor's credibility and be used as evidence of fraud.

Fraud and Abuse

Numerous federal statutes target kickbacks, overcharging, and other fraud and abuse issues. These laws are extremely complex, making it difficult for practitioners to follow the letter of the law. The U.S. Congress recently required the Secretary of Health and Human Services to provide advisory opinions to assist in clarifying whether an arrangement violates the law.[57]

A major area of enforcement activity concerns kickbacks and antireferral regulation, in which an individual receives payment for referrals to an entity in which he or she has a financial interest or simply for making a referral. These referral fees generally include another provider, an attorney, or even a "runner" who receives payment, discounted office space, income guarantees, or other benefits for referrals. At issue is the intent of the parties and whether the scheme is intended to induce referrals. Marketing plans can be deemed legitimate or else considered kickback schemes, depending on how they are structured. Kickbacks are also illegal when the provider refers to a laboratory or other venture in which the provider has a financial interest. The law provides "safe harbors" for many activities; any question about an activity should be addressed to counsel familiar with the area.

Overcharging is considered fraud, but it is important to recognize that this violation can occur in a variety of ways. Miscoding, upcoding to a higher fee, unbundling procedures normally billed together to bill the higher, separate amounts, and false reporting of time involved all incur serious penalties. Many of these practices are less of a concern to chiropractors given the few codes available to them, but as additional codes are developed for chiropractic use, chiropractors should familiarize themselves with these issues.

Some states regulate the waiver of copayments, a few outlaw the practice outright, and others require that the insurer be notified of the practice. Failure to disclose waiver of copayment can be interpreted as evidence that the provider is not disclosing to Medicare or the insurer the true amount of the ordinary and customary charge, and is therefore inflating the fee to the payer.[58–60] If waivers of fees are granted, they should be occasional, and the chart should reflect that the chiropractor did examine and base the waiver on the patient's financial circumstances, rather than giving an across-the-board waiver. Medicare has taken the position that the routine waiver of copayments is unlawful because it results in false claims, is essentially a kickback to the patient, and results in excessive utilization.[57–61]

Across-the-board cash discounts for those who are not covered by insurance is also considered fraud. Just as with the waiver of copayment, this conduct informs the insurer that they are being charged a premium, rather than the provider's usual and customary rate. This issue arises not only with health insurance, but also with personal injury, worker's compensation,[62] and other third-party payment arrangements.

The provision of unnecessary services is another major area of controversy for chiropractors, given professional differences of opinion among chiropractors, and especially between chiropractors and medical physicians who review many claims about the necessity of treatment.

Other Practice Issues

Health care practice is a complex business, requiring attention to numerous details beyond the central issues already described. Such an issue arises when a practitioner provides inadequate services because of a patient's limited resources or an insurer's restrictions on payment. Chiropractors should be cautious and should not give an appearance of expressly withholding treatment they believe is indicated due to financial concerns. Once they accept a patient, they become responsible for that patient's treatment.[63]

Advertising is another area that requires attention. An advertisement claiming "Whatever the Cause, We Can Help," for example, can be interpreted as a guarantee, creating liability on the part of the practitioner for a poor result.[64] It can also create disciplinary exposure for exceeding one's scope of practice.

HEALTH CARE FREEDOM

Recent advancements by chiropractic in the health care system are occurring within the context of an overall renaissance in natural health care. The acceptance and potential for integration of alternative and complementary medicine have been progressing rapidly over the past decade. While this public development is positive, considerations of the legal rights one has to practice or to access the care of one's choice still have a direct impact on the development of chiropractic. The accelerating acceptance of alternative care, and the gradual development of additional access to the range of alternative practice, has arisen from public demand rather than from a recognition of such a right in the law. Courts generally hold that the U.S. Constitution does not provide a right to choose one's form of health care.

Ninth Amendment and the Right to Privacy

The Ninth Amendment and the "penumbra" of the Constitution have been held to create a right to privacy. The most famous opinion in this regard is *Roe v. Wade*,[65] which established a constitutional right for women to have an abortion. This right of privacy has also been held to allow people the right to make end-of-life decisions.[66,67] Yet while the courts recognize that the right to privacy and autonomy in one's decisions allows freedom at the beginning and end of life, they have been slow to extend such autonomy to choice of modality of treatment for the life lived in between. Courts do not extend this right to the practice of unorthodox medicine[68,69] or to patient access to the care of their choice. The issue has been raised in areas such as the right of a provider to practice an unconventional approach[68] and to provide nutritional and herbal treatments for cancer.[70,71]

The argument that the Ninth Amendment grants the right to seek the health care of one's choosing has been advanced without success.[72] Terminal cancer patients have no constitutional right of privacy superior to the state's police power, that allows them access to laetrile; there is no right of privacy that requires the state to allow access to laetrile. The only rights courts have found within the meaning of the Amendment are those that survive scrutiny of the "traditions and [collective] conscience of our people" to determine whether a principle is "so rooted [there] … as to be ranked as fundamental."[73] While those seeking alternatives to conventional medical care would certainly rank such freedom as fundamental, the courts limit "retained" freedoms to such clearly, fundamentally, and universally held beliefs as the right to have a family, or, as in *Griswold* and its protection of birth control dissemination, to decide when to have a family.

The judicial opinions rejecting the Ninth Amendment as a constitutional right to medical freedom are consistent with a vast and definitive array of case law that allows states the greatest possible latitude in regulating public health and safety. Potential rights under the Ninth Amendment must be balanced against the Tenth Amendment, which reserves all nonenumerated powers to the states; this includes the so-called "police power," which allows the states virtually exclusive power to regulate matters of public health and safety. The state's police power almost always outweighs a call to what advocates of health care freedom might hope to see in the shadow of the Ninth Amendment.

One remarkable exception to this perspective is *Andrews v. Ballard*,[74] in which a Texas court found a statute restricting acupuncture to medical physicians irrational and unconstitutional. Whether chiropractors can practice acupuncture has been a frequent matter of dispute. In *Andrews*, the court found that the right to privacy includes the right to access the health care of one's choice, placing a limitation on the state's right to regulate health care practice and limit its practice to medical professionals. With rare exceptions,[75] other courts have generally declined to follow *Andrews*.[76]

It is instructive to note that a careful reading of *Roe v. Wade* and its progeny suggests that the Court was not as impressed with the right of a woman to have an abortion as it was distressed at the idea of the state having the right to limit the medical judgment of a physician. The courts have traditionally given great deference to medical physicians in virtually all areas of the law. This deference, even in the face of demonstrated monopolistic practices, has been a significant source of the difficulty faced

by unconventional and alternative providers. The courts turn to the very profession whose professional bodies have opposed chiropractic as well as other alternative and complementary approaches for guidance in how these matters should be addressed. It is not surprising that a privacy right to choose one's treatment from a diverse array of modalities has not been widely adopted by the courts.

Terminology

"any willing provider" laws
battery
CHAMPUS
copayment
current procedural terminology (CPT)
Dietary Supplement Health Education Act (DSHEA)
direct access laws
gatekeeper
indemnity insurance
independent medical examination (IME)
independent practitioner
informed consent
liability
malpractice
Medicaid
miscoding
National Institutes of Health
Ninth Amendment
peer review
scope of practice
standard of care
unbundling
upcoding
utilization review (UR)
Wilk case

Review Questions

1. In what year did the final state pass a chiropractic licensure law?

2. Does the fact that a procedure is taught in chiropractic training institutions mean that the practice will be within the chiropractor's scope in a particular state?

3. Are there any circumstances in which sexual contact with a patient is legally acceptable?

4. What criteria determine malpractice?

5. Is the creation of pain during a procedure by itself sufficient to create malpractice liability?

6. Does the practice of adjusting patients unaware of the impending adjustment violate the principle of informed consent?

7. What was the AMA's primary defense in the Wilk case? How did the chiropractor plaintiffs overcome this defense?

8. What are some limitations of the Wilk decision? Are there still legal ways discriminate against chiropractors?

9. How does Medicare define coverage for chiropractic services?

10. Name three fraudulent billing practices.

Concept Questions

1. Chiropractic scope of practice in the U.S., unlike other nations, is governed by state laws, which vary substantially from one another. What do you believe is the proper scope of practice for chiropractors?

2. What would be different now if the Wilk suit had never been filed?

References

1. Starr P: The Social Transformation of American Medicine. Basic Books, New York, 1982

2. Moore TG: The purpose of licensing. *J Law Econo* 8:93, 103, 1965

3. Peterson: Dynam Chiropr 13(2):3, 1995

4. Eisenberg, et al: Unconventional medicine in the United States. *N Engl J Med* 246 at 251 (Jan. 28, 1993)

5. *See*, e.g., *State, Ex Rel. Iowa Department of Health v. Van Wyk*. 320 N.W. 2d 599 (Iowa 1982)

6. *See*, e.g., *Jutkowitz v. Department of Health Services*, 596 A.2d 374, 384 (Conn. 1991)

7. *See*, e.g., *Attorney General on Behalf of People v. Beno*, 373 N.W.2d 544, 554 (Mich. 1985)

8. *See*, e.g., *Feingold v. State Board of Chiropractic*, 568 A.2d 1365 (Penn. 1990)

9. In Maryland, e.g., *see* 24 Op. Atty. Gen. 172 (1939)

10. *See*, e.g., *State, Ex Rel. Iowa Department of Health v. Van Wyk*, 320 N.W.2d 599 (Iowa 1982) Scope of practice would not be expanded to include acupuncture, the drawing of blood for diagnostic procedures, or nutritional consultation despite suit by chiropractic board against the department of health

11. *Matter of Sherman College of Straight Chiropractic*, 397 A.2d 362 (Sup. Ct. N.J. 1979) Chiropractors following "mixed" school of chiropractic sought to prevent accreditation of a school teaching "straight" chiropractic.

12. Acupuncture and Oriental Medicine Laws. National Acupuncture Foundation (1995 Ed)

13. *See*, e.g., *State Board of Chiropractic Examiners v. Clark*, 713 S.W.2d 621 (Mo. App. 1986) Laser stimulation of acupunture points acceptable as a "reflex technique"

14. *Stockwell v. Washington State Chiropractic Disciplinary Board*, 622 P.2d 910, 914 (Washington, Ct. App. 1981) (Chiropractor did meridian therapy as well as gave nutritional advice.)

15. Cf. *State v. Wilson*, 528 P.2d 279, 282 (Wash. 1974) (Galvanic stimulation "penetrates" skin and is therefore practice of medicine and barred to chiropractors).

16. *See*, e.g., *Spunt v. Fowinkle*, 572 S.W.2d 259, 264 (Tenn. 1978)

17. *Foster v. Board of Chiropractic Examiners*, 359 S.E.2d 877 (Ga. 1987)

18. *Norville v. Miss. State Med. Association*, 364 So.2d 1084 (Miss. 1978); (The American Chiropractic Association used the phrase "drugless profession" until 1974.)

19. *See*, e.g., *State v. Hinze*, 441 N.W.2d 593, 594 (Neb. 1989)

20. American Chiropractic Association Policy Ratified by the House of Delegates, June 1991

21. *See* 21 U.S.C. § 321(g)(1)(B)

22. Dietary Supplement Health and Education Act of 1994, codified at 21 U.S.C. §§ 321, 331, 342, 343, 343-2, 350, 350B; 42 U.S.C. §§ 281, 287C-11

23. 21 U.S.C. § 343(r)(6)(B)(i)

24. 21 U.S.C. § 321(g)(1)(C)

25. *See* American Chiropractic Association Policy on X-Rays Ratified by the House of Delegates, July 1993

26. *See*, e.g., *Tilden v. Board of Chiropractic*, 898 P.2d 219, 221 (Or. App. 1995)

27. *See*, e.g., *Wengel v. Herfert*, 473 N.W.2d 741, 742 (Mich. App. 1991)

28. *See*, e.g., Malpractice—No Virginia, Herbs and Oils Will Not Clear Up a Virulent Strep Infection, *Chiro Legal Update*, April–May 1994 at 1.

29. *Boudreaux v. Panger*, 481 So.2d 1382, 1387 (La. App. 5 Cir. 1986)

30. *Campbell v. F.H.P.*, No. 624061 (Orange County, Cal. 1994)

31. *Rogers v. Schulyer*, 551 N.Y.S. 2d 5 (A.D. 1 Dept. 1990)

32. *Pitre v. Hospital Service District*, 532 So.2d 501 (La.App 1 Cir. 1988)

33. *See, e.g., Jones v. Malloy*, 412 N.W.2d 837 (Neb. 1987) Referral for possible myeloma not followed-up by chiropractor who continued to see patient for two years.

34. *Boyle v. Revici*, 961 F.2d 1060 (2d Cir. 1992

35. *See, e.g., Clair v. Glades County Bd. of Commissioners*, 635 So.2d 84 (Fla. App. 1 Dist. 1994)

36. *Kerkman v. Hintz*, 406 N.W.2d 156, 161-62 (Wisc. App. 1987)

37. *See, e.g., Kelly v. Carroll*, 219 P.2d 79 (Wash. 1950)

38. *Salazar v. Ehmann*, 505 P.2d. 387, 388-89 (Colo. App. 1972)

39. *See, e.g., Mostrom v. Pettibon*, 607 P.2d 864, 867 (Wash. 1980)

40. *Wilk v. American Medical Association*, 895 F.2d 352 (7th Cir. 1990)

41. 15 U.S.C. § 1

42. American Chiropractic Association

43. Marion Merriell Dow, 1993

44. *See, e.g., Philip Solla et al. v. NYS Health Maintenance Organization Conference, Inc.* Civil Action CV 93-5473 (Eastern District of New York) This one action, for example, is being brought by the chiropractic Alliance for Equal Access to Health Care Organizations.

45. "Health Insurers Embrace Eye-of-Newt Therapy," *Wall St J* B1 (Jan. 30, 1995)

46. *Bumgarner v. Blue Cross & Blue Shield of Kansas*, 716 F. Supp. 493 (D. Kan. 1988) Alleged RICO violations, fraud, breach of contract, negligence, tortious interference with contractual rights, tortious interference with contractual rights, tortious interference with business relationships, and defamation.

47. *Guarantee Trust Life Ins. Co. v. Gavin*, 882 F.2d 178, 181 (5th Cir. 1989)

48. RCW § 48.43.045

49. Bulletin issued by the Washington Insurance Commissioner (Dec. 19, 1995)

50. *Blue Cross of Washington and Alaska v. Senn*, Washington, D.C., Super Ct., No. 96-2-00137-3 (Filed 1/8/96)

51. *See, eg., Prudential Insurance Co. of America v. Arkansas*, No. LR-C-95-514 (E.D. ark, 1995), arguing that the Patient Protection Act of 1995 is preempted by Federl law and is unconstitutional

52. *See, e.g., Clair v. Glades County Board of Commissioners*, 635 So.2d 84 (Fla. App. 1 Dist. 1994)

53. *See, e.g., Dutcher v. Allstate*, 4th Dist. No. 94-0169 (May 24, 1995) Error to instruct the jury to find a reasonable degree of "medical" possibility when one witness was a chiroractor.

54. *See, e.g., Corcoran v. United Health Care, Inc.*, 965 F.2d 1321, 1331 (5th Cir. 1992)

55. *See, e.g., Saari v. Litman*, 486 N.W.2d 813 (Minn. App. 1992)

56. *Rogers v. Coronet Insurance Co.*, 424 S.E.2d 338 (Ga. App. 1992)

57. Health Care Portability and Accountabilty Act of 1996, P.L. 104–191, 205 (b).

58. *See, e.g., Kennedy v. Cigna*, 924 F.2d 698 (6th Circ. 1991)

59. *Feiler v. New Jersey Dental Association*, 467 A.2d 276 (1983)

60. *Reynolds v. California Dental Services*, 216 Cal. Rptr. 331 (1988)

61. Office of Inspector General, Special Fraud Alert, Routine Waiver of Co-payments or Deductibles Under Medicare Part B

62. *See, e.g.,* California Labor Code § 1871.7

63. *See, e.g., Harris v. Friedman*, No. 75757 (Imperial County, Cal.)

64. *See,* Chiropractic Legal Update, April/May 1990 at 1

65. *Roe v. Wade*, 410 U.S. 113 (1973)

66. *See, e.g., Matter of Quinlan*, 348 A.2d 801 (N.J. Super. Ct. Div. 1975), *modified*, 355 A.2d 647 (N.J. 1976)

67. *In re Boyd*, 403 A.2d 744 (D.C. 1979)

68. *Guess v. Bd. of Medical Examiners*, 967 F.2d 998 (4th Circ. 1992) "there exists no protected privacy right to practice unorthodox medical treatment…".

69. *See, e.g., Majebe v. North Carolina Board of Medical Examiners*, 416 S.E.2d 404 (N.C. Ct. App. 1992) Dr. Guess, an M.D. physician, had no privacy right to practice acupuncture.

70. *Rutherford v. United States*, 442 U.S. 544 (1979)

71. *People v. Priviteria*, 591 P.2d 919 (Cal. 1979)

72. *U.S. v. Vital Health Products*, 786 F. Supp. 761, 777-78 (E.D. Wisc. 1992), *aff'd* 985 F.2d 563 (1993)

73. *Griswold v. Connecticut*, 381 U.S. 479, 493 (1965) (J. Golderg, concurring)

74. *Andrew v. Ballard*, 498 F. Supp. 1038 (S.D. Tex. 1980)

75. *See, e.g., Potts v. Illinois Department of Regulation and Education*, 128 Ill.2d 322, 538 N.E.2d 1140 (1989)

76. *See, e.g., Rogers v. State Board of Medical Examiners*, 371 So.2d 1037 (Fla. Dist. Ct. App. 1979)

16
Sports Chiropractic
Ed Feinberg

The sports chiropractic field provides challenging and rewarding experiences for the practicing doctor. Athletes develop a wide variety of needs and conditions, and they seek out chiropractic care for many reasons. In the treatment and rehabilitation of injury, the sports chiropractor provides accurate diagnoses, safe and appropriate management protocols, and many therapeutic options. The sports chiropractor also gives opinions about training techniques, nutritional programs, and coaching procedures. Athletes tend to be extremely cooperative patients. Their goals usually extend beyond the removal of pain as they strive constantly to improve their abilities. Most athletes can understand how a subluxation that subtly alters function can limit performance and how the elimination of subluxation can help them achieve optimal performance.

The influence of chiropractic in competitive sports has grown rapidly during the last decade. Chiropractors have participated at the Olympic Games in an official capacity since 1980, and chiropractic is now an integral part of the U.S. Olympic Committee sports medicine program. Sports chiropractors apply for 2-week rotations at the Olympic training centers. Those chiropractors who attend the Olympic games are selected from the 2-week rotation participants. Sports chiropractors have been supplying services at Wrangler Rodeos since 1993. More than 180 rodeos per year have specially trained and certified chiropractors available. Chiropractors also provide care for professional football through the National Football League (NFL), professional basketball through the National Basketball Association (NBA), and professional hockey through the National Hockey League (NHL). Professional volleyball tournaments have chiropractors available, as do professional auto-racing competitions. Chiropractic is also available at virtually every kind of sporting event at the local, collegiate, and high school levels.

Sports injuries provide a wide variety of patient presentations for the chiropractor. In addition to spinal injuries, the sports chiropractor handles extremity injuries, visceral injuries, and head injuries. The sports chiropractor must have the specific training and experience to handle these situations competently. This sometimes means being a participant in an athletic health care team. When treating elite or professional atheletes, it is often necessary for the sports chiropractor to communicate, and work closely with, orthopedists, physical therapists, athletic trainers, and/or coaches. This requires good communication skills and a current knowledge of the activities and value of those professional specialties.

The on-field activities at an athletic event are potentially the most exciting aspects of a sports chiropractic experience. At these events, the chiropractor must be prepared to see everything from bee-stings to broken bones to life-threatening emergencies. Each sport has different risks, and the chiropractor must be prepared for all the potential injuries prior to competition. Furthermore, the sports chiropractor must be prepared to interface with emergency medical services and other health care professionals who might participate at the event. In my experience, athletes are extremely appreciative of our presence at these events, and the chiropractors share in the competitive spirit. When a patient of mine wins an event, I can feel part of the victory.

To participate competently in all these activities, the sports chiropractor needs specialized education and experience. Sports chiropractic clubs at many colleges provide an excellent place to begin. Many colleges provide excellent postgraduate programs to further the training of the sports chiropractor. The American Chiropractic Association (ACA) Sports Council offers guidelines for these programs and provides testing procedures to certify the participants. In addition to formal instruction, practical experience is a vital part of the sports chiropractor's training, particularly regarding on-field event participation. First-aid and emergency procedures are taught competently at Red Cross and cardiopulmonary resuscitation (CPR) programs. Practical training may be attained while assisting an experienced sports chiropractor or other emergency health care practitioner. The sports chiropractor must know how to approach emergency situations calmly with a rational protocol before attending a sports event as the sole emergency care practitioner.

CHIROPRACTIC AND ATHLETIC PERFORMANCE: THE KINEMATICS OF SPORT

The kinematics of sports describes a fascinating and complex orchestration of body motion. The sports chiropractor requires a full appreciation for the complex coordination of properly functioning bones, joints, muscles, ligaments, and nerves. One basic principle of sports kinematics, found throughout all sporting activities, is the concept of the kinetic chain. The kinetic chain[1] includes all the musculoskeletal structures necessary to perform an activity. Each musculoskeletal structure has its particular function in the proper performance of a sport activity. As an example, the kinetic chain for throwing is not limited to the upper extremity. Proper throwing activities involve the acceleration of the lower extremity, pelvis, spine, shoulder girdle,

and upper extremity. All these structures are included in the kinetic chain for throwing. All these structures must be properly functioning and coordinated for throwing performance to be optimal. The principle of the kinetic chain can be demonstrated by comparing the mechanics of throwing to a roller skating whip[2] (Fig. 16-1). Just as each skater contributes to the speed and control of the final skater, each part of the kinetic chain contributes to the speed and control of a baseball.

A classic example of the influence of the kinetic chain on performance has been described as the Dizzy Dean Syndrome. Dizzy Dean was a professional pitcher during the 1930s. During an all-star game, his foot was hit by a line drive, fracturing his toe. He was subsequently given an oversized shoe so that he could continue to play. Although he was able to pitch, an abnormal alteration in the function of his kinetic chain resulted in a shoulder injury that ended his career. Thus, a change in one part of the kinetic chain produced dramatic effects at another part of the chain.

Subluxation at any part of the kinetic chain can result in poor performance or risk of injury from athletic activity. Treating that subluxation can improve performance and reduce risk. Subluxation is not the only disorder that can have an adverse result. The sports chiropractor must be familiar with all such disorders, treating those within the chiropractic scope of practice and referring others as necessary.

Sports chiropractors must study the mechanics of athletic injury and the ways in which injured components may adapt. Athletes often feel compelled to perform while injured. It is only with a complete understanding of these processes that we are able to determine safely when and how, or if, an athlete may return to practice or competition.

Elegant scientific studies are continually refining our understanding of kinematics in sports. Until recently, the precise kinematics of sport activity was not well understood. In the past, sport kinematics theories were developed by coaches and athletes by trial and error, using the quality of performance as an outcome measure. Over the years, speculation on the precise details of sport kinematics was prolific, yet it was never possible to eliminate the variables associated with a specific athlete's ability or motivation.

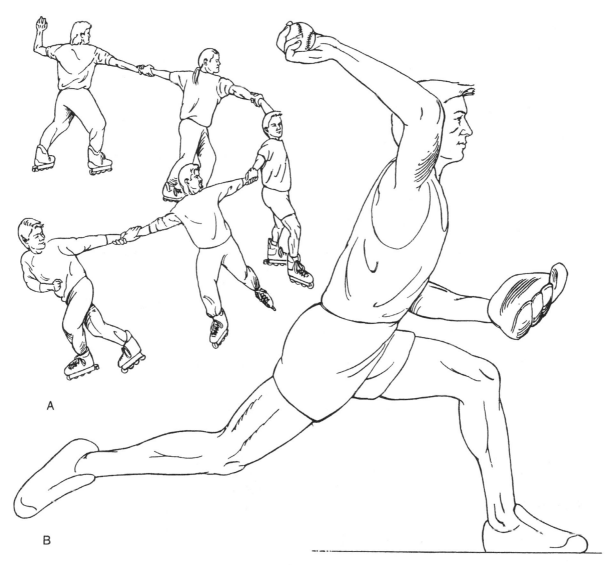

Figure 16-1. Kinetic chain. Examples of kinetic chains. **(A)** A chain of roller skaters executing a whip maneuver. **(B)** The body segments of a baseball pitcher. (From Zachazewski et al.,[2] with permission.)

Recent technologic developments have provided considerable advancement in the detail and accuracy of our understanding of sports kinematics. High-speed video photography and computer analysis have allowed scientists to observe, in detail, the position of the various body parts of an athlete during a sport activity. By comparing the mechanics of several different types of athletes within a sport, we

are developing a better understanding of the mechanisms necessary for optimal performance. This information has been even further developed by the simultaneously recording of muscular activity with fine-wire electromyography (EMG). These findings are then observed in various different athletic populations. It is now possible to distinguish amateur performance from elite performance with a kinematic point of view. It is also possible to compare athletes with various disorders to determine how they adapt, or possibly what mechanics caused the development of their complaints.

This type of information is invaluable to the sports chiropractor attempting to treat or prevent various disorders in the athlete. A good example is the relationship of shoulder instability to pitching or throwing sports. High-speed video and EMG techniques have demonstrated the presence of specific muscle activity imbalances in the pitcher with shoulder instability.[3] These studies can be used to tailor treatment for such patients. By strengthening and training those less active muscles, we promote improved performance with decreased risk of injury.

ON-FIELD EVENT PARTICIPATION

On-field event participation is the most exciting experience in sports chiropractic. Usually done on a volunteer basis, as a community service, it provides emotional rewards as well as name recognition and occasional referrals. Event participation can be dangerous, however, if done in a haphazard manner. Prudent event participation requires specific attention to preparation and safety protocol.

PRE-EVENT PREPARATION

Proper preparation before an event helps ensure a competent and beneficial experience for the sports chiropractor and the participating athletes. Event preparation begins with event-specific considerations. The needs of the athlete vary with the individual sports. For example, contact sports, such as football or rugby, lead to very different physical stresses and injuries than do racquet sports such as tennis or squash. It is important for the field chiropractor to have an intimate understanding of these specific stresses. It is also important for the sports chiropractor to understand the sports-specific terminology used by athletes, coaches, and referees. For example, if a player comes off a field and says, "I just got dinged," it is necessary to know exactly what he or she means.

Before the event, the sports chiropractor must ask whether other health care professionals will be present, such as paramedics or medical doctors. It is often our responsibility to make the first contact with these individuals. We work together as a team, without competition, for the benefit of the athletes. I inform them of the services I offer and of how I wish to enlist their help when conditions present that are more appropriate to their specialized skills. Interestingly, athletes often prefer working with chiropractors when they are injured. If other health care professionals are not present at the event, the chiropractor assumes greater responsibility and should participate only if training and experience allow competent performance. An improperly handled emergency can be a disaster not only for the athlete but for the chiropractor and our profession as well.

Proper equipment must be immediately available at the sports event. A sports event equipment bag is stocked with many items, some of which vary according to specific sports needs. Diagnostic tools are necessary to determine the extent and severity of injuries. Athletic tape, braces, and splints are often used. Rubber gloves, sterile dressings, bandages, and antibiotics are necessary for bleeding lesions. Emergency tools for artificial respiration and cervical stabilization may be appropriate. Other tools vary according to specific needs. A good pair of tweezers or forceps, or both, may be needed to remove gravel from road rash at a bicycle race. A ring cutter may be needed to remove a ring from a severely swollen finger at a football game. Remember that the local emergency medical system is available in most areas. In addition to a well-stocked equipment bag, portable chiropractic tables, towels and an ice chest with plastic bags are probably the most frequently used event equipment.

EMERGENCY PROCEDURES

Although severe medical emergencies are rare at most sporting events, the sports chiropractor must be expertly prepared for such a circumstance. Emergency medical training is available through many sources. Red Cross CPR and first-aid training can initiate this process and must be reviewed and updated regularly. Postgraduate sports chiropractic training programs expand on this training with in-depth regional protocols for management. Academic training, though vital, is not alone sufficient preparation for emergency care. On-field training with an experienced sports chiropractor or other emergency-trained practitioner is necessary before any individual can competently handle such situations. Assisting trained experienced chiropractors at events, as well as visiting emergency departments, and riding with paramedics, can help provide essential experience to the student.

A complete discussion of emergency procedures is beyond the scope of this text, yet some basic principles of emergency care can be introduced. The first task of the sports chiropractor in an emergency situation is to quickly assess the scene. Is there imminent danger to the injured, to other athletes, or to spectators? Perhaps competition must be stopped until the athlete is removed from the field. If the mechanism of injury is unclear, are there other individuals available who saw the trauma and are they capable of providing such information? Are competent individuals available to contact emergency medical services if necessary? Once a safe environment is established, the next step in emergency care is to perform a primary survey.

During a primary survey, the sports chiropractor assesses the immediate danger of mortality or morbidity. Over the years, a systematic approach has been developed, commonly described as the ABCs of emergency care[4-7] (Table 16-1). Airway assessment determines whether there is an open pathway from the mouth to the lungs. Blockage of this pathway must be addressed first—obviously, any other procedures will be futile if no oxygen can reach the blood. Tilting the chin back and removing foreign objects from the mouth are the simplest methods of airway management. If there is any possibility of cervical spine fracture, this procedure must be modified to protect the spinal cord.

Breathing assessment is simple. If breathing is absent, some form of artificial respiration must be provided. Pocket masks should be available and used to prevent disease transmission. Circulation assessment first determines the presence of a heartbeat, with a check of the pulse. The carotid pulse is most reliable for this purpose. Absent pulse requires the initiation of CPR. Circulation assessment continues with discovery and control of bleeding, usually accomplished by simple direct pressure of a sterile pad on the wound. Gloves are worn whenever blood is present to prevent possible disease transmission.

Spinal assessment for fracture or dislocation is most important in the cervical spine but must be considered in other areas as well. Careless management of spinal fractures can be disastrous, resulting in spinal cord damage that can cause permanent disability, or even death. For this reason, extreme caution must be used to rule out spinal fracture as part of a primary survey. The signs and symptoms of cervical spine fracture include loss of sensation or motor function in the extremities, spinal deformity, and extreme spinal pain. Not all cervical spine fractures are that obvious to diagnose, however. The general rule regarding cervical injury is to assume cervical fracture until proved otherwise. The precise protocol for on-field evaluation of possible cervical spine fracture is beyond the scope of this text but must be immediately available to the event chiropractor. Cervical spine stabilization with emergency transport to a hospital is the proper management of a suspected cervical spine fracture.

Immediate activation of the local emergency medical service is paramount to proper care of the severe medical emergency. A call to 911 should be made, if possible, from a hard-wired phone, not a cellular phone. In busy cities, cellular phone calls can be routed through neighboring communities and can reach a distant emergency service. These emergency services then need to call a closer service and verbally transmit directions to your location. This delay can be critical to the patient. Hard-wired phones, such as pay phones, are connected directly to the closest 911 service with the exact address immediately available to the 911 operator.

Following the primary survey, a secondary survey is performed to assess all other possible injuries to

Table 16-1. The Primary Survey: The ABCs of Emergency Care

Airway
   Tilt chin back, empty mouth
Breathing
   Initiate respirations if absent
Circulation
    Check pulse
    Initiate compressions if absent
    Bleeding
    Direct pressure if present
spinal
    Assess possible fracture/dislocation
    Immobilize and emergency transport

the patient. The competent sports chiropractor must clearly understand how to evaluate and manage all the musculoskeletal and organ systems that may be injured at a sporting event. Every potential danger requires its own protocol of management. Blunt head trauma can cause a mild concussion or a fatal hematoma. Second impacts following concussion can result in significant brain damage or death. Extremity injuries can cause compressive compartment syndromes that can result in permanent disability if left unattended. Hypothermia and hyperthermia are both potentially fatal and require close evaluation. A collapsed lung or a ruptured spleen must be recognized early to avoid potentially disastrous results. A chiropractor who is providing these services at a sporting event must be fully trained in all appropriate emergency protocols.

TYPICAL ON-FIELD EXPERIENCE

Although expertise in emergency procedures is necessary for the competent sports chiropractor to work at a sporting event, serious injuries are not commonplace. This is not to imply that the sports event chiropractor is idle, waiting for the serious injury to occur. On the contrary, he or she is usually quite busy providing various treatments to athletes. The usual athletic event treatment is either a pre-event treatment or some form of sports injury management.

Many athletes seek out pre-event chiropractic care. Subluxation of the spine or extremities can result in suboptimal biomechanics that reduce performance and increase risk of injury. Competitive athletes are usually quite sensitive to aberrations in their musculoskeletal system and seek remedies when available. Adjustments are not the only service provided by most event chiropractors. Some athletes are recovering from injuries and benefit from soft tissue therapies or from taping procedures to protect the injured tissues. Rodeo cowboys are an excellent example. After being bounced around on a bull or bronco, a cowboy will often drive for hours sitting stiffly in a truck to reach the next rodeo competition. This is the perfect recipe for stiff, sore muscles and subluxated joints. These athletes are extremely appreciative of the increasing availability of sports chiropractic at their events. Pre-event treatments are not only for the recently injured. These procedures may also be prophylactic for the uninjured athlete.

During competition, the occasional injury is bound to occur. If many athletes are competing at large events, injury management becomes a major aspect of the sports chiropractor's job. Most of these injuries are not medical emergencies, but early and proper management can minimize damage and quicken the athlete's return to competition. Assessment of the injury is always the most important initial step of management. The sports chiropractor must first determine whether the athlete can return to play or must remain sidelined for further evaluation. Fractures are not always remarkably painful and screening procedures should be routine to aid early discovery. Soft tissue injuries are appropriately managed with a proper combination of cryotherapy, mobilization, taping, and gentle adjustments. Potential complications such as myositis ossificans or compartment syndromes must be considered. Blunt trauma of large muscles presents the risk of developing myositis ossificans[7,8] (Fig. 16-2). Vigorous massage and ultrasound is avoided after such an injury. Cryotherapy to the injured muscle, while it is placed in a stretched position, is proper management. Compartment syndrome develops if swelling or

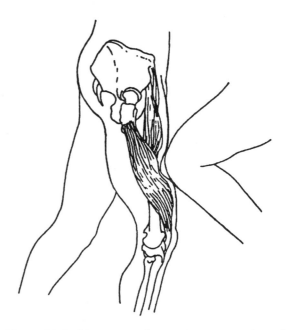

Figure 16-2. Myositis ossificans. Large anterolateral muscle mass of the thigh is exposed to direct trauma, leading to contusion. (From Reid,[7] with permission.)

bleeding cause excessive pressure that can result in vascular or neurologic compromise.[7,8] This is most common in the leg or forearm after significant trauma. Loss of a pulse and aberrant sensation are late findings of this condition. Early findings include palpable tightness, a patient feeling of pressure, and serious pain. Cryotherapy may prevent compartment syndromes but if one develops, immediate referral to a hospital may be necessary for surgical release of the pressure.

IN-OFFICE SPORTS INJURY MANAGEMENT

Sports injury management begins as soon as the injury is detected. Many athletes are familiar with injury and recognize that early intervention results in more rapid recovery. Some athletes resist intervention, especially if it involves loss of training or competition. It is important that the sports chiropractor clearly understand the natural process of wound healing and the interventions that can speed and improve the healing of tissues. If an athlete is returned to competition too early, the risk of additional serious injury is high. If an athlete is prevented from training or competition for too long a period of time, loss of performance may result. The influence of coaches, owners, team mates, fans, scholarships, and careers may also exert pressure on these decisions. Sports chiropractors must use their knowledge about the physiology of the healing process to determine the point at which active training and competition may be safely resumed. When working with an elite athlete, the chiropractor is often part of a health care team, including athletic trainers, physical therapists, physiatrists, and orthopedists. In difficult cases, obtaining opinions from additional professionals can confirm the sport chiropractor's suggestions as well as influence the athlete to follow recommendations.

Very mild injuries are common and require no professional intervention for rapid, successful recovery. Informed home use of ice, heat, and exercise can return an athlete to play without interruption. More significant injuries may benefit from a variety of therapeutic procedures available to the chiropractor. For borderline cases, I usually recommend that the athlete seek professional advice if symptoms of injury persist beyond 2 days. Sports chiropractors are uniquely prepared to provide benefit to the athlete who has sustained a sport injury. Training and experience in diagnosis, therapeutic procedures, rehabilitation, and adjusting techniques provide the sports chiropractor with all the skills necessary to manage most athletic injuries from beginning to end. The sports chiropractor must also identify those cases that require additional professional assistance.

THE NATURAL HISTORY OF SOFT TISSUE HEALING

The body's response to soft tissue trauma follows a predictable sequence of events. These events have been divided into three phases: inflammatory phase, repair phase, and maturation (or remodeling) phase.[9-11] The timing of these phases is generally predictable but varies with the severity, extent, and type of tissue injured, as well as the age, general health, and nutrition of the athlete. Patients with mild injuries may have a prolonged inflammatory phase if they do not modify those activities that cause continual irritation and repeated microtrauma. By contrast, patients with moderate injuries may swiftly cruise through an inflammatory phase if they strictly follow all recommendations regarding nutrition, therapy, and activity. For these reasons, it is necessary to examine patients regularly and directly evaluate the signs and symptoms of the various phases of tissue healing.

Inflammatory Phase

The inflammatory phase is the initial phase of tissue healing, typically lasting no longer than 72 hours if properly managed. It begins as injured or irritated tissues produce and release the chemical mediators of inflammation. These include histamine, prostaglandin II, leukotrienes, kallidin, bradykinin, and serotonin. These chemicals cause a variety of physiologic responses. They directly stimulate the nociceptors, causing pain. They also cause nociceptor facilitation, such that mild additional stimuli also cause pain. Palpation or movement will cause pain in an inflamed tissue that would not otherwise be uncomfortable. Capillaries become more permeable when exposed to the chemical mediators of inflammation. This greater permeability allows proteins and cells to leave the vascular system.

Vasodilation is another result of inflammation. Increased blood supply provides the cells and nutrients required for tissue repair. It also causes the tissue to appear red and hot on examination. Together, vasodilation and increased capillary permeability cause edema and the physical appearance of swelling. Gross edema can exert pressure on vessels and cells, inhibiting vascular flow; this will slow the repair process. Chemotaxis is also a part of the inflammatory process. Phagocytes are attracted to the inflamed tissues to perform the important function of removing cellular debris. Fibroblasts are also attracted to the area.

The degree of inflammation is clinically evaluated by determining the extent to which the above processes are occurring. This is done by examining for the cardinal signs of inflammation, namely redness, swelling, heat, pain, and functional loss (Table 16-2). When determining the degree of inflammation, the sports chiropractor must diagnose which tissue is injured and consider the anatomic location of that tissue. A very superficial tissue, such as the lateral ligaments of the ankle, will display very obvious signs of inflammation even with moderate severity. A deep tissue, such as a lumbar ligament, which is several muscle layers deep, will display only subtle signs of inflammation, even though the severity of injury and inflammation may be substantial.

Inflammation, though a necessary process, is typically greater than desired for optimal healing. Excessive edema causes congestion that diminishes fluid and nutrient exchange. Congestion prevents the rapid clearing of the chemical mediators of inflammation, prolonging the process. Prolonged inflammation allows fibrotic scar formation to develop in tissues adjacent to the injured tissues. Such scar, called *adhesions*, can alter biomechanic

Table 16-2. Evaluating the Degree of Inflammation: Cardinal Signs[a]

Redness
Swelling
Heat
Pain
Functional loss

[a]Remember: the depth of the tissue will determine the apparent degree of inflammation.

function, reduce range of motion, and increase the risk of recurrent injury. With the vast majority of sports injuries, the goal of treatment during the inflammatory phase is to diminish the degree of inflammation.

Repair Phase

The repair phase is the second phase of tissue healing. It begins with the resolution of the inflammatory phase and may last from a few days up to 6 months. Damaged tendons and ligaments heal by the formation of fibrotic scar; regeneration does not occur. Damaged muscle also heals by fibrotic scar but also has some limited capacity to regenerate muscle fibers. Fibrotic scar is composed of type III collagen, which is not as strong as the type I collagen found in healthy tendons or ligaments. Furthermore, the collagen fibers are disorganized. They are oriented in multiple directions unlike the precise regimented orientation of tendon or ligament tissue. As a result, fibrotic scar is always weaker than uninjured tissue. Like a weak link in a chain, if that tissue is injured again, it will be damaged at the site of the fibrotic scar.

One or 2 days after an injury, fibrocytes are chemically attracted to the injured region. These cells produce collagen fibers to help stabilize and strengthen the injured tissue. Weak hydrogen bonds between the collagen fibers provide some strengthening of the scar. Gradually, covalent bond cross-links form to replace the weaker hydrogen bonds and provide greater strength. Collagen fibers may also form within and between tissue adjacent to the injury. These adhesions can have deleterious effects.

Maturation (Remodeling) Phase

The maturation or remodeling phase is the final phase of tissue healing. This phase has been reported to last from weeks up to 1 year or more. During this phase, reorganization and continued covalent bond cross-linking of collagen fibers further increases scar strength. At this time, there is a balance of tissue anabolism and catabolism, with collagen fibers broken down and built up simultaneously. Though there is no net change in the quantity of tissue collagen, the quality may change in the right therapeutic environment. This is also true of adhesions that may be present adjacent to the injured tissue. Remodeling may reduce their deleterious effects.

REHABILITATION

Chiropractic management of soft tissue injuries must follow a progressive development that parallels the natural process of soft tissue healing. Procedures are individualized according to the needs and capabilities of the particular patient; progression is dependent on individual response. Sports chiropractic often demands a very personal approach because the pressure to return a patient to competition rapidly is high. Several types of therapy are used to this end. Zachazewski et al.[1] summarize some basic considerations in their rehabilitation pyramid (Fig. 16-3).

Controlling Inflammation

Once it is determined that an acute sports injury is stable and protected from further trauma, reduction of inflammation is the next step in management to prevent congestion and its associated dangers. If inflammation goes unchecked, excessive scarring can result with adhesions that can decrease range of motion, reduce function and power, and increase the risk of reinjury (Fig 16-4). Ice therapy, also called cryotherapy, is useful for this purpose. Cryotherapy causes vasoconstriction and controls pain to counteract the inflammatory process. Cooling the tissues immediately after injury also has the added benefit of reducing the production of the chemical mediators of inflammation. Heat should be avoided during the inflammatory phase because the result-

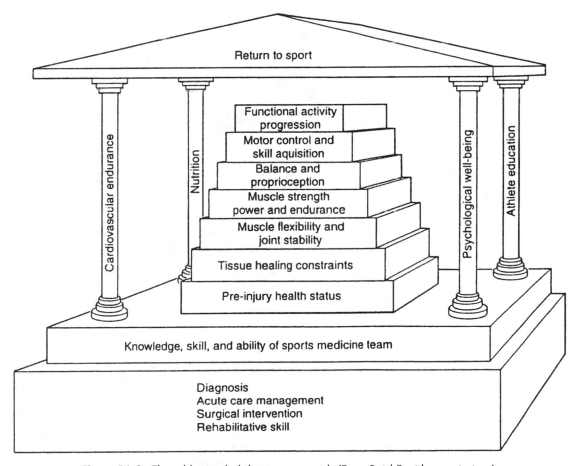

Figure 16-3. The athletic rehabilitation pyramid. (From Reid,[7] with permission.)

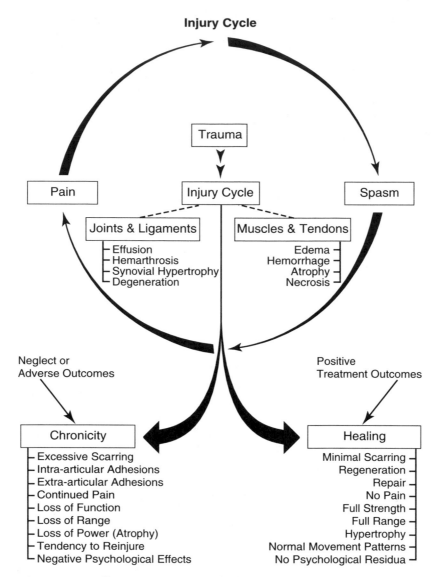

Figure 16-4. Inflammation. Injury cycle illustrates the range of outcomes of trauma in response to treatment. Inflammation should be minimized to assist in allowing the events of healing to assume positive pathways as rapidly as possible. (From Reid,[7] with permission.)

ing vasodilation can exacerbate congestion and damage fragile, developing capillaries. Nutritional supplements such as proteolytic enzymes, glucosamine sulfate, and vitamins A, C, and E, can also assist in the control of inflammation. (See Ch. 9)

If inflammation is severe, over-the-counter or prescription anti-inflammatory drugs may be necessary for optimal control. Excessive reduction of inflammation can have hazardous results, however. Cortisone injections have been shown to reduce tissue strength following injury when used excessively to control inflammation.[8] It has also been speculated that nonsteroidal anti-inflammatory drugs (NSAIDs) may have similar effects if abused in the early stages of tissue healing, but this has not been documented.[8] In the absence of strong medications excessive reduction of inflammation is not possible.

Motion Therapies

In the past, damaged tissues were always immobilized during the early healing stages. It was believed that immobilized tissues would heal faster with little risk of injury. Unfortunately, these tissues also healed with adhesions and weak scar, causing restricted range of motion and high risk of recurrent injury. We have since learned that early motion of soft tissue injury results in stronger, more organized scar with fewer adhesions, provided it can be performed without causing further tissue damage.[2,7,8] This is performed initially by carefully and repeatedly moving the body part through its full, pain-free range.

As the tissues strengthen, more aggressive stretching exercises are gradually initiated. Stretching exercises improve range of motion by lengthening adhesions that may be present either within or between involved soft tissues. Stretching also provides tension to the fibrotic scar. Improved remodeling of the tensioned scar results in enhanced organization and greater strength. Improved flexibility has other benefits. A more flexible tissue is less likely to be injured because of its elastic properties. Furthermore, a tissue that is not tight, except at end range, will produce proper stretch reflex responses that allow greater power generation. Tight hamstrings not only increase the risk of hamstring injury but also result in excessive hamstring stretch receptor stimulus, causing reflex inhibition of the quadriceps and a reduction of maximal quadriceps power.

Stretching must be achieved with controlled procedures that avoid damage to the developing scar. Static stretches are used with gradual forces for 20 to 60 seconds per repetition. Heat may be applied before the stretching exercise to increase effectiveness, provided the signs of inflammation are minimal. More aggressive ballistic stretches are avoided. High-velocity stretches activate the monosynaptic stretch reflex that contracts the muscle to be lengthened, thereby reducing effectiveness and risking potential damage. Proprioceptive neuromuscular facilitation techniques use neurologic reflexes to assist the stretching process. For example, prior contraction of a muscle antagonist causes neurologic inhibition of the stretched muscle, allowing greater relaxation and a more effective stretch. Other methods of proprioceptive neuromuscular facilitation are also available.

Adjusting a patient during the inflamed phase should only be performed with low force and extreme control. Removal of subluxation has many benefits for healing athletes. Greater range of motion allows more effective passive exercise, resulting in stronger scar formation with fewer adhesions. Reduced muscle tension facilitates vascular and lymphatic flow, speeding the resolution of inflammation. Improved vascular and neurologic flow allow for maximal trophic effects. These benefits do not outweigh the hazard of additional tissue injury. Adjustments during the inflammatory phase should be attempted only if they can be accomplished without causing further trauma. Delaying an adjustment for 1 or 2 days is not severely detrimental, yet the additional trauma from a high force adjustment at this stage may be devastating. It is important, when treating these patients, to remember that subluxations often occur in regions adjacent to the tissue injury or in any part of the kinetic chain. A patient with a shoulder rotator cuff tear, for example, could experience far-reaching complications. Pain and spasm can affect the entire upper quarter of the spine. Cervical, thoracic, and shoulder girdle subluxations should be evaluated and treated. As the tissues strengthen, the risk of adjustment diminishes, and subluxation treatment is pursued more aggressively.

Manual soft tissue therapies used to aid healing of sports injuries are described elsewhere in this text (see Ch. 9). In general, the more gentle procedures are used in the early stages of healing to assist reduction of inflammation and to encourage improved organization of collagen scar. More aggressive procedures are reserved for the later stages of healing to stretch and tear adhesions or collagen fibers that do not contribute to strength. Therapeutic ultrasound has also been shown to improve scar strength and soften adhesions. It is often beneficial when used in conjunction with the above techniques.

Tension Therapies

Resisted exercise is instituted early to provide tension to the developing scar. Gentle forces are used initially with the goal of improving scar strength, not muscle strength. If muscle injuries are severe, even gentle resisted exercises can cause damage and must be avoided in the early phases of healing. Resisted exercise is used only if it can be performed without causing further tissue damage. As healing progresses, a gradual increase in the resistant forces will strengthen muscle fibers as well as fibrotic scar. It is important to focus on specifically rebuilding the strength of any injured muscle. After resisted exercise, blood perfusion through the muscle is high, and muscle fibers are warm and supple. Stretching exercises are most effective at this time and should be incorporated into a cooldown program.

Isometric exercises cause muscle tension without any joint motion. Isometric is the safest type of exercise in the early phases of healing, especially if joint injury or instability has occurred. Following shoulder dislocation, isometric exercise is used as soon as tolerable. Isotonic and isokinetic exercises cause muscle tension that moves a joint through a range. These exercises increase muscle strength more effectively and are recommended when safe.

Athletes are often required to stop their usual training programs because of sports injuries. This causes declining performance capabilities and emotional distress. It behooves the sports chiropractor to prescribe exercises for the uninjured tissues to maintain maximal performance. Furthermore, whenever possible, aerobic exercise should be continued. Aerobic capacity rapidly decreases in the absence of training. Continued aerobic training can prevent this. Aerobic exercise has the added benefit of producing endorphins that can elevate an injured athlete's emotional status.

Proprioceptive Coordination Training

Just as it is vital to evaluate and adjust all parts of a kinetic chain, we must also train for proper coordination among those parts. After sports injury, athletes often develop altered mechanics due either to abnormal proprioceptive responses from damaged tissues or to fear of possible re-injury. Ignoring these factors can lead to diminished performance and increasing risks of new or recurrent injury.

Coordination development should begin as soon as it is determined safe. Combined movement patterns without resistance will initiate the process.[12] This is performed to train the simultaneous use of two or more muscle groups. At the ankle, active free movements between dorsiflexion with inversion and plantar-flexion with eversion, or dorsiflexion with eversion and plantar-flexion with inversion are examples. As tissues heal, resistance can be added to combined motion exercises. Early in rehabilitation, it is also important to perform closed-chain exercises. A closed-chain exercise is one in which the distal part of the limb puts pressure on a stable, unmoving surface.[8] This increases the proprioceptive stimulus, promoting proprioceptive training.

For an ankle injury, the seated patient may place the foot on a wobble board placed on a stable floor. Controlled ankle movements on the wobble board will help develop proprioceptive sense and coordination in the affected ankle following injury. As the patient improves, he or she may stand and balance on the wobble board with gradually increasing degrees of difficulty. Difficulty may be varied by using different types of wobble boards and different types of exercises. As the patient's ankle continues to improve, running and balance exercises are added to the conditioning program. Use of a trampoline may be beneficial. Running exercises must always begin on a smooth, flat surface free of divots or potholes. Running exercises can include running forward, running backward, making figure eights, sidesteps, and carioca crossovers (Fig. 16-5). Skipping and hopping may be included as well. An appropriate combination of these exercises can assist in the development of proprioceptive coordination necessary for safe sports activity.

Proper athletic form is required for optimal, risk-free performance. Improper form can cause injury in almost any sport. Even athletes with excellent form can develop improper form following sports injury as a result of muscle weakness, flexibility loss, proprioceptive alteration, or fear of re-injury. Assessment and training for athletic form constitutes the final step of rehabilitation before an athlete is returned to competition after a significant sports injury. Pitching is an excellent example of the need for proper form. I am amazed at how many high school and college pitchers I have met who have never been trained or evaluated for proper pitching form. Improper form is responsible for many types of pitching injuries, usually involving the shoulder or elbow, but potentially involving any part of the kinetic chain. Following injury, pitchers begin form

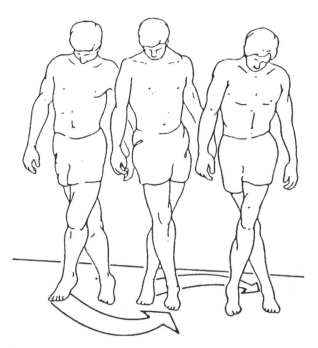

Figure 16-5. Carioca crossover drills produce increasing torque. (From Zachazewski et al.,[2] with permission.)

training with only gentle tosses, concentrating on body position, coordination, and accuracy. In later stages, form assessment includes all the various pitches at full force. High-speed video evaluation of pitching mechanics can be beneficial. Recognizing the subtleties of elite athletic form is beyond the ability of most sports chiropractors. Although basic common errors can be recognized and altered as a result of advice, input from a professional training coach may be required.

SPORTS CHIROPRACTIC TRAINING

At this point, the student may be asking, "How do I become a superb sports chiropractor?" The scope of this chapter is limited to basic concepts and procedures used by the sports chiropractor. For the interested student, sports chiropractic training can begin during chiropractic college. Many chiropractic colleges have student sports chiropractic clubs. If your school doesn't, consider starting one.

Sports chiropractic clubs can use several avenues to expose the student to pertinent topics. Sports chi-

ropractors are easily encouraged to give presentations on various aspects of their specialty. These presentations can often be designed to train the student in specific procedures with practical hands-on sessions. Some sports chiropractic clubs include event participation experience as part of their program. This provides an excellent opportunity for students to view, and sometimes participate in, the on-field experience. Students attend the sporting events with an experienced, licensed sports chiropractor. The exact student role and responsibility must be clearly delineated for this kind of experience to work. At these events, the licensed doctor has complete authority, and no procedure is performed without his or her sanction.

Students should have completed training in soft tissue therapies, emergency procedures, and public communication prior to event participation. Such training will ensure a valuable learning experience without the *faux pas* that could prove embarrassing or disastrous. Sports chiropractic clubs can also encourage the development of sports chiropractic elective courses to provide more in-depth training. Some colleges have very active sports chiropractic clubs. Their members and officers are available to assist club development at other chiropractic colleges.

The ACA sports council is also available to assist club development. Many excellent sports chiropractors can be contacted through this organization. Student membership is available at a reduced fee. Sports council publications provide current information on a variety of sports-related topics as well as a national network of sports event participation.

After graduation, one can enroll in postgraduate training programs in sports chiropractic. The Certified Chiropractic Sports Physician (CCSP) program includes 100 hours of training, usually provided one weekend per month, to avoid interruptions to a doctor's practice. The Diplomate of the American Chiropractic Board of Sports Physicians (DACBSP) program provides an additional 200 hours of training, plus a minimum of 100 hours of on-field experience and other requirements. These programs are presented by many chiropractic colleges. The ACA sports council provides general guidelines and administers certifying tests to ensure consistency. These programs initiate an excellent process of learning that continues when the sports chiropractor specializes in a particular sporting activity.

THE SPORTS CHIROPRACTIC PRACTICE

Embarking on a sports chiropractic career affects the way a doctor interacts with all patients. The athlete uses chiropractic treatment to strive for optimal performance. The elimination of pain is only one aspect of that process. Athletes also understand the value of exercise and tend to be very cooperative patients, performing home exercise activities consistently. Soon the sports chiropractor views every patient as an athlete. Some patients come to the office seeking only reduction of pain, but the sports chiropractor with an athletic attitude infuses the doctor–patient experience with a desire to strive for optimal performance as is appropriate to the individual patient. There is no patient, regardless of age or physical condition, who will not benefit from some appropriate form of physical conditioning. Physical conditioning programs have many advantages. Physically fit patients have fewer subluxations and less musculoskeletal pain. Additionally, physically fit patients have fewer strokes or heart attacks, the major causes of mortality in America.[13] Physically fit patients experience a better quality and longer life.

Physical conditioning is only beneficial if performed consistently. The exercise bike or treadmill gathering dust in the attic is of no benefit. Patients need to find conditioning programs that they enjoy to obtain an exercise benefit for the long term. Sports are exercises that patients can enjoy. Sports chiropractors should use every procedure at their disposal to help their patients enjoy sports activities and experience a high-quality, long life.

Terminology

adhesions
carioca
chemical mediators of inflammation
closed-chain exercise
cryotherapy
dinged
electomyography
kinematics
kinetic chain
pocket mask
proprioception
proprioceptive training
shoulder instability

Review Questions

1. Describe the various body parts involved in the kinetic chain of a baseball pitch.

2. Which of the following should be available for the treatment of bleeding injuries?

    A. Gloves

    B. Antibiotic ointment

    C. Bandages

    D. All of the above

3. Which of the following is the first step in the emergency evaluation of a seriously injured athlete?

    A. Scene assessment

    B. Airway assessment

    C. Fracture assessment

    D. Bleeding assessment

4. The first step in the control of bleeding in the injured athlete is to …

    A. Clean the wound

    B. Apply direct pressure

    C. Apply antibiotic ointment

    D. Glove the hands

5. During a football game, a player falls hard on his head and is rendered unconscious. Which of the following would be proper responses to this situation?

    A. Have several players carry the injured athlete off the field to allow resumption of play.

    B. Stop the game until proper assessment and stabilization are ensured.

    C. Unbuckle and remove helmet.

    D. Use ammonia ampules to revive the injured athlete.

6. A cellular phone is the best tool available for accessing the 911 emergency medical services in the event of a serious sports injury. True or false? Why?

7. The severity of pain following an athletic injury is a reliable indicator of fracture. If an athlete is not

experiencing severe pain, fractures are not present. True or false?

Concept Questions

1. How has chiropractic participation in sporting events helped the development of the profession?

2. How can sports chiropractors incorporate injury prevention into their work?

References

1. Bergmann TF, Peterson DH, Lawrence DJ: Chiropractic Technique. Churchill Livingstone, New York, 1993

2. Zachazewski JE, Magee DJ, Quillen WS: Athletic Injuries and Rehabilitation. WB Saunders, Philadelphia, 1996

3. Blousman R, Jobe F, Tibone J et al: Dynamic electromyographic analysis of the throwing shoulder with glenohumeral instability. J Bone Joint Surg 73B:389, 1991

4. Bergeron JD: First Responder Update. 3rd Ed. Prentice-Hall, Englewood Cliffs, NJ, 1993

5. Cantu RC, Micheli LJ: ACSM's Guidelines for the Team Physician. Lea & Febiger, Philadelphia, 1991

6. Roy S, Irvin R: Sports Medicine: Prevention, Evaluation, Management, and Rehabilitation. Prentice-Hall, Englewood Cliffs, NJ, 1983

7. Reid DC: Sports Injury Assessment and Rehabilitation. Churchill Livingstone, New York, 1992

8. DeLee JC, Drez D: Orthopaedic Sports Medicine Principles and Practice. WB Saunders, Philadelphia, 1994

9. Leadbetter WB, Buckealter JA, Gordon SL: Sports Induced Inflammation. American Academy of Orthopedic Surgeons, Rosemont, IL, 1990

10. Buckley P, Grana WA, Pascale M: The Biomechanical and Physiological Basis of Rehabilitation. p. 225. In Grana WA, Kalenak A (eds): Clinical Sports Medicine. WB Saunders, Philadelphia, 1991

11. Hubbel S, Buschbacher R: Tissue Injury and Healing: Using Medications, Modalities and Exercise to Maximize Recovery. p. 19. In Buschbacher R, Brandom R (eds): Sports Medicine and Rehabilitation: A Sports Specific Approach. Hanley and Belfus, Philadelphia, 1994

12. Kisner C, Colby LA: Therapeutic Exercise, Foundations and Techniques. FA Davis, Philadelphia, 1985

13. Shephard RJ, Miller HS: Exercise and the Heart in Health and Disease. Marcel Dekker, New York, 1992

17
Chiropractic Pediatrics

Joan Fallon

The care of children is among the most challenging aspects of chiropractic practice. Spinal subluxations can occur at any age. When subluxations are present and contraindications to chiropractic adjustment are absent, chiropractic intervention is used. The immature bone development in young children calls for creative modification of standard chiropractic techniques, with a minimal application of force. With children, as with adult patients, rigorous attention to diagnosis is essential, so that when referral to other practitioners is necessary, it is done in a timely fashion.

Pediatrics is the study and care of children from conception through adolescence. This chapter addresses the care of the pregnant woman, the child in utero, and the early years of postnatal life. Each period is covered with respect to examination, correction of subluxation, and adjusting procedures, as well as its particular hallmarks of growth and development.

Like others before them, contemporary practitioners of chiropractic pediatrics, such as Maxine McMullen and Larry Webster, have taught generations of chiropractors how to take care of children.

PRENATAL CHIROPRACTIC

Maintaining health during pregnancy is vital to a positive birth outcome. Chiropractic care during pregnancy can be valuable for both mother and child. Those aspects of health that need to be addressed during the prenatal period, in addition to chiropractic care, include proper diet, education, exercise, and high-quality obstetric care. Chiropractors should encourage pregnant patients to receive the best possible care in each of these areas.[1]

Hormonal changes that occur during the pregnancy, especially elevation of estrogen and progesterone, initiate significant changes in the body of the pregnant woman (Tables 17-1 and 17-2).

Among the most important changes that take place during pregnancy are those that affect connective tissue. Increased overall laxity of the connective tissue permits the baby to grow and develop in an environment that minimizes stress on the mother. In addition to allowing the baby to grow and the mother to gain weight, these connective tissue changes permit substantial changes in the cardiovascular, renal, musculoskeletal, and respiratory systems. They allow the body to accommodate increased vascularity, tissue growth, blood volume, and other factors. Without these changes, the body of the pregnant woman would be unable to support the pregnancy. These changes set the stage for the birth of the child.[1,2]

THE BIRTH

Birth is divided into multiple stages, each of which requires significant communication between the

Table 17-1. Changes Produced by Progesterone During Pregnancy

1. Decreases smooth muscle tone
2. Decreases vascular tone
3. Increases temperature
4. Increases fat storage
5. Produces overbreathing (increased depth of respiration) decreases PCO_2
6. With estrogen, enhances development of the breasts

(From Fallon,[1] with permission)

musculature of the uterus, the central nervous system, and the endocrine system. Interaction between the endocrine and nervous systems affects the "neuromuscular harmony" of the uterus,[3,4] enabling the uterus to contract properly and expel the fetus during delivery, increasing the likelihood of a positive birth outcome.

Figure 17-1 demonstrates the birth mechanism in an occiput anterior vaginal delivery. Malposition is one of the most common problems encountered during the birth process. When the baby deviates from the occiput anterior position, the likelihood of trauma to the baby during delivery increases.[5,6]

Malposition/Malpresentation

Six major malpositions are possible, along with additional compound presentations. The four significant malpositions are discussed below.

Table 17-2. Changes Produced by Estrogen During Pregnancy

1. Produces significant alteration in connective tissue by increasing the mobility of the joint capsules, spinal segmental motor unit, and the pelvis
2. Promotes the growth of the uterus and control of its function
3. With progesterone, helps promote breast development
4. Increases water retention/conservation
5. Reduces sodium excretion

(From Fallon,[1] with permission.)

Normal Birth

Engagement: Flexion Descent

Rotation, Beginning Extension

Complete Extension

Restitution (External Rotation)

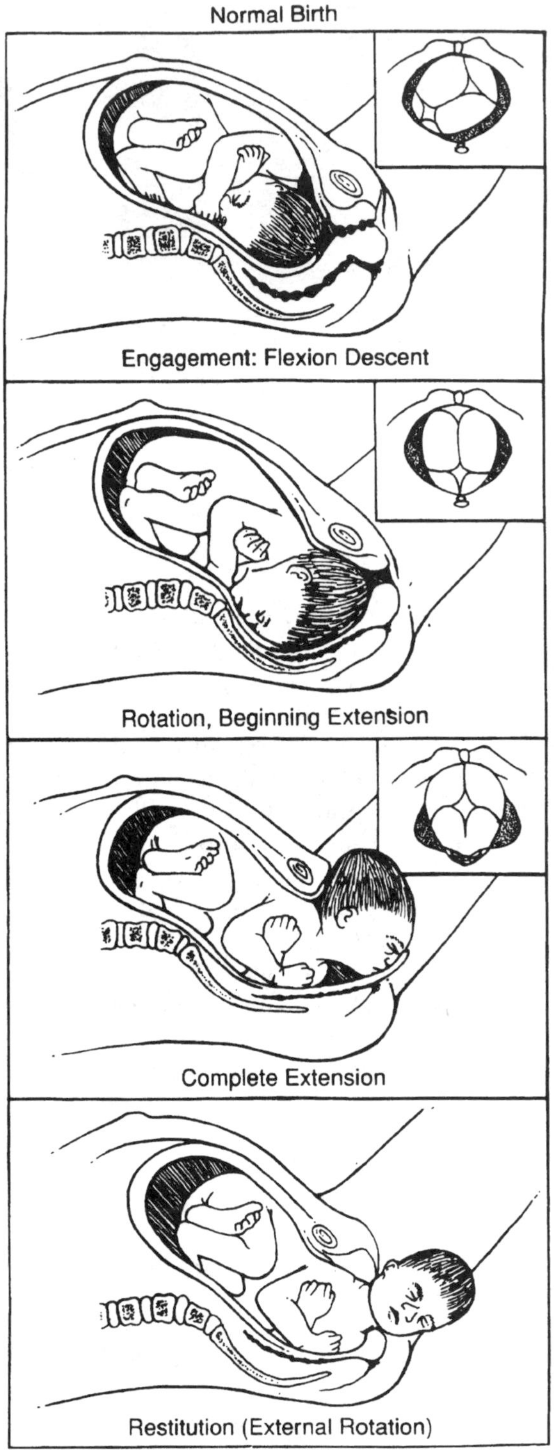

Figure 17-1. Normal birth mechanism. (From Fallon,[1] with permission.)

Occiput Posterior Presentation

The occiput posterior presentation is the classic "upside-down" presentation, in which the baby is born looking up at the ceiling (Fig. 17-2). It accounts for 13 percent of all head presentations in which the presenting part is the vertex and the denominator the occiput. The mechanism of the birth is such that the head of the fetus presses on the sacrum, applying pressure to the sacral plexus. Under these circumstances, the sacrum may subluxate, and labor may intermittently stop and start due to this mechanism.[1,6] *Back labor* is the hallmark of this presentation.

Breech Birth

In a breech birth, the presenting part is one or both feet or the buttocks, rather than the head (Fig. 17-3). It occurs approximately once in 40 births and accounts for the most significant number of vaginal birth-related traumas. The head is delivered last.

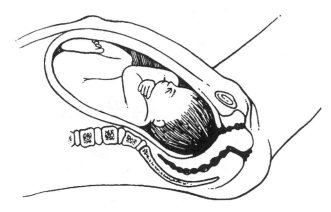

Figure 17-2. Occiput posterior birth. (From Fallon,[1] with permission.)

After the pelvis opens to deliver the shoulders, it closes down again on the head. Delivery of the head often requires significant force, which can traumatize the neonate.[1]

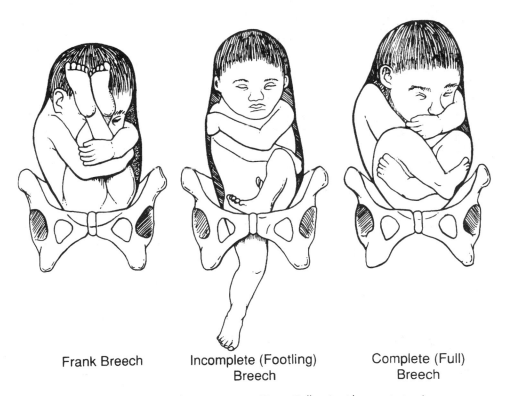

Frank Breech   Incomplete (Footling)   Complete (Full)
                              Breech   Breech

Figure 17-3. Breech presentation. (From Fallon,[1] with permission.)

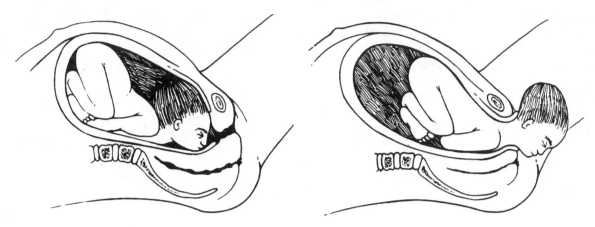

Figure 17-4. Face presentation. (From Fallon,[1] with permission.)

Face Presentation

In the face presentation, the presenting part is the face with the denominator the chin (Fig. 17-4). Face presentation occurs in approximately 1 in 300 births. Of special interest to the chiropractor is the extreme extension of the neck. This presentation can present with frank subluxation and abnormal molding of the cranial bones.[1]

Shoulder Presentation

Occurring in approximately one in 200 to 300 births, shoulder presentation is rare, often converting to a more stable presentation (Fig. 17-5). It occurs in a variety of conditions, such as twin

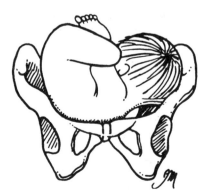

Figure 17-5. Shoulder presentation. (From Fallon,[1] with permission.)

birth, hydramnios, placenta previa, multiparity, and unusual fetal shape.[1,6]

In addition to helping the mother with musculoskeletal and neurologic problems that can develop during pregnancy and childbirth, there is anecdotal evidence of reduced time in labor as a result of chiropractic care. Experience in my practice indicates that, with chiropractic care, the mean time spent in labor decreases by approximately 25 percent.[7] Further research on this topic is warranted.

NEONATAL EXAMINATION AND CARE

The initial cursory examination of the child is done in the delivery room, assigning scores of 0 to 2 for heart rate, respiration, color, reflexes, and muscle tone. This calculation is called the *Apgar score* (Table 17-3). Scores are taken at 1 minute after birth and again at 5 minutes after birth, providing caregivers a statement about the newborn's overall status. A child with generalized musculoskeletal problems, central nervous system (CNS) depression, or respiratory failure will be identified in the first 5 minutes after birth.[8]

After the child leaves the delivery room, a more thorough examination should be performed in order to evaluate the reflexes, heart sounds, and gross anatomy. In certain cases, including home births, this examination may be performed by a chiropractor. The following discussion can serve as a guide in assessing the child's overall health status.

Table 17-3. Apgar Score

Sign	0 Points	1 Point	2 Points
Heart rate	Absent	Slow (below 100)	Over 100
Respiratory effort	Absent	Slow and irregular	Good, crying
Muscle tone	Flaccid	Some flexion of extremities	Active motion
Reflex irritability	No response	Grimace	Vigorous cry
Color	Pale	Cyanotic	Completely pink

(From Goldbloom,[20] with permission.)

Inspection

Generalized inspection of the child should be undertaken by examining the unclothed child. Skin color, skin texture, ear size and shape, and so forth, should be examined.

Figures 17-6 and 17-7 depict head abnormalities that may be discovered at the neonatal examination. Caput succedarum (Fig. 17-6) is caused by subcutaneous edema due to disruption of lymphatic drainage. Cephalohematoma is pooling of blood under the periosteum, which does not cross the suture line[1,8] (Fig. 17-7).

In addition, generalized inspection of the child will demonstrate whether the child presents as "floppy," often referred to as floppy baby syndrome, (Fig. 17-8) or rigid (Fig. 17-9). The presence of rigidity or a floppy-type syndrome will give the chiropractor clues about both subluxation and the overall health of the child's nervous system and the possibility of insult.[1,8,9]

ASSESSING SUBLUXATION IN THE NEONATE

Subluxation in the neonate can be induced by the birth process or by overt birth trauma. The most common subluxation sites in the neonate are in the upper cervical region (occiput, C1 and C2), although other areas of the spine may be involved as well.

Motion and static palpation as well as instrumentation may be useful in assessing subluxation in the neonate. In cases of extreme birth trauma or abnormal physical examination findings, radiography may also be appropriate. In addition, the McMullen reverse fencer reflex can be used to assess the presence and level of subluxation in the neonate.[10] This method uses the child's normal fencer reflex, which is reversed when the child is hung upside down. In the absence of a proper response, presence of a subluxation can be confirmed and the level determined by palpation and other standard methods of chiropractic analysis.[10]

Correction of the vertebral subluxation complex in the neonate may be accomplished by a variety of chiropractic techniques. Diversified, toggle, and Activator are among the most frequently used techniques for the neonate. It is crucial to remember that due to the cartilaginous nature of the child's vertebrae, low force is all that is required to make an osseous correction.

Primitive Reflexes

The primitive reflexes represent a key aspect of the chiropractor's neonatal examination. Presence of these reflexes demonstrates immaturity of the nervous system. Normally, they are present for approximately the first 6 months of life. Some of the more important primitive reflexes and signs are highlighted below.[8,9,11]

Palmar Grasp Reflex

- *Stimulus* — place examiner's finger in baby's hand

Figure 17-6. Caput succedarum. (From Goldbloom,[20] with permission.)

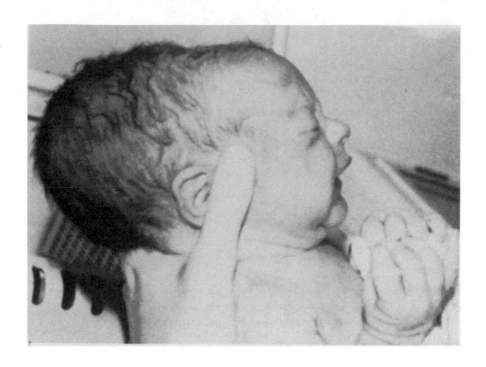

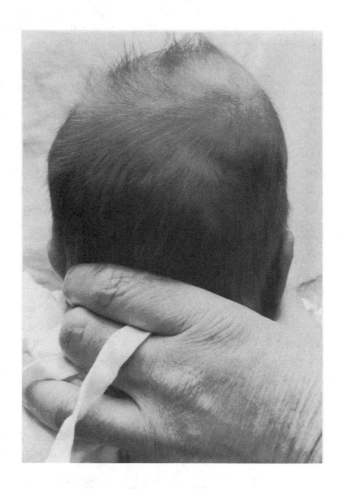

Figure 17-7. Cephalohematoma. (From Goldbloom,[20] with permission.)

Figure 17-8. "Floppy" infant. (From Goldbloom,[20] with permission.)

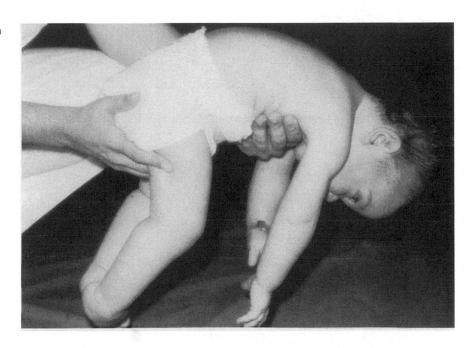

- *Response* — fingers curl to stimulus
- *Duration* — 3 to 6 months
- *Indications* — cerebral insult when persistent

Steppage Reflex
Figure 17-10 illustrates the steppage (placing) reflex, commonly known as the Babinski sign.

- *Stimulus* — with the baby held upright, the dorsum of the foot strikes the underside or top of the table
- *Response* — places foot down
- *Duration* — variable, 2 to 4 months

- *Indications* — possible neurologic insult when absent

Moro Reflex
Figure 17-11 demonstrates the Moro (startle) reflex.

- *Stimulus* — clap hands, make loud noise, begin to drop the child (taking care to maintain a firm enough grip that the child is not actually dropped)
- *Response* — extension of extremities followed by rapid flexion; opening of the eyes

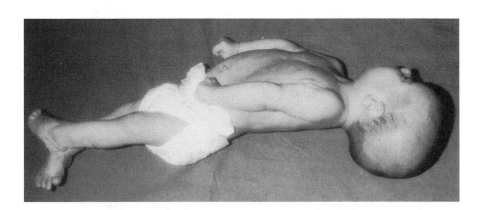

Figure 17-9. Rigidity with scissoring. (From Goldbloom,[20] with permission.)

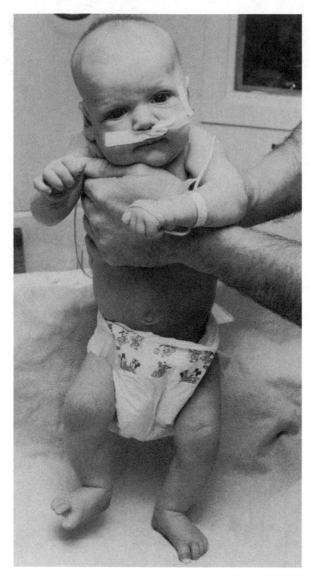

Figure 17-10. Steppage reflex. (From Goldbloom,[20] with permission.)

- *Duration* — 4 months
- *Indications* — if absent, possible neurologic insult; if asymmetric, points to a possible fracture

Tonic Neck Reflex
Figure 17-12 presents an infants with tonic neck (fencer reflex).

- *Stimulus* — baby placed supine with head turned to one side

- *Response* — extension of extremities on side to which head is turned
- *Duration* — 4 to 6 months
- *Indications* — if present beyond 6 months, possible neurologic insult

Rooting Reflex
Figure 17-13 demonstrates the rooting reflex.

- *Stimulus* — stroke baby's cheek
- *Response* — baby moves head to side of stroking
- *Duration* — 3 to 4 months
- *Indications* — if absent, possible severe CNS problem

Babinski Reflex
Figure 17-13 illustrates the classic Babinski reflex.

- *Stimulus* — stroke the sole of the foot medial to lateral and heel to toe
- *Response* — toes spread out; great toe dorsiflexes
- *Duration* — 16 to 24 months
- *Indications* — beyond 2 years, neurologic deficit

Physical Examination

The physical examination of the child should include a full musculoskeletal examination, including an Ortilani check for congenital hip dysplasia (Fig. 17-14) as well as inspection for talipes. Auscultation, percussion, height/length, weight, and palpation of the abdomen should all be performed.[8,10]

INFANCY

Infancy is marked by significant growth and development. This period is clearly defined by the child's ability to achieve certain milestones of growth and development.[8] Some significant milestones and their average achievement times are listed below:

Sitting up	4–5 months
Rolling over	3–5 months
Crawling	5–7 months
Creeping	6–9 months
Walking	11–14 months

Figure 17-11. Moro/startle reflex. (From Goldbloom,[20] with permission.)

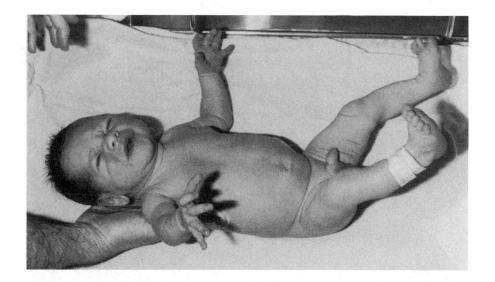

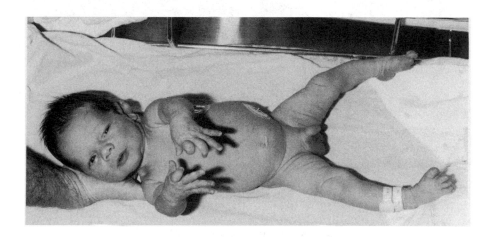

While infancy is marked by significant changes in the growth and development of the child, it is also marked by the beginnings of childhood illness. For the first time, the child must acquire his or her own immunity. An acute illness will activate the child's immune function.

At approximately 6 months, the child's immune system begins to function on its own without the help of maternal antibodies. Coupled with significant changes in the child's surroundings due to newfound mobility, this elicits changes in the child's immunologic status. At this time, childhood illness such as otitis media may appear.

Otitis Media

Because the eustachian tube parallels the horizontal plane to a greater degree in infancy than later in life, infants are highly susceptible to eustachian tube backup and to the formation of otitis media. As a result, otitis media is the most common diagnosis for physician office visits by children under age 15 and accounts for the largest number of office visits to pediatricians.[12] Questions regarding the effectiveness of antibiotics and other allopathic methods used to treat otitis media are raised with increasing frequency. In 1994, clinical practice guidelines on

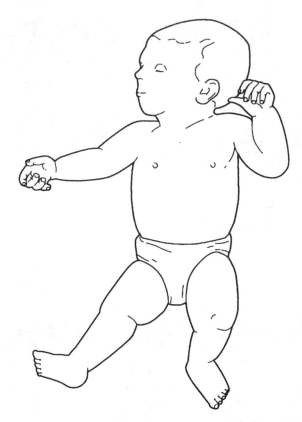

Figure 17-12. Tonic neck reflex. (From Goldbloom,[20] with permission.)

otitis media with effusion prepared by an expert panel for the Agency for Health Care Policy and Research stated that the medical literature on the subject is "voluminous but unenlightening" and called for further studies to clarify issues, including natural history, diagnosis, prevention, interventions, and long-term outcomes.[12] Dissatisfaction with conventional care has led many parents to seek out new ways to treat otitis, including chiropractic care.

Chiropractic research on otitis media includes a restrospective study by Froehle,[13] in which 93 percent of all otitis media episodes improved under chiropractic care; 75 percent of infants improved in 10 days or less, and 43 percent within one or two visits. Interestingly, Froehle's data indicated that a history of past antibiotic use was associated with a less favorable outcome. Of those patients with no history of antibiotic use, 60 percent improved with two chiro-

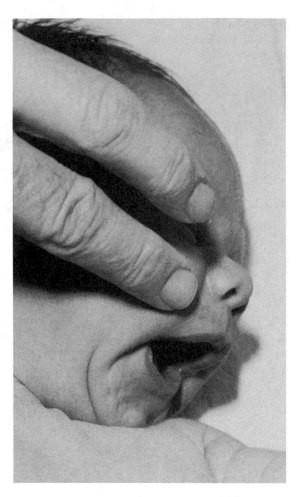

Figure 17-13. Rooting reflex. (From Goldbloom,[20] with permission.)

practic adjustments or less, while 65 percent of those who had taken antibiotics required more than two visits before exhibiting clinical improvement.

A case series by Fysh[14] reported the effects of chiropractic adjustments in five children with chronic recurrent otitis media, each of whom had been under the care of a medical pediatrician for at least 6 months without resolution. Four of the five patients exhibited some improvement after the first adjustment, and none required more than five visits for resolution. On motion palpation, all five patients had fixations involving the second cervical vertebra. Fysh states that children with otitis media generally exhibit signs of subluxation in the upper cervical region.

Figure 17-14. Ortilani check. (From Goldbloom,[20] with permission.)

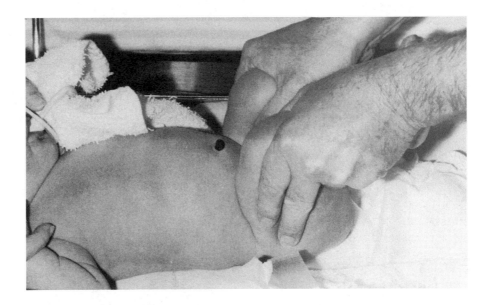

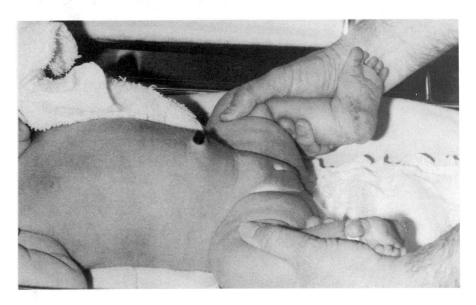

Determining Subluxation in the Infant

As the child explores new bodily movements associated with developmental milestones, subluxative changes occur most frequently in the areas used to perform these movements.[9] Holding the head up, sitting, creeping, and crawling involve successive parts of the spine. Since the neonate can only hold its head up, subluxative changes in this phase of life are most likely in the cranium and cervical spine. As the infant begins to crawl, the entire spine comes into play, and subluxations of the thoracic, lumbar, and pelvic levels appear more frequently. Adjustive procedures for the infant include all full-spine techniques, each of which is appropriately modified for the child's body.

TODDLER PERIOD

The toddler period is also marked by significant growth and development.[8,9] The child begins to walk and negotiate the world upright, experiencing for the first time what adults take for granted. Gait considerations are extremely important for the chiropractor to keep in mind in working with toddlers. Problems first encountered at this time include[8,11]:

Tibial Torsion

In tibial torsion, the child toes in, with normal positioning of the patellae. This problem usually occurs at 6 to 18 months and is abnormal only when it persists beyond that time

Femoral Torsion

In femoral torsion, the patellae point inward and the child toes in (Fig. 17-15). This problem may be the direct result of subluxation of the pelvis in an internally rotated position or an overcompensated externally rotated pelvis.

Genu Varus/Genu Valgus

Genu varus is characterized by significant bowing of the legs. This problem is often a normal physiologic step in the child's gait development. If it persists well beyond the age of 2 years, more problematic conditions need to be ruled out, including rickets and metaphyseal dysplasia. Similar considerations apply in genu valgus, in which the toe-out position is present (Fig. 17-17). This condition can develop in children who are obese, who have rickets, or who have other conditions, such as renal osteodystrophy.

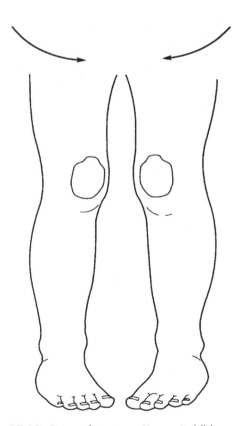

Figure 17-15. Femoral torsion. (From Goldbloom,[20] with permission.)

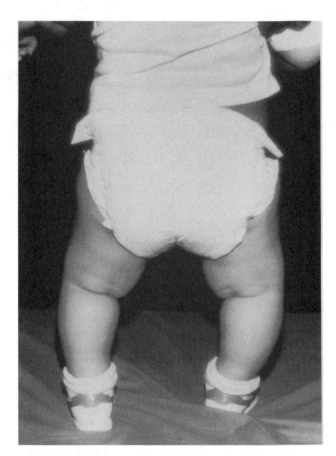

Figure 17-16. Genu varus. (From Goldbloom,[20] with permission.)

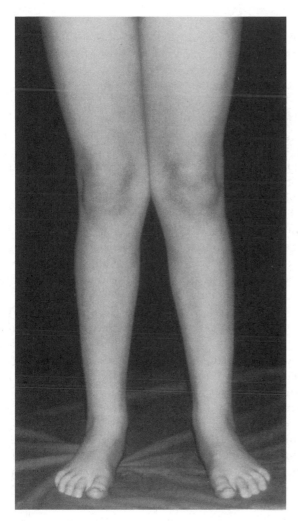

Figure 17-17. Genu valgus. (From Goldbloom,[20] with permission.)

Legg-Calvé-Perthes

Legg-Calvé-Perthes is an avascular necrosis of the femoral head that appears in children aged 2 to 10 years. It can present as frank pain at the femoral head or, more likely, as a limp or difficulty moving the hip joint or distal joints.

Chiropractic Adjustment Considerations for the Toddler

Full spine techniques are recommended due to more complex and accelerated movements of the toddler.

At this age, the child may not be fully cooperative, which requires the doctor to be artfully swift in palpation and chiropractic adjustment procedures.

SCHOOL-AGE CHILDREN/ADOLESCENCE

Care of the school-age child entails attention to physical, social, and behavioral development, including interaction with peers, parents, siblings. The average school-age child is free of illness to a greater extent than the toddler, infant, or neonate. With children now beginning school at increasingly younger ages, and with the advent of daycare for infants and early preschool during the past 20 years, the epidemiology of the child has changed. While the children of the 1960s and 1970s were often first exposed to their peers at ages 4 and 5 years, many children in the 1990s are in frequent close contact with peers as early as 6 months of age. As a result, they may develop immunity at an early age.

Scoliosis is one of the conditions that can present during this period. It is essential that the doctor of chiropractic bear this in mind when examining adolescents who present as patients. Scoliosis lies within the domain of chiropractic (Fig. 17-18), but both the etiology and the management of scoliosis remain controversial. Because this condition can be progressive, periodic radiographic evaluation is appropriate. Since the most severe cases of scoliosis can threaten heart and lung function, referral for medical evaluation is essential for cases in which progression continues unchecked.

Correction of the vertebral subluxation complex in schoolchildren and adolescents may be accomplished by the wide variety of techniques employed for adult patients, always bearing in mind the need for appropriate modification of the force of thrust. As with younger children, the school-age child's special needs must be addressed. Social and behavioral development, including interaction with peers, parents, and siblings is important to observe.

CURRENT STATUS AND FUTURE PROSPECTS

Chiropractic pediatrics is enjoying a renaissance in the 1990s. Attendance at postgraduate pediatrics courses is at an all-time high. The International Chiropractic Association (ICA) Council on Pediatrics

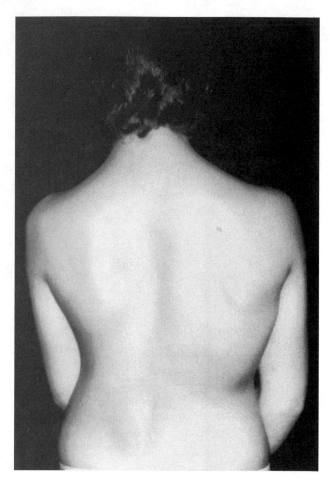

Figure 17-18. Scoliosis. (From Goldbloom,[20] with permission.)

offers a 3-year 300-hour diplomate program with a wide-ranging curriculum covering all aspects of pediatric practice for the chiropractor.

Research on pediatrics is accelerating but, like the overall field of chiropractic visceral disorders research, it is still in the early stages of development. Published reports such as the prospective study on infantile colic by Klougart et al.[15] provide a foundation for more definitive research projects in the future. In the Klougart study, 90 percent of infants improved within 2 weeks, and 23 percent improved after a single adjustment. Intriguing case studies on conditions, including myasthenia gravis,[16] attention-

deficit disorder,[17] head trauma,[18] and blocked atlantal nerve syndrome[19] also offer a foretaste of future advances.

The response of otitis media to chiropractic intervention is a particularly fertile area for research, in light of the poor track record of the allopathic approach to this condition and the previously cited examples of positive responses to chiropractic adjustments. The Foundation for Chiropractic Education and Research recently provided the funding for a study to be conducted by Charles Sawyer and colleagues at Northwestern College of Chiropractic, which will include retrospective and prospective investigations of otitis media, using tympanography protocols. Tympanography, which measures movement of the eardrum, offers an objective measure of patient response to supplement subjective reports of parents and doctors.

Over the past 25 years, the chiropractic research agenda has understandably focused on those conditions (low back pain, neck pain, and headaches) seen most frequently by chiropractors. Future research will focus more intently on conditions for which chiropractic shows great promise, but that comprise a smaller portion of contemporary chiropractic practice. If this research demonstrates conclusively that chiropractic offers significant, measurable benefits, chiropractic adjustments may eventually be included in the standard of care for pediatric conditions such as otitis media and infantile colic.

Terminology

Apgar score
Babinski reflex
breech birth
caput succedarum
cephalohematoma
developmental milestone
femoral torsion
genu valgus
genu varus
Legg-Calvé-Perthes
McMullen reverse fencer reflex
Moro reflex
neonate

otitis media
primitive reflexes
palmar grasp reflex
rooting reflex
steppage reflex
tibial torsion
tonic neck reflex
tympanometry

Review Questions

1. How do the hormonal changes of pregnancy affect connective tissue?

2. List four malpositions commonly encountered in the birth process.

3. What are the five areas evaluated in the Apgar score?

4. List three primitive reflexes and discuss their significance.

5. Why does otitis media occur with greater frequency early in life?

6. Discuss two studies indicating potential benefits from chiropractic care in cases of otitis media.

7. What subjective and objective measures have been used in chiropractic research on otitis media?

8. Which spinal levels are more likely to become subluxated in the infant than in the neonate?

9. Describe the McMullen reverse fencer reflex.

10. What were the key findings in the Klougart study on infantile colic?

Concept Questions

1. How would you respond to someone who states that no one under the age of 18 should receive chiropractic care?

2. What neurologic pathways might explain positive responses to spinal adjustments in cases of otitis media and infantile colic? What causative factors other than subluxations may be involved in these conditions?

3. What modifications of adjusting techniques are required in working with pregnant patients? With young children?

References

1. Fallon JM: Textbook of Chiropractic and Pregnancy. International Chiropractors Association, Arlington, VA, 1994

2. Ulfelder H: Mechanism of pelvic support in women. Am J Obstet Gynecol 72:856, 1956

3. Aminoff MJ: Neurological disorders of pregnancy. Am J Obstet Gynecol 132:325, 1978

4. Haldeman S: Interactions between the somatic and visceral nervous systems. ACA J Chiro 5:57, 1971

5. Levine MG, Holroyde J, Woods JR et al: Birth trauma: incidence and predisposing factors. Obstet Gynecol 63:792, 1984

6. Cruikshank DP, White CA: Obstetric malpresentations: twenty years experience. Am J Obstet Gynecol 116:1097, 1973

7. Fallon JM: Orthopedic and neurological conditions of pregnancy and chiropractic management of care. In Articles on Pediatrics. Vol. II. Int Rev Chiro, 1994

8. Barnes LA: Manual of Pediatric Physical Diagnosis. 4th Ed. Year Book, Chicago, 1972

9. McMullen M: Handicapped children and chiropractic care. Parts I and II. Articles on Pediatrics. Vol. II. International Review of Chiropractic, 1994

10. McMullen M: Assessing cervical subluxations in the infants under six months of age. Articles on Pediatrics. Vol. I. International Review of Chiropractic, 1994

11. Lovell WW, Winter RB: Pediatric Orthopedics. JB Lippincott. Philadelphia, 1978

12. Stool SE, Berg AO, Berman S et al: Otitis media with effusion in young children. Clinical Practice Guideline, No. 12. AHCPR Publ. No. 94-0622. U.S. Department of Health and Human Services, Public Health Service, Agency for Health Care Policy and Research, Gaithersburg, MD, 1994

13. Froehle RM: Ear infection: a retrospective study examining improvement from chiropractic care and analyzing for influencing factors. J Manipul Physiol Ther 19:169, 1996

14. Fysh PN: Chronic recurrent otitis media: case series of five patients with recommendations for case management. J Clin Chiro Pediatr 1:66, 1996

15. Klougart N, Nilsson N, Jacobsen J: Infantile colic treated by chiropractors: a prospective study of 316 cases. J Manipul Physiol Ther 12:281, 1989

16. Araghi HJ: Juvenile myesthenia gravis: a case study in chiropractic management. p. 122. In Proceedings of the International Conference on Pediatrics and Chiropractic, 1993

17. Arme J: Effects of biochemical insult correction on attention deficit disorder. J Chiro Case Rep 1:6, 1993

18. Hospers LA: EEG and CEEG studies before and after upper cervical or SOT category II adjustment in children after head trauma. p. 84. In Proceedings of the National Conference on Chiropractic and Pediatrics, International Chiropractic Association, 1992

19. Gutmann G: Blocked atlantal nerve syndrome in infants and small children. ICA Int Rev Chiro 46:37, 1990

20. Goldbloom R: Pediatric Clinical Skills, 2nd Ed. Churchill Livingstone, New York, 1997

18

Chiropractic in the Workplace

Prevention and Treatment

David P. Gilkey
Holly A. Williams

*C*hiropractic has long played a vital role in the treatment of work-related injury and illness, compiling a solid record of clinical effectiveness and cost-effectiveness. In recent years, development of a chiropractic specialty in occupational health has significantly expanded the range of work-related services provided by chiropractors. The profession's focus on treatment has been enlarged to include prevention and interdisciplinary case management.

Traditional roles of occupational health physicians, safety professionals, and industrial hygienists have been limited and generally separate, but the evolution of modern industry, regulatory overlap, and marketplace forces are bringing these disciplines closer together.[1] The chiropractic occupational health and safety physician is well equipped to offer a broad spectrum of needed services for a wide range of industry challenges.

INJURY AND ILLNESS PREVENTION
Prevention Paradigm and Safety Philosophy

The ultimate challenge to a physician is to prevent what he treats.

Joseph Sweere

According to Heinrich, 88 percent of accidents are the result of human behavior and are therefore preventable.[2] The American Public Health Association states that the cornerstones of prevention are anticipation of the potential for disease or injury, surveillance (accurate identification, reporting, and recording of occupational disease and injury), analysis of collected data, and control.[3]

Traditional methods of controlling or eliminating workplace hazards include engineering out, or removal of, the hazard; use of personal protective equipment; and training in the proper and safe use of equipment. Engineering is often quite costly and therefore cannot be used in many potentially hazardous environments. If the hazard cannot be engineered out, workers must be trained to minimize risk of injury or illness.

Corporate realities depend on the bottom line. Companies ask: if we commit to practicing prevention, can we stay in business, make a profit, and remain competitive? If the answer is yes, prevention and safety become part of the corporate culture. If not, prevention is reduced to after-injury record-keeping, accident investigations, and invocation of safety regulations. This results in increased accident rates and costly worker's compensation claims.

Industrialized nations are moving toward prevention strategies. In many cases, this is driven by the high cost of work-related injury and illness, although in some instances the desire to embrace prevention is an organic outgrowth of good management principles.

The Chiropractic Physician's Role in Industry

Duties of the occupational health physician are changing. Once largely limited to treatment services, occupational health physicians now perform roles ranging from purely administrative to highly interactive. Aside from treatment of occupational injury and illness, these include pre-employment and preplacement examinations, return-to-work and independent medical examinations, medical monitoring, health education and counseling, worksite analysis, job analysis, specific fitness evaluation, baseline health determination, evaluation of work influence, emergency planning, and rehabilitation programs. Experienced chiropractic occupational health specialists also participate in advising medical management, evaluating the effectiveness of medical programs, cost containment, and record management. In addition, they serve as advisors to employers or insurance companies and as patient advocates.[4–7]

ERGONOMIC IMPROVEMENTS AT SACO DEFENSE, INC.

Chiropractic occupational health consultant Robert Lynch was contacted by SACO Defense, Inc., a Maine firearms manufacturer, to assist in reducing musculoskeletal injury and lost workdays. After 3 months of detailed ergonomic analysis, Dr. Lynch advised implementation of a broad range of prevention strategies. Ergonomic improvements were made, where possible. More than 500 employees were trained in workplace safety measures. Included was a regimen of exercises designed by Dr. Lynch that employees performed for about 5 minutes, two or three times a day.

Lost workdays plummeted by 66 percent. SACO's workers compensation premiums dropped from $2 million in 1989 to $40,000 in 1993. In 1990, SACO experienced 44 lost-time injuries with 913 workdays lost. In 1994, there were two lost-time injuries, with a total of 3 days lost—an 82 percent improvement in lost-time injuries and 73 percent reduction in workers compensation costs per hours worked.[8]

OCCUPATIONAL ERGONOMICS

Ergonomic science is the study of people in relation to their jobs.[9,10] It includes environmental aspects of the workplace, such as temperature, light, noise, and the physical arrangement of the workplace. Because ergonomics is closely associated with neuro-musculoskeletal injury and disease, emphasis is placed on the design of the workplace as it relates to physical demands placed on the worker. Individuals have different physical capabilities and limitations. A key concept in applied ergonomics is to "fit the job to the worker," rather than force the worker to fit the job.[9–11] Applied ergonomics seeks to improve worker comfort through analysis and application of ergonomic principles.

Chiropractic education and training provide an excellent foundation for understanding the biomechanical basis of applied ergonomics. Anatomy, physiology, pathophysiology, posture, and biomechanics are fundamental aspects of ergonomics. The chiropractic postgraduate occupational health program includes problem-solving skills development, anthropometrics, safety engineering, risk factor identification and analysis, methods for passive and active analysis of the workplace, safety engineering, development and implementation of control strategies, ergonomic programs, and communication skills to increase effectiveness with industry.

Anthropometrics

Anthropometric data are used ergonomically to determine reach and clearance when designing the workplace. Data analysis shows variations between the sexes in average height, weight, reach, and other parameters. The following are examples of height and weight averages reported in U.S. populations[10–12]:

NASA   Male 70.8″/181 lb Female 61.8″/113.5 lb
Chaffin[10] Male 69″   Female 63.7″
Selan[11]   Male 69″   Female 63.9″

The "Golden Rule of Design" states that clearance allowances must be designed for the largest users and reach capabilities must be designed for the smallest users. It is important to incorporate adjustability whenever possible.

Back Pain Risk Factors

Physical and emotional risk factors associated with low back pain in the workplace are highly relevant to chiropractic practice. Correlations have been found between low back pain and the following factors[13]:

- Lack of job satisfaction
- Duration of employment under 5 years
- Time of day (6 AM to noon)
- Sense of monotony on the job
- Alcohol consumption
- Drug abuse
- Smoking tobacco
- Taller stature

Cumulative Trauma Disorders Risk Factors

Key risk factors associated with cumulative trauma disorders (CTDs) include repetition or frequency of motion, force of exertion, posture of the body, duration of task, recovery or cycle time, exposure to cold temperatures, and exposure to vibration.[9,14–20]

Gilkey and Williams[21] provide a detailed synopsis of key points in the proposed Occupational Safety and Health Administration (OSHA) ergonomic standards. Of particular importance are the following signal risk factors for CTDs:

- Performance of the same motion or motion pattern every few seconds for more than 2 continu-

ous hours, or for more than 4 hours total in the 8-hour work shift
- Fixed or awkward posture for more than a total of 2 to 4 hours
- Use of a vibrating or impact tool for more than a total of 2 to 4 hours
- Using forceful hand exertions for more than a total of 2 to 4 hours
- Unassisted frequent or forceful manual handling for more than a total of 1 or 2 hours

Other risk factors associated with the development of CTDs include age (50 percent of claimants are over age 50), hypertension, coronary heart disease, stroke, hyperlipidemia, genetic factors, alcohol and tobacco use, lack of exercise, and poor diet.[22]

Performing the Ergonomic Evaluation
Passive Analysis

The first step in ergonomic evaluation is passive analysis of workplace data, which should be performed every 2 years, to ensure the absence of negative trends in injury or illness. If available, documents describing types and patterns of worker injuries and illness should be thoroughly evaluated by the occupational health physician. Simple review and analysis of company documents can reveal significant clues to the presence of ergonomic hazards and related injuries.

Passive analysis begins with a review of OSHA logs for incidence and details of back injuries or CTDs.[11,23,24] This is followed by review of accident investigation reports for details about injuries and calculation of incidence rates (IR) and severity rates (SR) for CTDs and back injuries. Next comes detailed assessment of worker's compensation claims, health care costs related to CTDs and back injuries, absenteeism rates, and requests for job changes. Passive analysis calls for detective skills on the part of the analyst; the goal is to search for patterns contributing to injuries.

IR calculation can provide a comparison to a known industry standard. A high IR usually indicates a need for ergonomic and prevention intervention. SR calculation indicates the serious nature of injuries and potential costs associated with lost work days.

The calculation of IR and SR can be accomplished as follows[11,23,24]:

$$IR = \text{number of incidents for the time period} \times 200{,}000 \text{ hr/number of hours worked during the period}$$

$$SR = \text{number of days lost for the time period} \times 200{,}000 \text{ hr/number of hours worked during the period}$$

Active Analysis

Worksite evaluation affords the chiropractic occupational health physician the opportunity to observe, sample, measure, and record the presence of potential ergonomic hazards. This active analysis requires that the occupational health physician select the best tools for the job; no single form or checklist is applicable to all workplaces.[11] The specific nature of job tasks at each workplace determines the most appropriate approach for active analysis, which can include checklists, observations, interviews, videos, photographs, sampling, measuring, and monitoring.[11,23,24] The information gleaned from these various procedures is correlated with passive analysis findings to develop ergonomic prevention strategies.[11,23]

Active analysis should emphasize potential ergonomic hazards:

- Excessive force
- Frequent repetitions
- Awkward postures
- Fast cycle times
- Automated pace
- Monotony
- High stress
- Lack of worker control
- Excessive noise
- Excessive heat/cold
- Poor lighting

Ergonomic Intervention

Implementation of ergonomic controls endeavors to fit the job to the worker. Where possible, the first step is to engineer out the hazard. Today's technologic marketplace offers a wide array of ergonomic devices and equipment for both manufacturing and sedentary workplaces. Design solutions are specific to each worksite. Recommendations may include engineering interventions such as mechanical lift assist devices, power-driven hand tools, and adjustable workstations; ergonomic personal protection equipment such as friction enhancing gloves, protective eye wear, and hearing conservation wear; ergonomic training in proper work postures, proper lifting techniques, and fitness instruction; and administrative interventions, including job rotations and changes in break schedule and production rate.

Some ergonomic challenges require only simple intervention, while others entail complex and costly solutions. Communication with company management and all affected individuals is essential. Once intervention has been completed and an ergonomic program is under way, results may be measured by the same passive and active analysis methods used earlier. Programs should be monitored on an ongoing basis and audited every 2 years to document results and the need for further intervention.[11]

ERGONOMIC IMPROVEMENTS AT VARICON

Varicon, a glass manufacturing company with annual sales of more than $60 million, was suffering from an epidemic of low back injury cases when chiropractic physician and occupational health diplomate Joseph Sweere was called in to provide an ergonomic assessment. Dr. Sweere's recommendations included ergonomic improvements, safety training, wellness education, and worker preplacement selection and screening.

Following implementation of Sweere's prevention plans, Varicon's incidence of low back injury decreased by 80 percent.[25] The Varicon case established the efficacy of the biomechanical stress index (BSI), which is now widely used by chiropractic occupational health consultants.

NEUROMUSCULOSKELETAL ILLNESS AND INJURY

Scope of the Problem

Between 60 and 80 percent of the general population will suffer from low back pain at some point in their lives, and 20 to 30 percent are suffering from it at any given time.[26] The burden to social and financial systems is staggering.

Back pain is the most frequently cited reason for workers' filing injury claims. According to the National Safety Council (NSC), low back disorders make up 30 to 40 percent of all worker's compensation injuries.[27] The National Institute for Occupational Safety and Health (NIOSH) reports that 19 to 25 percent of all worker's compensation claims are for back pain.[28] Back pain is the second most frequently recorded reason for lost work days in America, the common cold being first.[29] The Bureau of National Affairs (BNA) reports that back pain accounts for more than 500 million lost workdays each year.[28] On any given day it is estimated that 6.5 million people are home from work, in bed, due to back pain. New back pain cases are generated at a rate of 1.5 million per month.[29]

Equally significant as the prevalence of back pain and injury are the costs associated with it. The average cost of a work-related lower back injury was $23,716 in 1990.[30] NSC reports that the total actual costs of all work-related injuries was $111.9 billion in 1993.[31] Most worker's compensation carriers agree that back injuries are the most expensive claims, comprising 65 to 90 percent of benefit costs.[32] The real economic impact of back pain also includes hidden costs, bringing total back pain expenses as high as $90 billion annually.[29] Because of the prevalence and costs, there has been a growing shift in awareness and concern about neuromusculoskeletal injury and illness in the workplace. While back pain clearly remains the number one challenge to industry, CTDs have emerged as a sleeping giant.

Cumulative Trauma Disorders

Rates and Costs

Review of the literature shows a sharp rise in the number of CTDs (Table 18-1).

A 770 percent increase in CTDs between 1983 and 1993 was noted, a trend attributed to increased

Table 18-1. Cumulative Trauma Disorders

Study	Year	Reported Cases of Occupational Illness	
		N	%
Sullivan[33]	1981	~20,500	18
Rigdon[34]	1982	~22,000	21
Chesler[16]	1988	115,000	48
Rigdon[34]	1990	147,000	50
Bureau of National Affairs[35]	1991	223,000	56
LaBar[36]	1992	282,000	60
Bureau of National Affairs[37]	1993	302,000	60

public awareness of CTDs, broader definitions of compensable claims, increased numbers of service industry workers, and increased use of video display terminals (VDT).[35]

CTDs are reported as occupational illnesses, not injuries. CTDs make up only 4 percent of the reported work-related injuries but constitute more than 61 percent of work-related illnesses.[27,38] Despite the alarming numbers, some experts feel that CTDs may be underreported, with incidence rates as much as 130 percent higher.[27]

CTDs are not only the fastest growing workplace illness but one of the most expensive occupational illnesses to treat. Cost estimates have recently been established at $20 to $27 billion per year in the United States.[36,39] The National Council on Compensation Insurance has stated that the average CTD case costs $29,000, including wage loss and treatment. Litigation and settlement costs exceed the medical and lost wage expenses, averaging $50,000 per case.[34] At the present time there is no indication of a decrease in CTD rates. OSHA has proposed an ergonomic standard, but compliance is voluntary, and utilization of the OSHA standard is sporadic at best. Greater efforts must come from industry before real reductions are seen in back injury and CTD illness rates.

Research on Causal Relationships

Only recently has serious research been undertaken to establish the relationship between workplace activities and exposures and specific ergonomic-related injury and illness.[20] This relationship is self-evident to many injured workers, and the existence of ergonomic hazards has long been recognized. Bernadini Ramazini, the father of occupational medicine, wrote in 1713[9]:

> So much for workers whose diseases are caused by the injurious qualities of the material they handle. I now wish to turn to other workers in whom certain morbid affections gradually arise from other causes, i.e. from particular posture of the limbs or unnatural movements of the body called for while they work. Such are the workers who all day long stand or sit, stoop or are bent double; who run or ride or exercise their bodies in all sorts of ways.

Despite this nearly 300-year-old warning, no formal study in ergonomics was undertaken until 1949, when the British Admiralty held the first ergonomics symposium.[40] A recent landmark in this evolving field came in 1995 when Silverstein and colleagues,[20] in an evaluation of the literature on work-related musculoskeletal disorders prepared for OSHA's ergonomics task force, stated, "The literature shows unarguably that certain jobs and certain work related factors are associated with the manifold risk of contracting a WMSD [work-related musculoskeletal disorder] compared to other population groups or groups not exposed to these risk factors." Though OSHA proposed an ergonomic standard in 1995, it has not attained legislative approval.

The literature search and evaluation process presented by Silverstein's group[20] focused on cumulative trauma rather than musculoskeletal accidents or back injuries. The basic cause and effect process for CTDs is described as follows[20]: "It is assumed … that repeated efforts (movements, postures, etc.), static work, continuous loading of the tissue structures, or lack of recovery time trigger or cause a pathological process that then manifests itself as WMSD [work-related musculoskeletal disorder]."

Strength of data was ranked for a variety of CTDs, based on the following criteria[20]:

1. Do the results of the studies show an association between disease and work exposure?
2. Do they show a temporal relationship?
3. Is there consistency in the association?
4. Can a change in disease be predicted by a change in work exposure?
5. Is there coherence of evidence?

Tendon Disorders

Tendon disorders include tendinitis, tenosynovitis, epicondylitis, De Quervain's disease, and Dupuytren's contracture. Silverstein's data review concluded that there is convincing evidence of a causal relationship between repetitive stress and tendinitis of the shoulder, hand, and wrist; that there is weakly convincing evidence for tendinitis of the elbow; that the evidence on Dupuytren's contracture is uncertain; and that the evidence for Achilles tendinitis is job specific. Associated risk factors include repetitive and overhead work for the shoulder; repetitive and forceful gripping for the hand and wrist; repetitive high force use for the elbow; and job-specific stresses such as ballet dancing for Achilles tendinitis.

Peripheral Nerve Disorders

Peripheral nerve disorders include carpal tunnel syndrome, thoracic outlet syndrome, and radiculopathy. Silverstein's data review concluded that there is strong evidence for carpal tunnel syndrome, weak evidence for thoracic outlet syndrome, and that there is no available evidence for cervical radiculopathy. Associated risk factors for carpal tunnel syndrome include repetitive and forceful gripping, repetitive movements, extreme positions, stretching, and contact pressure to the wrist. For thoracic outlet syndrome, risk factors include repetitive arm movements and manual work.

Muscle Disorders

Muscle disorders include neck tension syndrome, myalgia, and myofascial syndromes. It is stated that myofascial syndromes may also occur in the low back. A higher prevalence is reported related to repetitive work with constrained head and arm postures and to sustained and repetitive elevation of the arms. Silverstein's review of available studies found the data incomplete for establishing a strong association between muscle disorders and work exposure. Individual studies do support the relatedness of a portion of muscle disorders to occupational exposure. Specifically, fibromyalgia, traumatic myalgias, and muscle pain syndromes of unknown etiology are excluded from work-related myalgia syndromes. Examples of occupations affected are video display terminal workers, typists, and assembly-line workers. Associated risk factors include static loading and repetitive work.

Joint Disorders

Joint disorders include arthritis, osteoarthrosis, and spondylosis. Silverstein's group[20] concluded that evidence supports a moderate association of workplace risk factors and the development of osteoarthrosis. The one associated risk factor is continuous joint compression, which produces osteoarthrotic changes within joints.

Summary Conclusions for CTDs

- There is ample and consistent evidence to support the association of workplace risk factors of repetition, load, posture, and vibration to the development of CTDs.
- Related signs and symptoms increase with continued exposure.
- Related signs and symptoms decrease with diminished exposure.
- Expression of signs and symptoms is related to work organization, psychosocial, and personal mediating factors.

THE BACK AND SPINE

Initiating Factors in Workplace Injury

There is currently no risk factor and association ranking for low back pain comparable to Silverstein's influential work on CTDs. Many investigators offer lists of relative risk factors associated with low back pain, but no authority has firmly established strength of association. However, NIOSH reports the following hypothesized causes of low back pain and disability[41]: overexertion, strain, lifting, whole-body vibration, static posture, prolonged sitting, direct trauma, and psychosocial factors. The NSC identifies overexertion as the number one cause of back injury and lifting as the most frequently offending activity.[13,31]

Calculations of force are used as predictors of low back injury. The Utah Back Compressive Force Model is used to predict the compressive force brought to bear on the intervertebral disc. Evaluat-

ing factors include load, posture, frequency, and duration of lift. Assumptions are made for task characteristics and task posture. The NIOSH lifting equation considers a broad range of criteria[41]:

- Load weight
- Horizontal location—distance of the load away from the body relative to the feet
- Vertical location—distance of the hands above the floor
- Vertical travel distance—distance from origin to the destination
- Asymmetry angle—amount of deviation from a mid-sagittal plane
- Lifting frequency—average number of lifts per minute measured over a 15-minute period
- Lifting duration—the relative time engaged in lifting activity
- Coupling classification—the quality of load grip
- Significant control—the relative lifter control over load

Many factors are important in attempting to establish a cause-and-effect relationship between hazard exposure and a back injury. OSHA's proposed ergonomic standard has identified the following signal risk factors for lifting and back injury prevention[23]:

- Load weight over 35 lb
- Frequency of lifting more than 25 times in 2 hours
- Frequent forceful exertions greater than 10 lb in 2 hours

Epidemiologic studies of LBP show certain types of work have higher rates of incidence. Kelsey and Golden[13] report that the highest rates of low back pain occur in truck drivers, manual material handlers, nurses, and nursing aides.

Treatment Protocols for Spine-Related Injury

We propose the following as appropriate methods and practices for work-related neuromusculoskeletal conditions commonly seen in chiropractic practice. Initial diagnostic procedures include history-taking

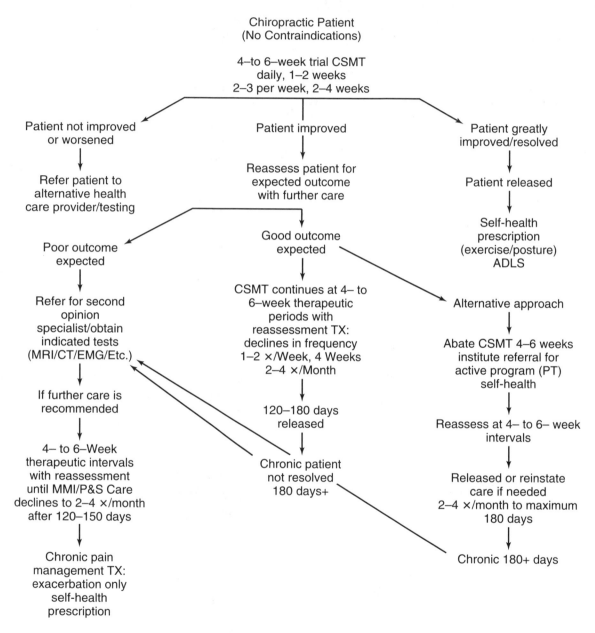

Figure 18-1. Algorithm for chiropractic spinal manipulation for somatic disorders. ADLS, activities of daily living; CSMT, chiropractic spinal manipulation therapy; CT, computed tomography; EMG, electromyography; MMI, maximum medical improvement; MRI, magnetic resonance imaging; P&S, permanent and stationary; PT, physical therapy; TX, treatment. (From Gilkey,[66] with permission.)

and physical examination, routine radiography, and indicated laboratory tests. Follow-up diagnostic and imaging procedures are performed only if indications for further testing exist after the therapeutic trial period. This follow-up testing, some of which requires referral to other health facilities, may include electromyelography (EMG), nerve conduction velocity (NCV), computed tomography (CT) scan, magnetic resonance imaging (MRI), discography, surface and electrode electromyography (EMG), and somato-sensory evoked potential (SSEP), thermography, functional capacity evaluation, and psychological assessment.[42–44]

Chiropractic spinal manipulation[45] (Fig. 18-1) is the foundation of the chiropractic physician's therapeutic approach. Where appropriate, adjunctive therapeutic procedures may include thermal treatments (hot and cold) and mechanically assisted traction or inversion therapy, which may be self-applied in chronic conditions. Other therapeutic options include ultrasound, electrotherapy, electrical muscle stimulation (EMS), interferential, galvanism, needle acupuncture, and nutritional therapy. The optimal therapeutic duration for these procedures is 1 to 3 months.[44,46–48]

Supervised exercise rehabilitation can play a crucial role in recovery from work-related injury or illness. The optimal therapeutic duration is 1 to 3 months as adjunct to other treatments. The patient's active participation in collagenous repair, tissue organization, and strengthening is essential.[40,49–53] Active exercise follows the acute phase of recovery and should continue through subacute to complete recovery. It is recommended that patients continue with exercise on a self-directed basis indefinitely.

The doctor's role is not limited to diagnosis and therapy. When necessary, carefully thought-out work restrictions should be instituted during acute and subacute phases of recovery as an adjunct to other treatments. Permanent restrictions must be judiciously applied. Workstation modification based on ergonomic analysis should also be considered.

The current consensus is that the greatest therapeutic impact is made on spinal conditions within the first 90 to 120 days and certainly by 6 to 9 months postinjury.[45,54] Chronicity, characterized by lack of improvement with time and treatment, can become evident by 4 to 9 months postinjury. Within the worker's compensation system, care offered for chronic somatic pain disorders, including spinal conditions, is frequently denied reimbursement due to alleged lack of appropriateness and cost efficiency. Collaborative efforts between disciplines are the best way to achieve true maximum therapeutic value and benefit.

OCCUPATIONAL CARPAL TUNNEL SYNDROME

History

Signs and symptoms of CTS include numbness, tingling, burning sensations, pain, and weakness in hand, wrist, and/or entire affected upper extremity. Symptoms may affect the cervical spine if the double crush syndrome is present. Work-relatedness of symptoms should be established: onset, provoking, quality, radiation, site, and timing (OPQRST).

Examination

Abnormalities of median nerve distribution in the affected extremity may include sensory and/or motor dysfunction, Phalen sign, Tinel sign, loss of vibratory perception, and isolated atrophy.

Laboratory Tests

Laboratory tests are not usually obtained on the initial visit but may be done on subsequent reassessment visits to rule out comorbid processes.

Radiologic Examination

Radiographs are appropriate if this condition has a traumatic history or suspected arthritic component. Wrist radiographs are not done routinely.

Electrodiagnostic Studies

EMG/NCV and quantitative sensory testing (QST) may be appropriate 6 weeks postonset if no improvement is obtained with initial therapeutic trial. Needle electrode EMG/NCV and QST studies are best facilitated through collaborative efforts with the appropriate specialist.

Therapeutic Procedures

1. Workstation modifications should be the first approach in an effort to remove ergonomic hazards.

2. Work restrictions would include reduced or eliminated repetitive and forceful gripping, repetitive movements, extreme positions, stretching, and contact pressure to the wrist and hand.

3. Cock-up splints may be worn to immobilize affected extremity with optimal duration of 1 to 3 months. Prolonged use is not recommended.

4. Cryotherapy and exercise should be undertaken with optimal duration of 1 to 3 months. In many cases, exercise should be concurrent with work activities.

5. Ultrasound may be applied directly to volar aspect of wrist with optimal duration of 1 to 3 months.

6. Electrotherapy may be used proximal and/or distal with optimal duration of 1 to 3 months.

7. Manual therapy techniques may be used both proximal and distal with optimal duration of 1 to 3 months.

8. Nutritional support of vitamin B_6 may be beneficial, optimal duration of 6 weeks.[6,44]

Patients with nonresponsive CTS should be referred for medical evaluation and care. Collaboration with appropriate medical specialists can be helpful in managing difficult cases of CTS. Because CTS may develop into a permanent disabling condition, it is crucial that the chiropractic physician not permit permanent neurologic decompensation to occur.

OCCUPATIONAL TENDINITIS/TENOSYNOVITIS

History

Signs and symptoms of tendinitis/tenosynovitis include intermittent dull, throbbing, aching pain progressing to sharp qualities. Numbness and weakness may also be reported. Work-relatedness of symptoms should be established: onset, provoking, quality, radiation, site, and timing (OPQRST).

Examination

Abnormalities are usually local. Tenderness to palpation, swelling, erythema, crepitus, and increased heat may be found.

Laboratory Tests

Laboratory tests are not usually obtained on the initial visit but may be done on subsequent reassessment visits to rule out comorbid processes.

Radiologic Examination

Radiology is not routine for tendinitis. Shoulder films may reveal calcific tendinitis or bursitis.

Therapeutic Procedures

1. Appropriate workstation modifications should be the first approach in an effort to remove ergonomic hazards.

2. Appropriate work restrictions can include reduction or elimination of the following:
   Hand and wrist—repetitive forceful gripping
   Elbow—repetitive high force use
   Shoulder—repetitive overhead work
   Achilles—high stress loading.

3. Splints may be worn to immobilize or restrict affected body part with optimal duration of 1 to 3 months. Prolonged use is not recommended.

4. Cryotherapy and exercise should be undertaken with optimal duration of 1 to 3 months. In many cases, exercise should be concurrent with work activities.

5. Ultrasound may be applied directly to the affected area, with an optimal duration of 1 to 3 months.

6. Electrotherapy may be used proximal with optimal duration of 1 to 3 months.

7. Manual therapy techniques may be used proximal with optimal duration of 1 to 3 months.

Patients with nonresponsive tendinitis/tenosynovitis should be referred for medical evaluation and care. Collaboration with appropriate medical specialties can be helpful in managing difficult cases of tendinitis/tenosynovitis.[6,27,44]

THORACIC OUTLET SYNDROME

History

Signs and symptoms of thoracic outlet syndrome may include neck pain, occipital headaches, intermittent arm pain, numbness, paresthesias, fatigue, and weakness. Work-relatedness of symptoms should be established: onset, provoking, quality, radiation, site, and timing (OPQRST).

Examination

Abnormalities are usually regional, affecting the neck and upper extremity. Symptoms and signs may include tenderness of the cervicothoracic musculature to palpation, hand blanching, positive neurovascular compression tests, and possible sensorimotor dysfunction. Postural defects may also be present, such as head carriage far forward beyond the gravity line (craning the neck forward).

Laboratory Tests

Laboratory tests are not usually obtained on the initial visit but may be done on subsequent reassessment visits to rule out comorbid processes.

Radiologic Examination

Radiology is routine for thoracic outlet syndrome. Relevant findings on cervical/thoracic films may include cervical ribs or hypertrophied transverse processes of C7.

Electrodiagnostic Studies

EMG/NCV are used only after a failed therapeutic trial of 6 weeks or more. These tests may be helpful to evaluate the presence of neurologic entrapment.

Therapeutic Procedures

1. Appropriate workstation modifications should be considered to remove ergonomic hazards.
2. Appropriate work restrictions include reduction or elimination of repetitive overhead work.
3. Cryotherapy and exercise should be undertaken with optimal duration of 1 to 3 months. In many cases, exercise should be concurrent with work activities.
4. Ultrasound may be applied directly to cervical/thoracic junction area with optimal duration of 1 to 3 months.
5. Electrotherapy may be used proximal with optimal duration of 1 to 3 months.
6. Traction of the cervical spine may be very helpful with optimal therapeutic duration of 1 to 3 months. Patient may do well with self-employed home traction.
7. Manual therapy techniques may be used locally at the cervical/thoracic junction with optimal duration of 1 to 3 months.

Patients with nonresponsive thoracic outlet syndrome should be referred for medical evaluation and care. Secondary diagnostic tests may include CT scan, MRI, EMG/NCV. Collaboration with appropriate medical specialists can be helpful in managing difficult cases of thoracic outlet syndrome.[6,24,44]

WORKER'S COMPENSATION

Historical Development

Worker's compensation is a system of benefits designed to protect and assist workers suffering adverse health affects as a result of their employment. The first worker's compensation legislation was passed in 1910 in New York but was soon declared unconstitutional. Successful enactment of a worker's compensation law occurred in 1914[55] and by 1948 all American states had enacted worker's compensation laws.[2] Worker's compensation covers medical care, compensation for wage loss, costs for vocational rehabilitation, compensation for permanent disability, and death benefits for heirs.[2,6,7]

Chiropractic care is recognized in all state workers compensation laws in the United States, but many states give employers great latitude in determining which provider will treat the injured worker. Since 1974, U.S. federal employee worker's compensation law has allowed injured employees to be treated by the chiropractor of their choice. Chiropractic coverage follows Medicare language, reimbursing for manual manipulation of the spine for subluxations demonstrated on radiography. Like Medicare, it does not cover adjunctive physical therapy procedures performed in the chiropractic office. However, unlike Medicare, federal workers compensation does mandate reimbursement for radiography, physical examinations, and appropriate laboratory tests.

Chiropractic Cost-effectiveness

Numerous studies have provided cost comparisons between medical and chiropractic services, with virtually all concluding that chiropractic demonstrates greater efficacy and cost-effectiveness. A 1988 Florida study[56] showed the average cost of a case managed by a doctor of chiropractic (DC) was $1,204 compared to similar cases managed by medical doctors (MDs), which averaged $2,213. The average total temporary disability for chiropractic patients was 39 days, compared to 58 for those under medical management. A 1991 Utah study[57] analyzed 3,062 back injury claims for comparison of DC to MD services. DC managed cases had one-tenth the lost time compared to MD managed cases. The average treatment cost per DC case was $526 compared to MD costs of $684. Additional worker's compensation studies from Montana, Wisconsin, Oregon, Iowa, California, and Kansas reiterate similar cost efficiency benefits of chiropractic services[56] (for further details, see Ch. 10).

Defining Accident and Illness

A work-related accident is an instantaneous event—anything else is considered an illness.[58] In determining eligibility for worker's compensation benefits, injuries must fit into 1 of 2 categories: arise out of employment (AOE), or arise in the course of employment (COE).[2,58] COE is the clear and simple work-related accident that is readily apparent to all parties. AOE can be an insidious disease that does not manifest for many years.[58] Examples of illnesses are asbestosis or CTD, in which the disease manifestation occurs long after the exposure. All back injuries are reported as accidents.[2]

Work-related injury cases entail significant paper work. Injuries must be reported to employers within a given statute-mandated time period. In many instances, the statute is 1 year's duration. In most instances, employers require immediate notification of work-related injury or illness. This can be difficult when injury or illness is not apparent to the worker. Disputes can erupt when communications are delayed. Prompt reporting is always a good practice.

Case Management Issues

Care and management of patients have historically been the responsibility of the treating physician. With work-related injuries, however, third-party payers, administrators, employers, and consultants often usurp this decision-making role, particularly in cases that fail to resolve as quickly as expected. Physician management has become more complex in recent years.

Cost has become the prime focus of most state worker's compensation systems, with efforts to reduce costs acting as the driving force behind changes in the way occupational health services are provided and paid. Unfortunately, prevention is not often pursued with the same enthusiasm as other cost containment strategies. Great efforts have been made to design treatment algorithms and standard protocols to guide the treating physician into uniform channels of service delivery, with some state worker's compensation divisions forming multidisciplinary panels of experts to develop treatment guidelines. These guidelines have empowered nonmedical personnel to question treatments deviating from prescribed treatment protocols.

Even without treatment, 80 to 90 percent of back pain cases resolve in 90 to 120 days and treatment guidelines generally provide satisfactory results for this group of patients. The challenge, however, is the remaining 10 to 25 percent, who account for 80 to 90 percent of the worker's compensation treatment expenditures.[32,59] The political and economic imperative of "appropriate care at a reasonable price" is difficult to apply fairly to recalcitrant neuro-musculoskeletal injury or illness syndromes. Managed care, with its cost-sensitive policies that reward providers for undertreating, can compound the problem in these cases. Credentialing and pre-authorization procedures often require adherence to worker's compensation consensus, or proprietary guidelines. Physicians who frequently depart from the guidelines place themselves in jeopardy of losing authorization to render service.

The chiropractic profession's Mercy Guidelines provide a standard by which other guidelines can be measured. While questions about frequency of visits, duration of care, and the number of treatments that will be reimbursed often receive the most attention, deeper issues including patient needs, therapeutic goals, necessity and appropriateness of care, indications and contraindications, safety, and effectiveness are strongly emphasized in the Mercy document.[43,45]

Frequency and duration of care become self evident as a by-product of good practice.

Reporting Requirements

The worker's compensation system places much of the onus for reporting on the occupational health physician. Occupational health care facilities and offices must file timely reports conveying useful, accurate information[7]:

- First report of injury—usually includes injured worker identification, time, date, place, description of accident or illness, diagnosis, treatment plan, and work status
- Employee ability to work—whether the employee is on temporary total disability, temporary partial disability, or able to return to work unrestricted
- Treatment plan—what services are necessary, how frequently the patient will be seen for treatment, and an estimate of the expected duration of care
- Interval status reports—progress reports, to be sent monthly and describe improvement, worsening, need for ongoing care, referral, special testing, expected release date, and ability to work
- Modified work—inform the employer if permanent or temporary changes are needed in the physical demands of the injured worker's job
- Maximum medical improvement—when all available forms of care have been offered and the condition ceases to improve, and 6 to 9 months have passed. When maximum medical improvement is reached, report the symptomatic plateau, and describe the nature and frequency of stationary state[45,46]
- Permanent disability—report persistent or recurrent pain and any permanent loss or restriction of physical activity
- Need for vocational rehabilitation—offer opinion regarding the worker's ability to perform his or her usual and customary pre-injury work and need for retraining in a less physically demanding job
- Release from care—notify the worker's compensation carrier and/or employer when releasing a patient from care

Litigation

A key indicator of workplace safety, health, and morale is the amount of litigation of worker's compensation cases. If more than 10 percent of worker's compensation injury cases are represented by lawyers, there is a problem in that workplace. Litigation in workers compensation occurs within the worker's compensation system itself and not in the civil courts.[60] However, evidence from a worker's compensation proceeding may be admissible in a civil action.[60] Cases of permanent disability and impairment may be litigated. Common issues in question may be:

- Causation—Is the illness or injury work related?
- Apportionment—What percentage of the illness or injury is related to this work situation?
- Benefits—Is the injured worker entitled to any or all of the worker's compensation benefits?
- Does any permanent disability or impairment exist? If so, how much?
- Is the injured worker entitled to vocational rehabilitation benefits?

Litigation generally delays benefit distribution to the injured worker while driving up the cost of its delivery. In recent years efforts have been made to reduce the amount of litigation in the worker's compensation system. One such strategy is the use of the independent medical examiner (IME). Ideally, this is a physician with specialty training in occupational health. Reports follow special formats established by worker's compensation courts or administrators.

IME Reports

Complete IME reports should contain the following[61]:

- History of injury or illness
- Past medical history
- Physical examination findings
- Review of medical records
- Diagnostic impression
- Opinion on causation and apportionment
- Opinion on maximum medical improvement status
- Residual subjective complaints

- Residual objective findings
- Opinion on the worker's ability to return to work
- Residual permanent disability and impairment
- Opinion regarding the need for future chiropractic/medical care
- Discussion of any unusual or conflicting issues, disagreements with other examiners, or special concerns about which the judge should know

WORKER REHABILITATION

Rehabilitation of workers focuses on 2 main areas: physical and vocational. Physical rehabilitation is largely addressed in the treatment paradigm. Physical rehabilitation goals are intended to achieve restoration of optimal strength, stability, and integrity in the injured worker through a planned functional program. Vocational rehabilitation is the successful return to work through a planned program.

In uncomplicated cases physical rehabilitation does not present a challenge—treatment leads to resolution and the patient returns to work. Serious, disabling, and prolonged illness and injury presents a formidable challenge. Physical and vocational rehabilitation may require interdisciplinary collaboration to facilitate return to work.

Strategies must be developed to overcome barriers to successful return to work. Several areas should be addressed[53]:

- Functional work capacity limits
- Musculoskeletal integrity and stability
- Behavior and attitude factors
- Cognitive factors
- Vocational status

Each component must be evaluated, measured, and assessed. This process calls for interdisciplinary referral and communication with the medical physician, occupational therapist, physical therapist, psychologist, counselors, and vocational or case management specialist. The injured worker should be encouraged to cooperate and participate actively in his or her rehabilitation. There should also be an effort to involve the employer liaison and worker's compensation insurance representative. A team approach is most likely to yield optimal results.

Assessing Physical Capabilities and Limitations

The physical capabilities and limitations of workers can be assessed with numerous techniques. Useful methods include the following[6,49,59]:

- Static strength testing (isometric)
- Dynamic strength testing (isotonic and isokinetic)
- Job analysis
- Work simulation testing
- Manual materials handling testing
- Aerobic capacity testing
- Posture tolerance testing
- Anthropometric measures

The assessment of musculoskeletal stability and integrity is measured in part by the above tests. Such tests are indicators of functional capacities but may not reflect the seriousness, nature, or outcome of the pathophysiologic process of the injury or disease. In cases in which the chiropractic occupational health physician is evaluating a patient but is not the treating doctor, it is essential to obtain the opinion of the treating physicians as to the patient's relative risk of injury, re-injury, exacerbation, or regression from such testing or involvement in work activities.

Specific concerns regarding behavioral and attitudinal factors may include the following[59]:

- Abnormal illness behavior, such as delayed recovery, hypochondriasis, hysterical neurosis, functional overlay, functional illness, nonorganic pain, and malingering
- Abnormal treatment behavior, such as frequently changing doctors, frequent disagreements with the treating doctor, self-prescription for care, self-directed use of splints, braces, and medical equipment
- Chronic pain syndrome development postinjury is a complex disorder characterized by physical and mental stress, including disproportionate subjective complaints to objective findings, psycho-

logical findings, lack of motivation, and continuing beyond 6 months

- Psychosocial stressors such as anxiety over possible reinjury, marital problems, or child-related concern at home
- Dependency and addiction to prescription, over-the-counter, or illegal drugs, or alcohol
- Employment dissatisfaction with an underlying desire to change jobs or careers, or punish the boss
- Secondary gain impeding recovery for a monetary settlement for injuries or disabilities

Vocational Status Assessment

Vocational status assessment can be a key indicator of success in physical rehabilitation and vocational rehabilitation programs. Lack of job satisfaction is strongly associated with occupational injury; workers who dislike their jobs are 2.5 times as likely to suffer industrial injuries.[62] Understanding how the worker feels about his past and potential employment is critical. Questions to be answered in this assessment process include the following:

- Is there job satisfaction?
- Have there been negative work appraisals from supervisors?
- Is there work available at the same company?
- What has been the length of disability?
- What type of disability status does the worker have?
- What pay scale will the patient return to?
- Does the worker agree with the job description?
- Have there been changes in the company?
- Is this a new company or career?
- Is the job description compatible with the injured worker's physical capabilities and limitations?
- What is the relative risk of re-injury or new injury with the proposed new job?
- Are there health insurance benefits on the new job, and do they cover the injured worker's residual needs from past injuries?

Worker's compensation systems vary from state to state with respect to vocational rehabilitation services. Some states provide vocational rehabilitation benefits for injured workers who are unable to return to their usual jobs. Costs may be capped at levels that significantly limit resource use. Some states have entirely eliminated the vocational rehabilitation benefit.

Return to Work

Early return to work is highly desirable. As many as 80 to 90 percent of injured workers return to their employment within the first month after injury.[13] Protracted total temporary disability drastically reduces the likelihood of ever returning to work. Only 50 percent of those remaining out of work for 6 months ever return. Of injured workers remaining out of work for more than 1 year, only 25 percent eventually return to work. The likelihood of return for workers off the job more than 2 years is negligible.[63]

Total temporary disability beyond 6 weeks is critical, as workers begin to decondition both physically and emotionally. Negative reinforcers associated with prolonged total temporary disability include loss of self-esteem, tax-free disability income, attention and sympathy from family and friends, relief from responsibilities, and revenge against the company.[64]

To authorize return to work, the occupational health physician should evaluate the following[59,63]:

- Are impairments stable?
- Are there potentially exacerbating work activities required?
- Is the injury/illness condition progressive?
- Is the condition characterized by remission and exacerbation of symptoms likely to cause additional total temporary disability?
- Does the impairment cause a direct threat of new injury to the worker or their coworkers?

Factors Encouraging Return to Work

Aronoff and colleagues studied the characteristics of injured worker's compensation patients who returned to work in spite of their pain. Based on case analyses done retrospectively 5 years postinjury, correlation was found with the following[63]:

- Early intervention and physical rehabilitation
- Positive hospital course of care
- High motivation
- Mastery of pain
- Stress-reduction strategies
- Positive work history
- Employment-centered purpose, identity, and satisfaction
- High incentive to return to work
- No psychopathology
- No medication dependency
- No secondary gain factors
- No litigation factors

Physical Improvement Strategies

Preparing a patient for return to work may include physical improvement strategies such as work hardening and back school.[47,50–53] The goal of increasing tolerance to work activities is based on the specific adaptation to the imposed demand (SAID) principle. This process involves 1 to 2 hr/day of physical rehabilitation including aerobic, flexibility, and strength training.[53] Fitness evaluation techniques may also be used in conjunction with work hardening.

Back school protocols, which offer education and training in proper posture, movement, strength assessment, and work safety hygiene, can enhance the injured's ability to accommodate actual employment. Protocols function to assess worker capability and increase tolerance to work activities. Goals are accomplished through work simulation in conjunction with other worker's compensation services.

DIPLOMATE PROGRAM IN OCCUPATIONAL HEALTH

Postgraduate education in occupational health trains chiropractors as consultants and advocates to industry with the ultimate goal of injury and illness prevention. Specific educational goals are intended to develop skills and knowledge for interdisciplinary problem solving and language development, team interaction, and application of illness and injury prevention in the workplace.

The occupational health diplomate program is taught as a series of postgraduate seminars at Council on Chiropractic Education (CCE) accredited chiropractic colleges. The curriculum is divided into 3 major phases of 100 hours each, with 24 learning modules. Upon completion of various topic modules, students take examinations and must achieve a minimum grade requirement. At the completion of all 3 phases of study, they become eligible for the American Chiropractic Board of Occupational Health diplomate examination.

Topics covered in the occupational health diplomate program include the following[65]:

- The field of occupational health
- Preplacement/biomechanical stress index
- Biomechanics/ergonomics
- Injury prevention
- Sitting in the workplace
- Physical rehabilitation
- Stress management
- Cumulative trauma disorders
- Chemical and environmental hazards
- Chronic pain
- Narrative report writing
- Occupational multidiscipline teams
- Legal considerations in occupational health
- Independent medical examiner's role
- Communications
- Safety engineering

The diplomate program also requires a class project of 1 academic year. Projects to date have focused on ergonomic problem solving of neuromusculoskeletal-related injury and illness in a specific industry setting.

Terminology

active analysis
carpal tunnel syndrome
chronic pain syndrome
cumulative trauma disorder (CTD)
ergonomics

hypochondriasis
malingering
maximum medical improvement
NIOSH
OSHA
passive analysis
physical rehabilitation
thoracic outlet syndrome
video display terminal worker
vocational rehabilitation
worker's compensation

Review Questions

1. What is the main reason that companies sometimes decide not to engineer out workplace hazards?

2. Name four duties of the occupational health physician.

3. What are the main risk factors associated with lower back pain?

4. What are the main risk factors associated with cumulative trauma disorders?

5. What is the most frequently cited reason for filing worker's compensation claims?

6. What explains the recent dramatic rise in incidence of CTD claims?

7. What is the optimal duration for the use of manual procedures in carpal tunnel syndrome and thoracic outlet syndrome?

8. True or false? In all states in the United States, workers injured on the job can choose to be treated by a chiropractor, with the assurance that the bill will be paid by worker's compensation insurance.

9. What are several methods of assessing physical capabilities and limitations?

10. What are several behavioral and attitudinal factors that may influence recovery from an occupational injury?

Concept Questions

1. How can specific training in occupational health expand the nature of a chiropractor's practice?

2. How can a chiropractor determine whether a patient is malingering?

References

1. Gilkey DP, Williams HA: The comprehensive environmental, health, and safety program: a new trend in industry. J Am Chiro Assoc 31:22, 1994

2. Tiffin J, McCormick EJ: Industrial Psychology. Prentice-Hall, Englewood Cliffs, NJ, 1965

3. Weeks JL, Levey BS, Wagner GR (eds): Preventing Occupational Disease and Injury. American Public Health Association, Washington, DC, 1991

4. LaDou J (ed): Occupational Health and Safety. 2nd Ed. National Safety Council, Chicago, 1994

5. Plog BA (ed): Fundamentals of Industrial Hygiene. 3rd Ed. National Safety Council, Chicago, 1988

6. Herington TN, Morse LH (ed): Occupational Injuries Evaluation, Management, and Prevention. CV Mosby, St. Louis, 1995

7. Sweere JJ: Role of the chiropractic physician in occupational health. p. 21. In Sweere JJ (ed): Chiropractic Family Practice—A Clinical Manual. Aspen, Gaithersburg, MD, 1994

8. Lammert G: Maine DC works with company and union to reduce injuries. J Am Chiro Assoc 8:41, 1994

9. Pheasant S: Ergonomics, Work and Health. Aspen, Gaithersburg, MD, 1991

10. Chaffin DB, Andersson GB: Occupational Biomechanics. 2nd Ed. John Wiley & Sons, New York, 1991

11. Selan J: The Advanced Ergonomics Manual. Advanced Ergonomics, Dallas, 1994

12. International Business Machines Corporation: Ergonomics Handbook. IBM, Purchase, NY, 1987

13. Kelsey JL, Golden AL: Occupational and workplace factors associated with low back pain. p. 9. In Deyo RA (ed): Occupational Back Pain, Spine: State of the Art Reviews. Vol. 2. Hanley and Belfus, Philadelphia, 1987

14. Carson R: Key ergonomics tips. Occup Hazards 8:43, 1994

15. Gilkey DP, Williams HA: Ergonomics and CTDs: the problems, causes, enforcement and solutions. J Am Chiro Assoc 31:27, 1994

16. Chesler L: Repetitive motion injury and cumulative trauma disorder: can the wave of products liability litigation be averted? Comput Lawyer 9:13, 1992

17. Keyserling WM, Armstrong TJ, Punnett L: Ergonomic job analysis: a structured approach for identifying risk factors associated with overexertion injuries and disorders. Appl Occup Environ Hyg 6:353, 1991

18. Kroemer KH: Avoiding cumulative trauma disorders in shops and offices. Am Ind Hyg Assoc J 53:596, 1992

19. Sandler HM: Are we ready to regulate cumulative trauma disorders? Occup Hazards 6:51, 1993

20. Hagberg M, Silverstein B, Wells R et al: Work Related Musculoskeletal Disorders (WMSDs): A Reference Book for Prevention. Taylor & Francis, Bristol, UK, 1995

21. Gilkey DP, Williams HA: Injury prevention in the workplace: a closer look at OSHA's proposed ergonomic standard. Occup Health Briefs 2:1, 1995

22. LaDou J: Cumulative injury in workers' compensation. p. 611. In Larsen RL, Felton GS (eds) Occupational Medicine: State of the Art Reviews. Vol. 3. Hanley and Belfus, Philadelphia, 1988

23. Occupational Safety and Health Administration: Draft of proposed regulatory text. (Internet, ErgoWeb, http://www.tucker.mech.utah.edu), 1995

24. American National Standards Institute: Z365—Control of Work Related Cumulative Trauma Disorders. ANSI, New York, 1994

25. Sweere JJ: Chiropractic in industry. Todays Chiro 5:10, 1988

26. Cassidy DJ, Wedge JH: The epidemiology and natural history of low back pain and spinal degeneration. p. 3. In Kirkaldy-Willis WH (ed): Managing Low Back Pain. 2nd Ed. Churchill Livingston, New York, 1988

27. Edril M, Dickerson OB, Glackin E: Cumulative trauma disorders of the upper extremity. p. 48. In Zenz C (ed): Occupational Medicine. 3rd Ed. CV Mosby, St. Louis, 1994

28. Bureau of National Affairs: Ergonomics: back pain identified as major problem for U.S. workers in NIOSH study of 1988 data. Occup Saf Health Rep 22:2068, 1993

29. Kahlil TM, Abel-Moty EM, Rosomoff RS et al: Ergonomics in Back Pain. Van Nostrand Reinhold, New York, 1993

30. Bureau of National Affairs: Statistics: back injuries blamed for half of claims filed by health care workers, cab drivers. Occup Saf Health Rep 23:484, 1993

31. National Safety Council: Accident Facts. 1994 Ed. NSC, Itasca, IL, 1994

32. Snook SS: The costs of back pain in industry. p. 1. In Deyo RA (ed): Occupational Back Pain, Spine: State of the Art Reviews. Vol. 5. Hanley and Belfus, Philadelphia, 1991

33. Sullivan K: Apple split keyboard gets tepid reaction. San Francisco Examiner, San Francisco, January 20, 1993

34. Rigdon JE: How a plant handles occupational hazards with common sense. The Wall Street Journal, September 28, 1992

35. Bureau of National Affairs: Ergonomics: repeated trauma claims of upper extremities most prevalent in meatpacking jobs, study says. Occup Saf Health Rep 24:846, 1994

36. LaBar G: Ergonomics can't wait any longer. Occup Hazards 4:33, 1994

37. Bureau of National Affairs: Ergonomics: 770 percent increase. Occup Saf Health Rep 24:1794, 1995

38. Bureau of National Affairs: Ergonomics: focus on cumulative trauma disorders said to cause "misdirection of resources." Occup Saf Health Rep 24:1181, 1994

39. White L: Back school. p. 325. In White L (ed): Back School, Spine: State of the Art Reviews. Vol. 5. Hanley and Belfus, Philadelphia, 1991

40. Oborne DJ: Ergonomics at Work. 2nd Ed. John Wiley & Sons, New York, 1992

41. U.S. Department of Health and Human Services, Public Health Services: Revised NIOSH Lifting Equation. Centers of Disease Control–National Institute of Occupational Safety and Health, Cincinnati, 1994

42. Haldeman S, Chapman-Smith D, Peterson D (ed): Guidelines for Chiropractic Quality Assurance and Practice Parameters. Aspen, Gaithersburg, MD, 1993

43. Vear HJ (ed): Chiropractic Standards of Practice and Quality of Care. Aspen, Gaithersburg, MD, 1992

44. Division of Workers' Compensation: Medical Treatment Guidelines. Department of Labor and Employment, Denver, 1995

45. Gilkey DP: Issues concerning chiropractic standards of practice. p. 22. In Sweere JJ (ed): Chiropractic Family Practice—A Clinical Manual, suppl. Aspen, Gaithersburg, MD, 1993

46. Schafer RC (ed): Basic Chiropractic Procedural Manual. 4th Ed. American Chiropractic Association, Arlington, VA, 1984

47. Mayer T, Politin P: Spinal rehabilitation. p. 533. In Haldeman S (ed): Principles and Practice of Chiropractic. 2nd Ed. Appleton & Lange, Norwalk, CT, 1992

48. North American Spine Society: Common diagnostic and therapeutic procedures of the lumbosacral spine. Spine 16:1161, 1991

49. Tramposh AK: The functional capacity evaluation: measuring the maximal work abilities. p. 437. In White L (ed): Back School, Spine: State of the Art Reviews. Vol. 5. Hanley and Belfus, Philadelphia, 1991

50. Mooney V: Preface. p. xiii. In White L (ed): Back School, Spine: State of the Art Reviews. Vol. 5. Hanley and Belfus, Philadelphia, 1991

51. Martin L: Back basics: general information for back school participants. p. 333. In White L (ed): Back School, Spine: State of the Art Reviews. Vol. 5. Hanley and Belfus, Philadelphia, 1991

52. Robinson R: The new back school prescription: stabilization training. Part I. p. 341. In White L (ed): Back School, Spine: State of the Art Reviews. Vol. 5. Hanley and Belfus, Philadelphia, 1991

53. Bronston LJ, Gehri DJ: A return to work protocol for mechanical low back pain. p. 214. In Sweere JJ (ed): Chiropractic Family Practice—A Clinical Manual, suppl. Aspen, Gaithersburg, MD, 1993

54. Gilkey DP: Chiropractic care: how much is enough? J Am Chiro Assoc 29:29, 1992

55. National Safety Council: Accident Prevention Manual for Business and Industry. 10th Ed. NSC, Itasca, IL, 1992

56. American Chiropractic Association: How to Help Your Employees and Your Company With Chiropractic. American Chiropractic Association, Arlington, VA, 1995

57. Jarvis KB, Phillips RB, Morris JD: Cost per case comparison of back injury claims of chiropractic versus medical management for conditions with identical diagnostic codes. J Occup Med 8:847, 1991

58. Gilkey DP, Williams HA: Occupational illness or injury. Int Acad Chiro Occup Health Consult Newsl 7:4, 1994

59. Scheer SJ, Wickstrom RJ: Vocational capacity with low back pain impairment. p. 19. In Scheer SJ (ed): Medical Perspective in Vocational Assessment of Injured Workers. Aspen, Gaithersburg, MD, 1991

60. Railton WS: OSHA Compliance Handbook. Government Institutes, Rockville, MD, 1992

61. Division of Industrial Accidents: Guidelines for Medical Examination and Report. Division of Workers' Compensation, State of California, San Francisco, 1985

62. Bureau of National Affairs: Hand surgeon correlates disability with negative job satisfaction, anger. Occup Saf Health Rep 24:398, 1994

63. Aronoff GM, McAlary PW, Witkower A et al: Pain treatment programs: do they return workers to the workplace? p. 123. In Deyo RA (ed): Occupational Back Pain, Spine: State of the Art Reviews. Vol. 2. Hanley and Belfus, Philadelphia, 1987

64. Imbus HI: Clinical aspects of occupational medicine. p. 3. In Zenz C (ed): Occupational Medicine. 3rd Ed. CV Mosby, St. Louis, 1994

65. American Chiropractic Board of Occupational Health: American Chiropractic Board of Occupational Health Curriculum Learning Objectives and Content Guidelines. American Chiropractic Association, Washington, DC, 1996

66. Gilkey DP: Issues concerning chiropractic standards of practice. p. 11. In Sweere JJ (ed): Chiropractic Family Practice—A Clinical Manual, suppl. Aspen, Gaithersburg, MD, 1993

19

Chiropractic in Hospitals and Integrated Settings

Robert S. Francis
Jon Buriak
C. Jacob Ladenheim

While the vast majority of chiropractic health care is delivered in freestanding private practices, a small but growing number of DCs work in multidisciplinary settings, including hospitals. According to current estimates by the American Chiropractic Association's (ACA's) Hospital Relations Committee, approximately 200 hospitals in the United States now offer chiropractic services. With the removal of American Medical Association (AMA) restrictions on medical physicians cooperating with chiropractors, MD-DC collaboration in the form of joint practices has also begun. Complex professional, legal, and interpersonal issues must be considered before entering into such arrangements. The rewards of offering integrated health care services to patients make such efforts worthwhile.

The movement toward multidisciplinary health care is part of several broader trends. Old biases against chiropractors are breaking down at the same time that attitudinal shifts toward team management and respect for diversity are pervading the society at large. The public is increasingly supportive of alternative forms of treatment, and more patients are seeking a partnership model to replace older authoritarian forms of the doctor–patient relationship. The traditional health care delivery model is undergoing changes of significant proportions.

INTERDISCIPLINARY COOPERATION

Chiropractic has traditionally been separate, distinct, and autonomous from the orthodox health care delivery system. This arrangement developed partly as a result of its alternative, non-allopathic model, and partly due to a bias in conventional medicine against non-allopathic practitioners.[1] The wall of separation stood largely unscathed until the late 1960s, when the chiropractic profession began a historic shift toward an explicitly scientific approach, gradually de-emphasizing its traditional philosophy-based practice and teaching models. Scientific clinical investigation of chiropractic procedures and theories provided the impetus for further research, which in turn led to increased interaction between the chiropractic and allopathic communities.

As the chiropractic profession sought greater inclusion in the mainstream health care system, its academic and clinical wings sought similar relations with the scientific community at large. As the research community brought forth evidence supporting chiropractic efficacy, a slow but steady increase in interaction between the allopathic and chiropractic communities developed.

Collaborative academic projects between a few chiropractic colleges and medical schools, aided significantly by the clinical curiosity of individual medical school faculty, began during the 1980s. In this era, gradually increasing numbers of chiropractic and allopathic private practitioners sharing the same patient populations developed cooperative relationships, exchanging records and reports, and in some cases referring patients to one another. Chiropractors have referred patients to medical physicians since the profession's beginnings. Increased medical referral to chiropractors is a new development.

Eventually, relations beyond mere referral began. Chiropractors needing access to advanced diagnostic procedures such as magnetic resonance imaging (MRI), computed tomography (CT), bone scans, and laboratory studies reached out to medical doctors specializing in these procedures. The need for consultation with other specialties created further interaction. Business partnerships between medical and chiropractic physicians developed as a natural consequence of this deepened interaction, which further encouraged clinical and academic communication and sharing.

Multidisciplinary professional associations on the local, state, and national levels have arisen since the mid-1980s, bringing together doctors sharing similar professional interests. Organizations such as the American Back Society and the American Association for Pain Management joined practitioners of medicine, chiropractic, osteopathy, psychology, physical medicine, and other disciplines under one common professional umbrella. Such linkages mark a significant shift in which previously isolated disciplines, inside and outside orthodox health care, move toward an integrated multidisciplinary model not only in new professional associations but in the delivery of health care services.

Training Models

Medical and chiropractic training evolved separately, with little interaction. This is changing. For example, since the mid-1980s, at Texas Chiropractic College, chiropractic interns have participated in rotations in medical facilities and private services during their final year of training. This began as an elective and is now a requirement for graduation. Services available to interns include orthopedics, family practice, radiology, rheumatology, neurology, neurosurgery, and physical medicine. Interns have the opportunity to experience the medical community at work in both didactic and clinical settings. From these interactions, professional referrals and working relationships naturally develop, along with the mutual respect and understanding necessary to sustain the dynamics of a multidisciplinary facility.

Chiropractic Role in Integrated Settings

Most opportunities for chiropractors to practice in integrated settings currently involve family practice, orthopedic, and pain management groups. Other multidisciplinary groups include acupuncturists, naturopaths, massage therapists, psychologists, and practitioners of mind–body medicine and other mental health disciplines. The focus of most integrated settings involving chiropractors is the musculoskeletal management of spinal and soft tissue conditions. Since such cases are commonly treated by family practitioners, orthopedists, and physical medicine specialists, these are the ideal professionals with which to develop integrated practices and facilities.

Chiropractors with hospital privileges who use procedures requiring hospital facilities, such as manipulation under anesthesia (MUA), have a ready-made environment in which to develop the interprofessional relationships necessary to initiate an integrated practice. MUA patients must be admitted to a hospital or ambulatory surgical center (ASC), a process that requires a medical or osteopathic physician as co-admitter, and thus directly involves the chiropractor with a full-scope physician in co-managing these patients. Such interaction forms the basis for developing trusting professional relationships where the medical co-admitter has an opportunity to observe and appreciate the clinical

COLORADO CARE CLINIC, P.C., BOULDER, COLORADO

Type of practice: Family practice, physical medicine, chiropractic, herbal medicine

Staff: Osteopathic physician, chiropractic physician, acupuncturist, nutritionist

Ownership: Osteopathic physician

Decision making: All administrative and management decisions made by the medical director, an osteopathic physician; effort toward clinical consensus regarding patient care maintained.

Dr. Miller [the osteopathic physician] and I have a synergy that transcends the politics of the chiropractic and medical communities. The patient's best interest is foremost in the decision making process. We have worked together referring patients to each other for quite a while and now enjoy treating and co-managing our patient population in the same facility. We have achieved a truly integrated health care program for our patients.

Mark Testa, DC

expertise, diagnostic ability, and training of the chiropractor. Multidisciplinary settings require that each specialist understand the clinical approach and expertise of his or her other colleagues. Experiencing another doctor's case management in a clinical setting is the ideal avenue for this.

Overcoming Challenges

Challenges faced by participants in multi-service facilities include quality assurance, risk management, legal issues, and the politics of clinical hierarchy. When physicians with a limited scope of practice and expertise join with those enjoying an unlimited scope and greater or different clinical training, a hierarchy may be established by default. This can lead to professional territorialism. Since certain clinical decisions may be deferred to the medical director of the facility, it is essential that the circum-

stances under which this is to occur be understood in advance by all involved parties. Assumptions that are not fully voiced and understood should not be made. The psychodynamics that come into play when chiropractic and medical physicians work together must not be underestimated. The degree to which the patient is truly co-managed depends upon mutual respect and understanding that grows out of the opportunity to observe and work with members of other professions.

SUMMIT INJURY AND WELLNESS CENTER, OAKLAND, CALIFORNIA

Type of practice: Chiropractic, medicine, physical injury and rehabilitation, homeopathy, acupuncture, and nutrition

Staff: Chiropractic physician, medical physician, and exercise physiologist practicing in two clinics

Ownership: Chiropractic physician

Decision making: Consensus process, but with approval of chiropractic gatekeeper

We have been able to provide the best of both medicine and chiropractic to our patients through a winning combination of concern for the patient's best interest and what is most clinically beneficial and cost effective.

Mark Miller, DC

GUIDELINES FOR COLLABORATION

Recognizing that chiropractors are increasingly involved in multidisciplinary case management, the Mercy Guidelines[2] offer suggestions to facilitate collaborative care:

1. Primary health care providers should supply sufficient information to enable the patient to make an informed decision regarding choices in treatment/care and of providers. Chiropractic practi-

tioners should be familiar with medical procedures and terminology as needed, so as to effectively understand and relate medical care delivered to or recommended to the patient.

2. Questions about care decisions made or recommendations made by another provider should be addressed directly to that provider in a constructive manner. Relying on the patient to be an effective messenger of critical information is inappropriate.

3. In a collaborative or cooperative care setting, every effort should be made to develop and present to the patient a consensus among all participating practitioners on the recommended course of care.

4. Practitioners should seek access to other health care facilities and institutions as necessary to meet the needs of their patients. This may include authority to admit or co-admit the patient into the appropriate clinical setting or hospital.

5. In the process of concurrent care, each professional party should be aware of the care decisions made by other participants, and fully coordinate activities and information for the patient's benefit.

The Business of Integrated Practice

With new approaches to pain management, DCs and MDs are increasingly working in concert managing the same patient population. Practices offering multidisciplinary services facilitate the treatment of common patients, combining essential care components of separate disciplines.

This arrangement benefits both patient and physician, offering the patient convenience and access to physician consults in a timely manner. This is the foundation of the infrastructure found in physician group practices and hospital-based practices. Access to other specialties allows for complete management of the patient in one setting and relieves the patient of the burden of separately seeking out the various practitioners needed.

Sharing expenses can also make good business sense. The advantages of shared overhead can allow a group of doctors to rent a space that is larger, better located, and better equipped than a single practitioner could manage alone. The sheer enormity of the task of obtaining and efficiently transferring information between offices weighs in favor of geographically consolidating the various disciplines. The beleaguered patient, shuttled from doctor to diagnostic facility to specialist and back again, is appreciative of any alliance designed to streamline this process.

A variety of professional multidisciplinary entities have been developed to allow DCs and MDs to co-manage the same patient population. These range from sharing a single office space to more complex legal and corporate arrangements that allow physicians to share the revenue from a jointly owned health care facility.

Ambulatory Surgical Centers

Opportunities for chiropractors performing MUAs can be among the easiest to establish, especially if the MUAs are performed at an ambulatory surgical center, which is the case for the vast majority of MUAs. These facilities are excellent environments for offering multiple services in an integrated setting. Even the smallest ASC is likely to have additional space where an initial pilot project may be undertaken to determine the efficacy of establishing a larger multidisciplinary practice.

Some integrated practices include anesthesiologists and chiropractors practicing together in an ASC where not only MUAs, but epidural steroid injections, facet blocks, sympathetic blocks, and other injection and pain management techniques, are performed in conjunction with spinal and extremity manipulation. Patients with both acute and chronic pain syndromes can be managed with a simultaneous approach utilizing these medical procedures in conjunction with chiropractic soft tissue and osseous techniques. This arrangement affords the chiropractor an opportunity to become integrated into a broader avenue of the medical community. Patients seen for pain management in this setting include not only those who self-refer, but also those referred by their medical physicians, most frequently orthopedists and family practitioners. This allows the chiropractor, as a member of the pain management team, to interact with these physicians as a peer and specialist in pain management and manual medicine. Furthermore, the DC's role need not be limited to pain management. Chiropractors with broader skills in nutrition, lifestyle management, and other areas can apply these for the patient's benefit when appropriate.

In the experience of one of us (R.S.F.), as a consultant establishing chiropractic services in ASCs and hospitals, most chiropractors who have been fully accepted into integrated facilities began with staff privileges either in a hospital or ASC. Through association with the hospital and the medical staff essential relationships are established that naturally lead to referrals and co-management of patients. This peer acceptance into the medical community fosters the growth of these relationships, eliminates bias, affords an opportunity to appreciate the expertise of those with different clinical training, and cultivates a milieu conducive to establishing business opportunities in integrated health care delivery.

VAX-D MEDICAL GROUP

Type of Practice: Multidisciplinary spine specialty clinic

Staff: General surgeon, chiropractor, anesthesiologist, internist, speech pathologist, and affiliated medical staff

Ownership: Equal partnership between chiropractor and medical physician

Decision making: MD gatekeeper and medical director triages patients to appropriate health care provider

Our clinic provides the only Vax-D (vertebral axial decompression) equipment in Arizona. Our holistic approach specializes in the rehabilitation of disc-related conditions of the neck and low back. Our protocol allows for initial chiropractic management and referral for medical management when appropriate.

Thomas Blankebaker, DC

If one accepts that collaborative care is the delivery system which makes the best economic sense for providers, meets cost containment requirements of payors, and yields the most efficient and psychologically satisfying care for the patient, additional questions soon arise. Crucial among these are: Which provider services should be included, and what is the best way to combine them? Team members must be identified and all clinical logistics must be agreed upon, including basic treatment guidelines, triage, and routing. Once these initial hurdles are cleared, the breadth of possibilities is enormous.

Independent Practices in a Common Facility

The informal, patient-friendly combining of independent practices into common facilities is the simplest and accordingly least expensive option. Regardless of which doctor(s) or corporate entity owns the physical plant, the convenience of sharing common space is significant. When given the choice between visiting an imaging facility across town or one in the same building, most patients will do what is fastest and easiest. When minimized travel is coupled with a warm assurance that arrangements will be made for the patient, compliance increases.

LEGAL CONSIDERATIONS

If the goal is to increase patient flow across practice boundaries by making services more attractive through the convenience or ease of scheduling that a multidisciplinary practice offers, no laws or regulations should threaten this arrangement. More complex situations arise, however, when doctors wish to pool their risk (investment, capital, patient bases) by sharing in practice income. Most states have some form of fee-splitting prohibition.

Statutes regulating health care providers and health care facilities vary greatly from state to state, a situation that has spawned a variety of business arrangements. Because of certain state-mandated restrictions on referral of patients, ownership of health care facilities, billing procedures, employment regulations regarding physicians, and many other rules and regulations, different states may

LAWNDALE MEDICAL CLINIC, HOUSTON, TEXAS

Type of practice: Family practice, including chiropractic, pediatrics, and physical medicine

Staff: Five medical physicians, 1 chiropractic physician, multiple affiliated staff

Ownership: Medical physician

Decision making: All administrative and patient management decisions made with approval of medical director; significant autonomy accorded to all doctors

I have always been supported by the medical doctors in this clinic regarding my patient care recommendations. It is refreshing to be able to totally manage my patient population and have the support of the five medical doctors in this facility. We have been able to forge a bond that serves the best interest of the patients.

Terry Moore, DC

require different types of legal entities to conduct business as a multispecialty health care facility. Federal guidelines must also be considered.

Problems and Risks
Self-referral

It is not surprising that practitioners order or perform more tests, procedures, and treatments when they expect to reap personal financial benefit from doing so. Controversy has arisen over referrals in which the referring doctor has an ownership interest in an ancillary facility to which he or she makes referrals.

In 1989 the first of a series of amendments to the Medicare law prohibited doctors from referring Medicare patients to clinical laboratories with which the doctor had a financial relationship. Beginning in 1995, the self-referral prohibition was applied to various health services covered by Medicare or Medicaid, including radiography, physical therapy services, MRI, CT, ultrasound, durable

medical equipment, and inpatient and outpatient hospital services. It is now unlawful for a doctor with a financial relationship with a provider of any of those services to refer a patient to such a provider or to bill for such services if performed pursuant to a referral.

Financial relationship is defined to include ownership or investment interest by the physician or "an immediate family member." It applies to any compensation arrangement that involves remuneration directly or indirectly, overtly or covertly, in cash or in kind.

Because a growing number of states have enacted their own anti-referral laws, generalizations found in written materials and educational programs often overlook regulatory and statutory provisions peculiar to the state in which the practice is operating. Furthermore, there are various exceptions under which referrals are permitted in specified, limited circumstances. These exceptions generally reflect a grudging recognition that some referrals are actually inspired by legitimate patient care concerns rather than economic benefit for the doctor. The exceptions are formulated, however, to render the economic impact of entering into such arrangements less desirable. Exceptions include restrictions such as having at least a 1-year term on rentals or leases, with compensation in accord with fair market value and what is deemed commercially reasonable.

Among the types of exceptions are the following:

- Group practice referrals for physicians' services if rendered by or under the personal supervision of another doctor in the same group
- Services provided by an entity in a rural area to residents of that area
- Rental or lease of office space or equipment (written, 1 year)
- Bona fide employment relationships
- Personal service arrangement
- Physician incentive plan

Penalties for violation of these rules go far beyond non-payment. They include:

1. Refunds for bills already paid

2. Civil money penalty of up to $15,000 for each service
3. Civil money penalty of up to $100,000 for each "circumvention scheme" whereby referrals are made if the physician "knows or should know" that a principal purpose is to secure referrals
4. Civil money penalty of up to $10,000 per day for failing to submit the proper reports.

Before attempting to scale this slippery slope, state laws must also be carefully considered and analyzed. New York, for example, adds a disclosure requirement. Doctors must reveal to patients, on a form specified by regulations, any financial relationship with facilities to whom they refer, even when such referrals are not prohibited. In addition to the disclosure of the financial relationship doctors must also advise of alternative sources of the same items or services.[3]

Fee Splitting

Statutory fee splitting prohibitions are common throughout the country and portend additional quicksand for joint venturers. Florida, for example, prohibits: "Paying or receiving any commission, bonus, kickback, or rebate, or engaging in any split fee arrangement in any form whatsoever with a physician, organization, agency, or person, either directly or indirectly, for patients referred to providers of health goods and services."[4]

If given their ordinary meaning, these words would prohibit most forms of joint practice. A recent court of appeals decision interpreting that statute illustrates the hazards. A Florida medical physician sold his practice to Integrated Home Health Care (IHHC). Although he acquired no ownership interest in IHHC as part of the sales agreement, IHHC hired the doctor to provide medical services for those patients it had acquired from him. He maintained exclusive control over the medical diagnosis and treatment for which he was compensated by flat salary. Patients were advised of the new arrangement. All services he rendered after the sale were for patients of IHHC and all fees were paid to it.

To that point the arrangement is straightforward enough. The problem arose over the plan for subsequent years. The doctor professed a desire to be relieved of business management responsibilities but to retain economic incentives. Toward that end, he and IHHC agreed in principle to a salary and bonus arrangement tied to the doctor's production. His base salary each subsequent year was to be equal to 35 percent of the prior year's practice revenues from services he personally performed, or that were performed under his direct supervision. He was also to receive a year-end bonus equal to 40 percent of the amount by which practice revenues exceeded a preset annual target.

Uncertain of the propriety of such an arrangement, the doctor sought a Board of Medicine declaratory statement on whether such an agreement would constitute a fee-splitting arrangement in violation of the statute. The Board issued an opinion under the auspices of the Agency for Health Care Administration concluding that "a salary based on a percentage of the previous year's revenues and year-end bonus based on current year revenues would each be in violation of the anti fee splitting statute."

Florida law allows an appeal from such an agency final order. Pursuing that review, the doctor argued that since all services which formed the basis for his compensation were going to be performed in house by IHHC there was no referral involved and the statute therefore did not apply. The court, however, agreed with the Board of Medicine that this interpretation was too narrow. Instead, the Board and the court decreed that salary and bonus could only be based on fees generated by services rendered personally by the doctor or by physician's assistants or nurse practitioners under his direct supervision. Since the proposed agreement tied his compensation to "total revenues generated" by him for IHHC, other income generating possibilities existed. For example, salary and bonus based on ancillary services ordered by the doctor and billed by IHHC constitute prohibited fee splitting. The doctor's protestations that the declaratory statement exceeded the question raised illustrates the hazard in asking for clarification from regulators ... sometimes you receive more guidance than you expect or desire.

Anti-Kickback Provisions

The term *kickback* strongly connotes bribery, corruption, and organized crime. However, running afoul of such prohibitions may be accomplished through a surprising number of seemingly innocent activities. Cost containment and fraud and abuse avoidance efforts have spawned statutory and regulatory efforts which make honest as well as dishonest doctors vulnerable.

The Medicare act includes an anti-kickback provision that prohibits offering, paying, soliciting, or receiving of any form of direct remuneration intended to induce referrals. Violation is a felony punishable by a fine of up to $25,000 and 5 years in jail. The onerous penalties are all the more intimidating in view of decisions holding that the government need only show that "one purpose" of such a payment is to induce referrals. It need not even be a substantial or primary purpose.[5]

However, a recent decision of the Ninth Circuit Court of Appeals will make criminal enforcement of this law much more difficult. That court held since a conviction requires that the defendant's act be done "knowingly and willfully," to be convicted a defendant must know that the anti-kickback statute prohibits the conduct and that he or she engaged in the prohibited conduct with the specific intent to disobey the statute.[6] This creates a very high burden of proof for prosecutors. Nonetheless, this impediment to successful criminal prosecution is no guarantee that regulatory zeal will ease. It may ironically cause more vigorous prosecution of civil charges which require a far less demanding burden of proof than the "beyond a reasonable doubt" standard required in criminal cases.

Business Structure

Professional corporation acts in many states allow only those licensed to render the services being offered by a professional corporation to hold stock in that entity. Under such a statute, a chiropractor and a podiatrist, for example, could not form a joint venture by issuing themselves shares in a new professional corporation.

Limited liability corporation acts in many states, however, afford broader allowable options for nonclinical support services. These states permit separately licensed professionals to cooperatively acquire real estate, equipment, and provide administrative services such as billing and management to a group of professionals sharing space.

False Claims Act

A law called the False Claims Act sounds as though it would be of concern only to unscrupulous doctors who bill for services or modalities never rendered, bill missed appointments as office visits, or fabricate nonexistent office visits. But the federal False Claims Act (FCA)[7] includes many less heinous activities, and encourages private citizens to bring claims against doctors on behalf of the government by rewarding them with up to 30 percent of any amounts recovered.

The expectation that this would entice private action has proved well founded. In a recent federal case in Tennessee, a private individual brought a claim alleging that physicians were referring their Medicare and Medicaid patients to a medical center in violation of anti-kickback and self-referral statutes. The District Court granted the defendants' motion to dismiss, since the plaintiff did not allege that any damage had been caused to the government.

On reconsideration, however, the court allowed this claim to proceed. In language that should be chilling to the honest provider, the court found that even if the medical services billed were necessary and actually rendered, the doctors were still liable under the False Claims Act. "Apparently, the government would have paid these health care charges regardless of who performed the services and regardless of the reason the patients chose the provider. There is no contention that government funds were lost or put at risk by Defendants' activities." The reasoning behind this holding was that "by submitting its claims, Defendants implicitly stated that they had complied with all statutes, rules, and regulations governing the Medicare Act, including federal anti-kickback and self-referral statutes."[8]

BENEFITS OF MULTIDISCIPLINARY PRACTICE

Enhanced Collaboration and Convenience

Despite the legal complexities inherent in the multidisciplinary practice, many have concluded that the benefits of such an arrangement outweigh its liabilities. Any pattern of practice that serves patients with increased convenience and serves doctors through cost-effectiveness and interdisciplinary coordination, is likely to thrive in an era of cost containment and interdependence. Most of all, if managed by caring, competent, and compassionate people, the multidisciplinary practice holds forth the possibility of a more integrated, patient-centered model.

The need for multidisciplinary integration was well articulated in *The Lancet*:

> In truth, compassion is often lacking in the traditional model of medical care. How could it be otherwise when the patient is progressively fragmented while coursing from one specialist to another? Working separately, specialists do not understand the subtleties of their clinical interface. Consultation is a potential passing of care, not a collaboration.[9]

By contrast, interdisciplinary practice fosters the emergence of true collaboration on many levels:

> Patients would know that their care is provided by a team ... and that at any given appointment, irrespective of the team member reviewing their case management is coordinated—one stop shopping.[9]

Moreover,

> The process is information driven. ... The necessary investment in data handling infrastructure and learning time for the professional may be considerable. Once learned, the end result is efficiency, (fewer patient visits over the course of an illness), patient satisfaction, and a culture of comprehensive management, injury and progress.[9]

Research and Training Opportunities

Multidisciplinary environments provide an excellent source of data for retrospective studies as well as more formally designed clinical trials. The research possibilities in integrated settings can prove valuable to academic institutions staffing outpatient facilities where chiropractors participate in the delivery of integrated services. Integrated settings also offer opportunities for chiropractic intern rotations. If delivery of better and more comprehensive health care in integrated settings is a goal, training models must reflect that objective.

Training is a significant issue in assessing the integrated practice movement. Having been involved in chiropractic academic administration in a number of capacities, including Dean of Clinical Sciences and Director of Institutional Research, and having participated in the accreditation process for chiropractic colleges, it is my (R.S.R.) perception that chiropractic college administration and faculty generally remain reticent to embrace a didactic and clinical teaching model that relies upon medical teaching institutions for a portion of the training of chiropractic interns. This mindset prevents and deters integration at the most crucial level—during the student's training. Perspectives on practice develop directly from what is experienced as a student. If chiropractic schools display institutional resistance to the integrated model, students will not be exposed to this concept while their belief systems about clinical practice are in the formative period.

This is particularly pertinent today as the health care delivery system evolves toward interdisciplinary collaboration. Continued avoidance of opportunities currently available for integrated training with medical teaching institutions will encourage the segregation of chiropractic from the rest of the health care delivery system.

Only a few chiropractic colleges have made significant strides in adopting joint clinical training with medical teaching institutions and private medicine services. Students at these colleges derive many benefits from the experience, including opportunities for collaborative practices, understanding the intricacies of medical specialties and facilities, and exposure to a fuller range of technology and teaching perspectives. This results in a broader learning experience than is available in an isolated institution. It also brings increased opportunities to expose the medical community and its patients to chiropractic, along with the most significant benefit of all—an enhanced ability to render quality health care to the patient.

CHIROPRACTIC IN HOSPITALS

Chiropractors have often faced a difficult dilemma: would a particular patient benefit most from the specialized care available in the office-based chiropractic practice, or should that patient be referred to an allopathic physician for care in a hospital setting? This question arises most urgently with non-ambulatory patients whose health status poses a risk to themselves or others, and those with life-threatening conditions or major complications such as head injuries. In such cases, continued outpatient treatment may pose unacceptable risks and the most prudent course is to arrange for the patient to be treated in the controlled environment of a hospital.

Because DCs were denied professional access to hospitals for so many years—due primarily to the AMA's anti-chiropractic policies[1]—patients usually could not receive concurrent care. Referral for allopathic hospital treatment meant that the patient would be denied the benefit of further chiropractic care for the duration of the hospital stay. Sadly, this is still the case in most areas.

Impact of the *Wilk* Decision

The influence of the AMA as a senior member of the Joint Commission on Accreditation of Hospital Organizations (JCAHO) was crucial in maintaining the decades-long boycott of chiropractic services. *Wilk v. AMA et al.*, the landmark chiropractic antitrust suit, sought among its other goals to gain chiropractic access to hospital facilities and services. Included in the court's decision was a requirement that prohibitions against chiropractic participation at JCAHO-accredited hospitals be eliminated. Hospitals were to proceed at their own discretion in the appointment of chiropractic physicians to staff positions on the same basis as other qualified health care professionals.

Following Judge Susan Getzendanner's 1987 decision in the *Wilk* case, the American Hospital Association changed its policy, as follows[10]:

> It is the policy of the American Hospital Association that individual hospitals themselves determine whether chiropractic services are to be provided in a hospital setting. This determination is made by the hospital's governing board taking into consideration, among other legitimate factors: state law, the needs of the patient constituency of the hospital, and appropriate procedural rules and regulations, having in mind protection of the legit-

imate interests of the patient and the hospital. Such considerations are no different with other licensed health care professionals. The American Hospital Association notes that, in line with such considerations, hospitals that are members of the American Hospital Association have incorporated chiropractic care into a hospital setting, where other licensed health care practitioners and doctors of chiropractic work in a common setting.

> The American Hospital Association specifically disavows any unlawful effort by any private, competitive group to "contain," "eliminate," or to undermine the public's confidence in the profession of chiropractic.

> The Association has no objection to a hospital granting privileges to doctors of chiropractic, where consistent with law, for the purpose of: (1) administering chiropractic treatment to patients who wish to have such treatment, whether administered in conjunction with or separate from other health care treatment or services administered by medical doctors or other licensed professional health care providers; (2) furthering the clinical education and training of doctors of chiropractic; or (3) having new diagnostic x-rays, clinical laboratory tests, and reports thereon, made for doctors of chiropractic and their patients, and/or previously taken diagnostic x-rays, clinical laboratory tests, and reports thereon made available to them, by individual pathologists or radiologists employed by or associated with such hospital upon request or authorization of the patient involved.

The AMA continued to resist Judge Getzendanner's ruling, appealing to the United States Supreme Court, which in 1990 upheld the decision of the lower court.

Meanwhile, several hospitals in the United States began providing chiropractic services on an inpatient basis, seeking increased facility utilization and greater patient benefits from combining two different but often complementary therapeutic approaches. The addition of chiropractic services did not supplant services already being provided by other hospital medical staff members, and provided a new source of patient referrals previously unavailable to the hospitals when those services were provided exclusively in an office-based environment.

Role of Chiropractors in Hospitals

In the hospital environment, the role of chiropractic physicians involves four main areas:

1. *Differential diagnosis:* In partnership with the patient's medical physician, the chiropractor arranges for appropriate diagnostic testing to determine the full nature of the patient's condition.
2. *Spinal adjusting and manipulation:* This is the hallmark of chiropractic practice, in both hospital and outpatient settings. Adjunctive physical therapy procedures, which many DCs use in their office-based practices, are provided by physical therapists in hospitals. DCs in hospitals can order physical therapy where appropriate.
3. *Manipulation under anesthesia:* This procedure can only be performed in hospitals or ambulatory surgical centers.
4. *Physical rehabilitation:* Rehabilitation programs in hospitals have grown substantially in recent years, and are expected to expand further as the focus in health care evolves from disease management to prevention.

While DCs should have no difficulty learning hospital operational protocol, assuming a rightful position on a team that has not previously included chiropractic physicians may require considerable time and patience. Therefore, as DCs begin to enter hospital practice, it is important that they do so with the intent of becoming cooperative members of the hospital health care team, rather than assuming an attitude of therapeutic invincibility. Because the hospital environment is unfamiliar to chiropractic clinical training, it is particularly important to understand its organizational structure, governance, medical staff organization, rules, and regulations.

Practical Steps Toward Inclusion

The American Chiropractic Association's (ACA) Hospital Relations Committee is composed of chiropractic physicians who practice in hospital environments and have expertise helping other DCs to acquire hospital privileges. It serves as a liaison for member chiropractors and hospitals, conducts surveys, and distributes information relevant to hospital practices. The committee has also performed a comprehensive examination of hospital bylaws, rules, and regulations as well as credentialing considerations such as privilege delineations. This information can serve as a template for implementing a program including chiropractic services in hospitals.

On the basis of experience at hospitals which have implemented staff privileges and medical staff membership for chiropractic physicians, three levels of inclusion of chiropractic services have proved effective depending upon the organization of the hospital in question:

1. Appointment to the general medical staff on an individual basis
2. Appointment to a chiropractic service under the jurisdiction of an existing department, such as the Department of Family Practice or Department of Surgery
3. Appointment to a separate Department of Chiropractic.

Chiropractic physicians who wish to utilize hospital facilities should thoroughly examine their personal and professional aspirations, practice logistics, and the needs of the particular hospital. Success at obtaining hospital privileges will primarily depend upon whether the bylaws of the hospital specifically provide for the granting of such privileges in accordance with the requirements of the Joint Commission on Accreditation of Healthcare Organizations. If so, the process of acquiring privileges at that hospital is greatly simplified.

However, most hospitals do not have provisions in their bylaws for granting privileges to DCs, and in such cases it is necessary that the bylaws be amended. While some hospitals are quite agreeable to granting privileges to chiropractors in order to take advantage of a new source of patient referrals, others are resistant.

If the hospital is genuinely interested in assigning privileges to chiropractic physicians, the process of amending its bylaws is a relatively easy, as there are no longer any JCAHO restrictions to granting such privileges. Hospitals that currently utilize chiropractic services can be used as models. Sample bylaws are available from ACA for use by the hospital's governing body in making appropriate revisions on the recommendations of the administrative chief executive and medical chief of staff.

Whether a particular hospital already has provisions in their bylaws for granting of privileges to chiropractic physicians, is amenable to the revision of their bylaws to accommodate this, or is resistant to the allowing of such privileges, the initial action by the interested DC is one and the same—submission of an application for privileges.

Before submitting an application, it is advisable to obtain as much information as possible about the hospital's demography, governance, composition of its governing board, administrative philosophy, corporate ownership, accreditation status, departmental organization, services provided, and its financial and legal status. Some of this information may be readily available in publicly distributed hospital literature or advertising, such as patient or employee-directed informational pamphlets, newsletters, telephone directories, employment opportunity bulletins, and continuing education offerings. Some may be available from friendly medical or osteopathic staff physicians; and some may require the services of a personal attorney, such as the hospital's present financial and accreditation stays, and present or past malpractice or medical staff litigation.

DCs should obtain as much information as possible in order to select the most appropriate hospital at which to apply for privileges, prepare and submit a well-developed application, and be sufficiently informed to assist the administrator, chief of staff, and governing board to amend the hospital's bylaws and governing protocol. Moreover, they must be prepared to make an appeal if the first attempt is unsuccessful, and have some prior working knowledge of the hospital's environment after acceptance.

Traditionally, chiropractors have had fewer local, state and federal guidelines and regulations imposed upon their practices than medical doctors. An in-depth understanding of rules and regulations governing hospital-based practices is essential for any chiropractic physician acquiring hospital privileges.

Levels of Clinical Privileges

JCAHO standards recommend that the medical staff of an accredited hospital "should be composed of physicians and other licensed individuals permitted by law and by the hospital to independently provide patient care." These persons must have delineated clinical privileges, must be subject to hospital and medical staff bylaws and governing protocol, and must be subject to the hospital's quality assurance review. The extension of privileges is based on professional criteria and designed to provide quality patient care. At a minimum, criteria include evidence of training, licensure, and current professional competence.

Depending on how a particular hospital chooses to interpret and apply these JCAHO standards relative to their requirements for clinical privileges and legal scope of practice requirements, hospital medical staff affiliations may be divided into the following four categories:

- Fully qualified physicians
- Partially qualified physicians
- Nonphysicians
- Staff affiliates

JCAHO standards specify that only medical and osteopathic physicians licensed for the practice of medicine in all its branches may be granted full active "staff membership" and relatively unrestricted patient-admitting privileges in a general hospital. Full active membership and admitting privileges are usually considered in terms of whether the physician is permitted by credentials, law, and JCAHO policy to assume primary and full responsibility for the overall care of patients. Full active membership also generally requires a specified number of admissions on an annual basis, and mandatory medical staff committee participation as a voting member.

Medical or osteopathic physicians who apply for general hospital privileges on the basis of a board certified specialty are usually not considered for full active membership inasmuch as they are not taking full responsibility for the overall care of patients. In these cases, "courtesy" or "consulting" privileges may be granted, along with patient admission privileges which are contingent on taking a complete history and performing a comprehensive physical examination within 24 hours of patient admission by a medical or osteopathic physician holding full active membership. Exceptions to this rule are sometimes made for oral surgeons who may be permitted to take a complete history and perform a comprehensive physical examination to determine a patient's fitness to undergo oral surgery.

Individuals other than medical or osteopathic physicians who are licensed to independently practice a limited branch of medicine in terms of body region, or a scope of practice less than all its branches (e.g., dentists, podiatrists) are ordinarily categorized by the JCAHO standards as "nonphysicians." In most cases, nonphysicians granted some degree of clinical privileges are required to co-admit with a medical or osteopathic physician having full active staff membership and admission privileges. This MD or DO is required by JCAHO standards to remain responsible for the overall care of the patient during hospitalization. In some cases, chiropractic physicians have been accorded a status that is essentially equivalent to that of a partially qualified physician.

Medical staff affiliates (or allied health practitioners) are licensed, registered, or otherwise certified professionals trained to perform a select group of activities under the direct supervision of a member of the medical staff. Included in this group are clinical psychologists, registered nurses, nurse anesthetists, nurse midwives, nurse practitioners, and professional medical assistants. Medical staff affiliates may or may not be allowed admission or co-admission privileges and may or may not write medical orders, depending on individual hospital policy.

In hospitals where the bylaws already accommodate chiropractic services, the nature of these privileges varies. Examples include the following:

1. Outpatient diagnostic referral privileges
2. Allied health practitioner status without admitting or patient order-writing privileges
3. Nonphysician status with co-admitting or courtesy privileges
4. Partially qualified physician status with courtesy admitting and patient order-writing privileges
5. Membership in a separate chiropractic department, or in a chiropractic service of another established department with courtesy admitting privileges contingent on the taking of a complete patient history and the performing of a physical examination within 24 hours by a full member of the medical staff

Team Approach to Securing Privileges

Policies on granting of clinical privileges to chiropractors also vary considerably from hospital to hospital. A team, rather than an individual, approach to the securing of hospital privileges is advisable for several reasons:

1. If the hospital's management is interested in granting privileges to chiropractic physicians in order to expand use of its facilities and support services, it may not be eager to expend the time and effort necessary to make the required bylaw changes for the limited benefits that one or a few staff chiropractic physicians might bring.
2. Each member of the team can provide unique contributions of knowledge and experience, which can have a cumulative benefit toward achieving the desired objective.
3. A team effort is more likely to result in the hospital's formation of a separate chiropractic department, or service within an existing department, thus opening the possibility of a more desirable staff membership level with courtesy admitting privileges, than if an individual chiropractor applies for clinical privileges as a nonphysician or allied health practitioner.
4. All members of the team will have acquired the same basic knowledge of hospital protocol necessary to productively function as members of the hospital's medical staff team, as well as among themselves in a chiropractic department.

In the long run, developing the spirit of cooperation required for work in hospitals and other interdisciplinary settings may yield an additional result. Aside from the benefits to patients and participating chiropractors already discussed, it is possible that this cooperative spirit will eventually help to decrease the intraprofessional acrimony that has divided the chiropractic profession for so long. Learning to collaborate with one's former opponents is good training for learning to more fully cooperate with those in the chiropractic family.

Terminology

admitting privileges
ambulatory surgical center
clinical privileges
fee splitting
full-scope physician
JCAHO
kickback
medical staff affiliates
manipulation under anesthesia (MUA)
non-physicians
self-referral

Review Questions

1. In which departments at medical facilities have chiropractic students participated in clinical rotations?

2. The majority of opportunities for chiropractors to practice in integrated settings are currently in which types of practices?

3. In what settings is manipulation under anesthesia performed?

4. What are the potential advantages of a multidisciplinary practice? What are some potential disadvantages?

5. What legal difficulties are posed by multidisciplinary practice? How can the participating chiropractor shield himself or herself against such liability?

6. How can multidisciplinary environments be helpful for education and research?

7. Which court case had the most significant impact on chiropractic participation in hospitals?

8. In what kinds of cases is it appropriate for chiropractors to treat patients in a hospital?

9. How do hospital privileges for chiropractors differ from privileges for full scope physicians?

10. Why is a team, rather than an individual, approach advisable for securing hospital privileges?

Concept Questions

1. If multidisciplinary practice becomes the norm rather than the exception, how will this effect the unique nature of the chiropractic profession? Do you see this as a positive development?

2. What changes in chiropractic education are needed to prepare chiropractors for multidisciplinary and hospital practice? Should these be incorporated on an elective or required basis?

References

1. *Wilk v. AMA*, 895 F2D 352 Cert den, 112.2 Ed 2D 524 (1990)
2. Haldeman S, Chapman-Smith D, Petersen DM: Guidelines for Chiropractic Quality Assurance and Practice Parameters. Aspen, Gaithersburg, MD, 1993
3. 10 Knocker Sec. 34.1 et seq., 1993
4. Florida Statutes Section 458.331 (1)(I)
5. *See*, e.g., *US v Greber*, 760 F2nd 68 (3rd Cir. 1995)
6. *The Hanlester Network v Shalala*, 51 F3rd 1390 (9th Cir. 1995)
7. 31 U.S.C. 3729–3733 (1983 & Supp. 1995)
8. *United States ex rel Pogue v. American Healthcorp, Inc., et al*, 914 Fsupp 1507 (1996)
9. Shipper H, Dick J: Herodotus and the multidisciplinary clinic. The Lancet 346:8986, 1995
10. JCAHO: The 1991 Joint Commission Accreditation Manual for Hospitals, Vol. 1: Standards. Joint Commission on Accreditation of Heathcare Organizations, Oakbrook Terrace, IL, 1990

20
Pathways for an Evolving Profession
Daniel Redwood

*H*ow can chiropractors and chiropractic students help the profession evolve so that it more fully reflects our noblest aspirations? For students immersed in mastering large quantities of technical information and field practitioners focused on day-to-day matters of patient care and practice management, such questions are usually crowded out by the press of immediate responsibilities. In the long run, however, they are crucial.

To survive for many generations, a healing art must be grounded in a system of enduring principles. Lacking that, the centrifugal force of new developments exerts too strong a destabilizing pull, eventually leading to loss of fundamental identity. To remain a distinct profession well into the future, chiropractors must hold fast to certain core principles. These include concepts shared with other natural healing arts along with unique chiropractic contributions to the overall body of healing arts principles and practice.

In addition to upholding the vital concepts of chiropractic and natural healing, individual chiropractors can influence the future path of the profession by:

- Distinguishing clearly among the proven, the probable, and the speculative
- Taking care to diagnose and prognose in ways that empower patients

- Minimizing patient dependency
- Serving those who cannot afford chiropractic services
- Making healthy lifestyle choices and thereby serving as a good example to others
- Modeling qualities of tolerance and openmindedness
- Learning about other healing traditions and interacting constructively with their practitioners

Although externally driven events will always exert an influence, the destiny of chiropractic is primarily in our own hands.

FOUNDATIONAL PRINCIPLES

Chiropractic could not have survived for a century without largely adhering to the tenets of natural healing enunciated by Daniel David Palmer and other chiropractic pioneers. These include the following principles drawn from the common domain shared by all natural healing arts, along with core chiropractic principles.[1]

Natural Healing Principles

1. Human beings possess an innate healing potential, an inner wisdom of the body.

2. Maximally accessing this healing system is the goal of the healing arts.
3. Addressing the cause of an illness should in most cases take precedence over suppressing its surface manifestations.
4. Pharmaceutical suppression of symptoms can in some instances compromise and diminish the body's ability to heal itself.
5. Natural, nonpharmaceutical measures (including chiropractic spinal adjustments) should in most cases be an approach of first resort, not last.
6. A balanced, natural diet is crucial to good health.
7. Regular exercise is essential to proper bodily function.

Endorsed and elucidated by chiropractors for a full century, these precepts are recognizable today as the foundation of the emerging holistic health or wellness paradigm.

Core Chiropractic Principles

The following constructs comprise the theoretical underpinning of chiropractic:

1. Structure and function exist in intimate relation with one another.
2. Structural distortions can cause functional abnormalities.
3. The vertebral subluxation is a significant form of structural distortion and dysfunction, and leads to a variety of functional abnormalities.
4. The nervous system occupies a preeminent role in the restoration and maintenance of proper bodily function.
5. The subluxation influences bodily function primarily through neurologic means.
6. The chiropractic adjustment is a specific, definitive method for the correction of the vertebral subluxation.

While the precise definition of the subluxation has changed over the years (see Ch. 3), emphasis on the interplay between subluxation, the nervous system, and human health has been at the core of chiropractic concerns since the birth of the profession, and remains so today.

TOUCHSTONES FOR FUTURE ADVANCEMENT

For individual chiropractors and the profession as a whole to rise to the challenges we face, we must draw on the best of our history, look inward with rigorous self-analysis, and then act based on a sense of higher purpose. To accomplish this, let us consider the following points:

1. *Distinguish clearly among the proven, the probable, and the speculative.* Some of the most justifiable criticism of chiropractic has been in reaction to the tendency of some chiropractors to "globalize,"[2] making broad overarching claims on the basis of limited, though powerful, anecdotal evidence. Anecdotal information and case studies can be of genuine value in formulating the basis for further research; we should not mistake them for scientific proof. Chiropractic's integrity and credibility, as well as its compliance with regulatory agencies, depend on its practitioners consistently making this distinction. To do so, we must stay well acquainted with current research. Keating (Internet communication, 1996) has noted that all health professions use unproven methods (only 15 to 20 percent of conventional medicine's methods are proven)[3,4] but that it is *never* acceptable to make inaccurate claims about these methods and techniques.

2. *Recognize the power of your diagnoses and prognoses.* Doctors have the power to dramatically shape patients' views of their own health. We have a responsibility to tell the truth, and a further responsibility to frame that truth in the manner most empowering to the patient. A patient once came to me with neck and shoulder pain, and related that she had been told by her previous chiropractor that on a scale of 1 to 10 (10 being the ideal) he rated her overall health at three. My own judgment was that this was a healthy, vibrant young woman who happened to have some musculoskeletal pain. However, it took time and effort to convince her that she was basically well. In our role as healing arts professionals, we need to be careful not to unthinkingly alter our patients' self-perception for the worse. We can convey to them that they are fundamentally ill people, or that they are healthy people who currently have certain symptoms or imbalances. There is a world of difference. It is essential to convey confidence in patients' strength and healing potential.

Even with severely ill patients, it is important to temper honest evaluation with hope.

3. *Minimize patient dependency.* Most chiropractic cases require multiple visits. However, as J.F. McAndrews noted earlier in this text, "depending on which chiropractor a patient sees, the recommended course of care for the same condition may vary drastically, from several visits with one doctor to several dozen—sometimes hundreds—with another. Such variations appear in all regions, among graduates of all chiropractic colleges, and in urban, suburban, and rural settings." Driven in some cases by perceived or real financial pressures and in others by a sincere belief that most or all patients require long-term, visit-intensive chiropractic care, chiropractors may discourage patient independence by scheduling more visits and performing more procedures than truly required for patients' well-being.

Because some of these subliminal motivations reside in us all, it is essential that we make a conscious effort to recommend only that treatment which is truly needed. We can encourage greater patient self-sufficiency through "active prevention," teaching exercises and other self-care methods, and decreasing frequency of treatment as soon as appropriate. Kingsbury[5] notes that in the early days of the profession, doctors spoke with pride of how *few* visits it took to resolve a patient's condition, and how long a patient could go without needing another adjustment. Such a mindset reflects a deep connection to the true purpose of chiropractic, and is emblematic of a patient-centered practice. It contrasts sharply with those who include in their definition of success maximizing the number of visits per case.

4. *Promote a healing partnership and patient-centered approach.* Doctor–patient relations are imbued with certain inherent inequalities. These include the doctor's social status and specialized knowledge, as well as the patient's sense of insecurity resulting from his illness and disability.[6] Doctors should offer patients opportunities for empowerment, so that the inequality created by their specialized knowledge is not generalized to all aspects of their relations with patients. Gordon argues persuasively for a "healing partnership,"[7] where the usual hierarchical model is transformed into a more egalitarian one where patients assume a significantly more active, responsible role. Gatterman makes a similar case within the context of chiropractic education and health care delivery.[8] Both Gordon and Gatterman call for a pattern of doctor–patient interaction that moves beyond the "men in white coats" hierarchical model that has become a cliché in our time. They embrace a mutually respectful relationship that calls on patients to relinquish powerlessness and doctors to surrender some of their power.

5. *Do everything possible to create a positive public perception of the chiropractic profession.* Many people still retain negative stereotypes about chiropractors, and it is imperative that chiropractors not act in ways that reinforce these ideas. We can better serve our patients and our profession by asking ourselves the following questions:

- Do I continue to treat patients who are showing no clinical progress after a reasonable (1 month in most cases) trial of care?
- Do I use radiography only when clinically necessary?
- Do I perceive patients as spines to be adjusted or do I also connect with them as people?
- Do my patients feel that I rush through their office visits?
- Do I encourage patients' questions and take time to answer them in sufficient depth?
- Is my primary focus the depth of the patient's healing or the size of my income?
- Do I have honest billing practices?
- How informed am I about the latest research relating to chiropractic?
- How open to and knowledgeable about alternatives to chiropractic am I?

In recent years, the medical profession has faced a burgeoning grassroots movement seeking alternatives to conventional care; chiropractors are not immune to a comparable response to our own less enlightened practices. We can move proactively to avert this by clarifying our ideals through a process of serious self-examination, and then changing those actions and attitudes that fail to measure up.

6. *Serve those who cannot afford your services.* In keeping with the spirit of healing and service that underlies the decision to pursue a career in chiropractic,

we can serve people in our communities by offering sliding scale or no-fee services to those whose financial status would otherwise prohibit them from seeking chiropractic care. This longstanding tradition in chiropractic dates back to the Palmers and other guiding lights of the profession's early years. Less universal now than in the past, it is scorned in some chiropractic circles. When I was a new graduate, a colleague advised me to discourage poor people from becoming patients, because "welfare refers welfare," a concept he had been taught at a practice management seminar. Aside from the fact that the basic premise is incorrect (poor people sometimes refer full-paying patients), this attitude is so insidious and uncompassionate that it deserves to be exposed to the cleansing light of day. Every spiritual tradition in the world speaks of the need to serve those less fortunate than ourselves. The admirable example of our chiropractic forebears calls us to do no less.

7. *Model a healthy lifestyle.* Actions speak louder than words—we must walk our talk. Doctors whose lifestyles offer an example of health-affirming choices are in the best position to influence patients to do likewise. This does not mean that we must be in perfect health before we can legitimately offer advice; it means that we need to make a sincere effort to choose a healthy lifestyle. This reflects on our own integrity as well as that of our profession. Honest self-evaluation is required. It should include questions like these:

- Is my diet consistent with what I know to be good nutrition?
- Do I smoke?
- Do I use alcohol or caffeine immoderately?
- Do I use other drugs?
- Do I exercise regularly?
- Do I get adequate rest?
- Do I utilize stress reduction methods?

If we find areas where our actions are inconsistent with our beliefs as chiropractors and natural health care practitioners, the relevant question is: why not make a change for the better today? We should not expect our patients to do for themselves what we are unwilling to do for ourselves.

8. *Cultivate tolerance and openmindedness.* In developing the clarity of awareness needed to attain mastery in healing arts practice, tolerance and openmindedness are among the most valuable tools. In health and healing, many questions have more than one correct answer. Back and neck pain, for example, can be remarkably responsive to chiropractic care, but not in all cases. In certain instances, other methods including acupuncture,[9,10] mind–body interventions,[11–13] or surgery[14,15] bring improvement or resolution. In a time of worldwide interchange of health information,[16,17] we chiropractors should educate ourselves about other healing methods and traditions in order to deepen our understanding of alternative practices and paradigms, to know when to refer patients to practitioners of these healing arts, and to incorporate into our own practices aspects of this knowledge compatible with our role as chiropractors. Calling on other qualified practitioners for assistance is sometimes precisely what the best interest of the patient requires. Informed people in all disciplines know that no method has all the answers, and that those claiming to possess a panacea are unaware of their own blind spots.

9. *Acknowledge nonphysical causation of illness.* Contemporary chiropractic practice is largely geared to the assumption that physical symptoms have physical causes. This is not the whole truth. Musculoskeletal pain and impairment can be strongly influenced by emotional stress and belief patterns.[18–21] Chiropractors can help in such cases by teaching patients to practice stress management techniques, and referring to mental health professionals where appropriate.

10. *Recognize the hand of friendship when it is offered.* To develop cooperative relationships with other health professionals, a spirit of mutuality is essential. Chiropractors have made commendable efforts in recent years to build such bridges with both conventional and alternative practitioners. As we reach out to others, we must not allow fear to dominate our perception of those who reach out to us. An anecdote from former U.S. Surgeon General C. Everett Koop recounted to me by Marc Micozzi may be instructive here. According to Koop, during the 1950s, he and I. S. Ravdin, then the leading figure in surgery at the University of Pennsylvania, had concluded that drugs and surgery were proving inadequate for some lower

back pain patients. They believed that chiropractic might be helpful and approached chiropractors in Philadelphia about doing research on chiropractic, with the hope that this might lead to including chiropractic as part of standard care for low back pain. The chiropractors refused to participate. Koop believes they had been persecuted for so long by organized medicine and local medical physicians that they had concluded that all MDs were their enemies.

It may not be easy for today's students and younger practitioners to fully appreciate the mindset of those 1950s-era chiropractors, who had grown so accustomed to hostility from the medical profession that they were unable to recognize a sincere hand of friendship. Rather than judging them harshly, we should acknowledge that whatever challenges we now face pale in comparison with theirs. We can empathize with their situation and honor the legacy of their struggle for professional survival, from which we all have benefited greatly.

At the same time, however, we must remember that opportunity does not always knock twice on the same door. As we stride with backs unbent into a new century filled with potential, we must be willing to let go of old grievances against individuals and professions that have wronged us in the past. Openings will be presented to us in the coming years beyond what we can currently conceive. Let us evaluate them with clear minds, assuming that people are sincere unless they prove otherwise, and then move forward together toward a future that fulfills D.D. Palmer's vision.

Terminology

active prevention
dependency
globalize
healing partnership
nonphysical causation
patient-centered approach
self-care

Review Questions

1. List seven common domain principles of natural healing shared by chiropractic and other natural healing arts.

2. List six core chiropractic principles.

3. How can a chiropractor's prognoses affect patients' self-perception of their own health?

4. What are the consequences of dependency?

5. How can chiropractors encourage greater self-sufficiency on the part of patients?

6. Why is it especially important for health practitioners to live in a healthy manner?

7. What reasons justify seeing some patients on a sliding scale or no-fee basis?

8. What are three reasons to learn about other healing traditions?

9. Name three methods other than spinal adjustments than can be helpful for some cases of lower back pain.

10. Do all physical symptoms have primarily physical causes?

Concept Questions

1. Why is it important to distinguish clearly among the proven, the probable, and the speculative? Have you seen cases where chiropractors failed to make this distinction? What are some possible negative consequences?

2. What are some stereotypes about chiropractors? What steps can the individual chiropractor take to overcome these stereotypes?

References

1. Redwood D: Chiropractic. p. 91. In Micozzi M (ed): Fundamentals of Complementary and Alternative Medicine. Churchill Livingstone, New York, 1996

2. Gellert G: Global explanations and the credibility problem of alternative medicine. Advances J Mind Body Health 10(4):60, 1994

3. Smith R: Where is the wisdom …? the poverty of medical evidence. BMJ 303:798, 1991

4. Office of Technology Assessment: Assessing the efficacy and safety of medical technologies. U.S. Government Printing Office, Washington, DC, 1978

5. Kingsbury GM: Does net worth equal self-worth? J Am Chiropr Assoc 33(8):23, 1996

6. Brody H: The Healer's Power. Yale University Press, New Haven, CT, 1992

7. Gordon JS: Manifesto for a New Medicine: Your Guide to Healing Partnerships and the Wise Use of Alternative Therapies. Addison-Wesley, Reading, MA, 1996

8. Gatterman MI: A patient centered paradigm: a model for chiropractic education and research. J Alt Comp Med 1:371, 1995

9. Coan R, Wong G, Ku SL et al: The acupuncture treatment of low back pain: a randomized controlled study. Am J Chin Med 8:181, 1980

10. Coan R, Wong G, Coan PL: The acupuncture treatment of neck pain: a randomized controlled study. Am J Chinese Med 9:326, 1982

11. Caudill M, Schnable R, Zuttermeister PC et al: Decreased clinic utilization by chronic pain patients: response to behavioral medicine intervention. Clin J Pain 7:305, 1991

12. Kabat-Zinn J, Lipworth L, Burney R: The clinical use of mindfulness meditation for the self-regulation of chronic pain. J Behav Med 8:163, 1985

13. Kabat-Zinn J, Lipworth L, Burney R, Sellers W: Four year follow-up of a meditation-based program for the self-regulation of chronic pain: Treatment outcomes and compliance. Clin J Pain 2:159, 1986

14. Albert TJ, Mesa JJ, Eng K, McIntosh TC, Balderston RA: Health outcome assessment before and after lumbar laminectomy for radiculopathy. Spine 21:960, 1996

15. van den Bent MJ, Oosting J, Wouda EJ et al: Anterior cervical discectomy with or without fusion with acrylate. Spine 21:834, 1996

16. Bodeker G: Traditional health systems: policy, biodiversity, and global interdependence. J Alt Comp Med 1:231, 1995

17. Bodeker G: Global health traditions. p. 279. In Micozzi M (ed): Fundamentals of Complementary and Alternative Medicine. Churchill Livingstone, New York, 1996

18. Drottning M, Staff PH, Levin L et al: Acute emotional response to common whiplash predicts subsequent pain complaints: a prospective of 107 subjects sustaining whiplash injury. Nordic J Psychiatry 49:293, 1995

19. Klapow JC, Slater MA, Patterson TL: Psychosocial factors discriminate multidimensional clinical groups of chronic low back pain patients. Pain 62:349, 1995

20. Lackner JM, Carosella AM, Feuerstein M: Pain expectancies, pain, and functional self-efficacy expectancies as determinants of disability in patients with chronic low back disorders. J Consult Clin Psychol 64:212, 1996

21. Riley JF, Ahern DK, Follick MJ: Chronic pain and functional impairment: assessing beliefs about their relationship. Arch Phys Med Rehabil 69:579, 1988

Glossary

Accessory motion — small, specific movements of a joint, independent of voluntary muscle action

Accreditation — the process through which the quality of educational institutions is evaluated; the Council on Chiropractic Education is the accrediting agency for chiropractic colleges in the United States

Active analysis — worksite evaluation in which the chiropractic occupational health physician observes, samples, measures, and records the presence of potential ergonomic hazard (see Passive analysis)

Active prevention — preventive measures that rely primarily on the active commitment and participation of the individual (e.g., dietary changes, exercise, and stress management practices)

Active release technique — a soft tissue technique in which pressure and tension are maintained by the practitioner while the patient moves the tissue from a shortened to a stretched position. This technique is used for the examination, diagnosis, and treatment of cumulative injury disorders

Adhesions — the abnormal adherence of biologic structures due to scar development

Adjustive lesion — the complex clinical entity that serves as a basis for treatment by adjustive procedures, as identified by observation, palpation, diagnostic imaging, and other procedures

Adjustment — 1. a maneuver specific in direction, point of contact, amplitiude, and velocity intended to partly or wholly correct a subluxation; 2. any chiropractic therapeutic procedure that uses controlled force, leverage, direction, amplitude, and velocity directed at specific joints or anatomic regions

Admitting privileges — privileges extended to physicians by a hospital, permitting them to admit patients to the facility; admitting privileges are generally based on whether the physician is permitted by credentials, law, and JCAHO policy to assume primary and full responsibility for the overall care of patients

Afferent — the sensory function of neural elements

Allodynia — pain due to a stimulus that does not normally induce pain; describes an objective response to clinical stimuli, when the normal stimulus can be tested elsewhere in the body; a loss of specificity of any sensory modality, with the final perception being pain; a simple example of allodynia is pain following light brushing after a sunburn

Allopathy — the practice of medicine based on using substances or procedures to counteract symptoms

Alternative therapy — a treatment method not commonly taught in allopathic medical schools, practiced in hospitals, or reimbursed by third-party payors; an unconventional therapy

Ambulatory surgical center — a free-standing medical or multidisciplinary facility where surgical and other procedures are performed; may include epidural steroid injections, facet blocks, sympathetic blocks, other injection and pain management techniques, and spinal and extremity manipulation with or without anesthesia

Anatomic barrier — the limit of anatomic integrity or movement, as imposed by an anatomic structure; forced movement beyond this barrier results in damage to the limiting tissues

Antidromic — conducting impulses in a direction opposite the normal

"Any Willing Provider" laws — statutes requiring that if a procedure is covered by an insurance policy, any provider licensed to perform that procedure within his scope of practice must be covered under the contract

Apgar score — a qualitative test developed by physician Virginia Apgar, used to determine the status of a newborn child at 1 minute and 5 minutes after birth; scores between 0 and 2 are assigned for heart rate, respiration, color, reflex irritability, and muscle tone; 10 is a perfect score; children with scores between 0 and 3 at 5 minutes tend to have higher rates of morbidity and mortality

Apposition — the condition of being placed side by side

Articulation — a joint; the point at which two bones meet

Ataxia — defective muscular coordination, especially manifested when voluntary muscular movements are attempted

Atonia — loss of normal muscular tone

Atrophy — decrease in size of a structure

Auscultation — the act of listening to the sounds generated in the body

Axon reflex — action potential propagation in an efferent direction on an afferent axon

Axoplasmic flow — an intracellular transport system that carries large molecules formed in the nerve cell body down the full length of the axon to the nerve fiber terminals

Axoplasmic transport — an intracellular transport system that carries large molecules formed in the nerve cell body the full length of the axon to the nerve fiber terminals and back again, at a rate faster than axoplasmic flow

Babinski reflex — spreading of the toes and dorsiflexion of the great toe in response to stroking the sole of the foot; this is normal up to 24 months of age; beyond that point it indicates a neurologic deficit, as in lesions of the pyramidal tract

Basic science laws — laws passed by some state legislatures beginning in the 1920s, requiring that chiropractors seeking licensure demonstrate proficiency on basic science tests

Battery — unlawful touching

Bifurcate — to split into two parts

Biomechanics — the application of mechanical principles to living structures

Blepharoptosis — drooping of the upper eyelid

Botanic medicine — a system of healing that uses plants as medicines

Boycott — an organized refusal to do business with an individual or group; the *Wilk v. AMA* lawsuit reversed the medical profession's boycott of chiropractic

Breech birth — a birth wherein the presenting part is one or both feet or the buttocks

Bruit — turbulence generated in an artery due to loss of laminar flow

Calor — localized increase in temperature; a cardinal sign of inflammation

Caput succedarum — an edematous swelling of the scalp at the point of birth presentation resulting from interruption of the lymphatic supply to the area; can result from a brow or breech presentation

Carioca — a crossover, side-stepping exercise in which one foot crosses in front of and then behind the other

Carpal tunnel syndrome (CTS) — a complex of symptoms resulting from compression of the median nerve in the carpal tunnel of the wrist; signs and symptoms of CTS can include numbness, tingling, burning sensations, pain, and weakness in hand, wrist, and/or entire affected upper extremity

Cauda equina syndrome — injury to the nerve roots of the lumbosacral region as they pass through the lower spinal canal. Usually caused by compression of the nerve roots from a large anteriomedial disc protrusion or spinal stenosis

Causalgia — burning pain, sometimes accompanied by trophic skin changes, caused by injury to a peripheral nerve

Caveat — the suggestion of caution

Cephalohematoma — unilateral or bilateral pooling of blood between the periosteum and the underlying bone; this pooling usually does not cross the suture line; the parietal bones are the most common site, but it can occur anywhere on the scalp

Cerebrovascular accident — a general term applied to conditions involving either ischemic or hemorrhagic lesions of the blood supply to the brain, usually resulting in injury or death of cerebral tissue

CHAMPUS — the health insurance plan for dependents of active members of the U.S. armed services

Chemical mediators of inflammation — histamine, prostaglandin II, leukotrienes, kallidin, bradykinin, serotonin

Chiropractic analysis — clinical assessment of a patient's state of biologic and neurologic integrity, primarily for the purpose of characterizing subluxation in general and vertebral subluxation complex in particular

Chronic cervical syndrome — a condition marked by paroxysmal deep or superficial pain in parts of the head, face, ear, throat, or sinuses; sensory disturbances in the pharnyx; vertigo; tinnitus, with diminished hearing; and vasomotor disturbances (including sweating, flushing, lacrimation, and salivation)

Chronicity — extended duration of a condition

Cineradiography — a fluoroscopic technique whereby the image is recorded on motion picture film

Clinical hypothesis — a reasonable conjecture about the cause of a patient's problem

Clinical privileges — delineation of the roles of various members of hospital staffs; categories of clinical privileges include fully qualified physicians, partially qualified physicians, nonphysicians, and staff affiliates

Closed-chain exercise — exercise in which the distal part of an extremity (hand or foot) is supporting some or all of the body weight on a solid, though sometimes unstable surface

Collimator — a device that limits the area of the x-ray beam

Common domain — principles and practices shared by various healing arts

Compensation — the counterbalancing of a defect in structure or function

Computed tomography (CT scanning) — a procedure which produces cross-sectional images of the body by directing an x-ray beam through the structures of interest; the x-ray attenuation is measured by detectors surrounding the patient; axial images are produced using computer techniques, data from the axial images may be reformatted to produce sagittal and coronal images

Conduction velocity — the speed at which action potentials are transmitted along a neuron

Consanguinity — genetic relationship; of the same bloodline

Consolidation — an increase in tissue substance that causes a structure to become more solid

Contraindication — any symptom or circumstance denoting the inappropriateness of a form of treatment that would otherwise be advisable

Contraindication, absolute — a set of circumstances in which a particular treatment is always inappropriate

Contraindication, relative — a set of circumstances where a particular treatment may be appropriate only if it is modified or applied in an unusual manner

Copayment — the percentage of services a patient covered by a health care insurance or managed care plan is responsible for paying out-of-pocket, generally due the provider at the time services are rendered

Council on Chiropractic Education (CCE) — the accrediting agency for chiropractic colleges

Counterstrain — a system of evaluation and treatment of joint pain, in which treatment involves moving a muscle or joint to a position of comfort, holding it in that position for at least 90 seconds, and then slowly returning it to the neutral position

Crepitus — creaking or crackling sounds, as in a joint

Cryotherapy — the application of cold as therapy

Cultism — membership in a group characterized by unquestioning loyalty to the principles of a founder or leader, unwillingness to analyze objectively any information that conflicts with the received precepts of that founder or leader, and unwillingness to change one's beliefs even when a preponderance of new evidence contradicts them

Cumulative trauma disorder (CTD) — a group of musculoskeletal disorders caused by repeated trauma to the body. Examples are carpal tunnel and thoracic outlet syndromes

Current Procedural Terminology (CPT) — a system developed by the American Medical Association to code health care procedures for billing purposes

Degeneration — breakdown; deterioration; falling from a higher to lower level

Denervation — the complete disruption of nerve supply to a cell, tissue, or organ

Dependency — a doctor–patient relationship in which the patient inaccurately believes that he or she requires ongoing intervention by the doctor or requires more frequent or intensive care than is actually necessary

Descriptive study — a research report used to illustrate, initiate, disconfirm, or support a clinical hypothesis; included are nonexperimental research designs (e.g., case studies) and case series, as well as quasi-experimental approaches (e.g. time-series designs)

Developmental milestone — a specific point in a child's development, identified by the accomplishment of various psychomotor skills, such as sitting up, rolling over, crawling, creeping, and walking

Dietary history — an extensive history of a patient's dietary habits, including not only foods and beverages but also medications and vitamin, mineral, and herbal supplements

Dietary Supplement Health Education Act (DSHEA) — 1995 U.S. law addressing the issue of health claims which may be made by supplement manufacturers; it allows claims regarding the impact on processes of the body, but not with regard to disease or illness

Dinged — the symptom of being dazed and confused following a head injury, indicating a mild concussion

Diplopia — double vision

Direct access laws — statutes requiring managed care plans to permit their members to access specialty care without referral from a primary care gatekeeper

Direct inquiry — a method in which the examiner seeks particular information

Disease — any morbid process altering the normal state of living tissue; it may be functional or physiologic, and may affect the organism as a whole or any of its constituent parts

Dis-ease — a lack of physiologic efficiency due to disruption of coordination by the nervous system; aberrant tone

Dislocation — the displacement of a bone; a luxation

Dolor — localized pain; a cardinal sign of inflammation

Doppler ultrasonography — a diagnostic modality whereby a high-frequency sound wave is transmitted through tissue until it reaches an acoustic barrier, usually some other type of tissue; a portion of this pulsed sound wave is then reflected back toward the source, where it can be imaged or measured. Doppler ultrasonography can detect blood flow within arteries by measuring the frequency shifts of sound waves reflected off moving blood cells

Duplex ultrasound scanning — a diagnostic imaging modality that combines Doppler ultrasonography with a complementary modality called real-time B-mode ultrasonography; allows an image to be created from the reflected sound wave, where the brightness of each picture element is dependent on the amplitude of the returning sound echo; the image is updated rapidly enough to allow the examiner to see real-time physiologic changes, such as the motion of blood vessel walls

Duration of care — the length of professional treatment

Dysafferentation — abnormal afferent input as a result of joint restriction, involving a functional decrease in the activity of large diameter mechanoreceptor afferent fibers and a simultaneous functional increase in activity of nociceptive afferent nerve fibers

Dysmenorrhea — painful menses

Dysmetria — inability to judge distance during purposeful muscular movements

Dysponesis — a reversible physiopathologic state consisting of unnoticed, misdirected neurophysiologic reactions to various agents (environmental events, bodily sensations, emotions, and thoughts) and the repercussions of these reactions throughout the organism; these errors in energy expenditure, capable of producing functional disorders, consist mainly of covert errors in action potential output from the motor and premotor areas of the cortex and the consequences of that output (Dorland's Illustrated Medical Dictionary)

Efferent — the motor or other effector function of neural element

Electromyography (EMG) — the recording and study of electrical muscular activity; it is most accurately performed with needle electrodes placed in the desired muscle

Empiricism — reliance on direct experience

End organ — an organ supplied, or affected, by a nerve

End play (End feel) — the short range movements, or quality of resistance of a joint, determined by springing a joint at the limits of its passive range of motion

End play zone — the area of joint movement past the physiologic barrier but before the anatomic barrier

Entrepreneurship — the art of developing and expanding a business in a private enterprise economy

Ergonomics — the study of people in relation to their jobs

Facilitation — lowered threshold for firing in a spinal cord segment, resulting from afferent bombardment associated with spinal lesions

Faye model — a theoretical model of the vertebral subluxation complex proposed by L. John Faye; components of this five-part model include neuropathophysiology, kinesiopathology, myopathology, histopathology, and a biochemical component

Fee splitting — paying or receiving any commission, bonus, kickback, or rebate, or engaging in any split-fee arrangement in any form whatsoever with a physician, organization, agency, or person, either directly or indirectly, for patients referred to providers of health goods and services

Femoral torsion — a gait abnormality in toddlers; both the patellas and the toes point inward; may result from pelvic rotation

Fencer reflex — see Tonic neck reflex

Fixation — 1. a dysfunctional state of restricted and decreased joint motion; 2. any physical, functional, or psychic mechanism that produces a loss of segmental mobility within an articulation's normal physiologic range of motion

Flexner report — 1909 report on the status of medical education in the United States, which resulted in the closing of almost half of medical schools and virtually all "sectarian" or nonallopathic institutions

Food frequency questionnaire — a questionnaire that can be self-administered by patients, which provides information on the frequency of consumption of various foods; useful in determining whether a single nutrient or food group is deficient or missing but is not inclusive of all specific foods and therefore may offer an incomplete picture of the patient's total food intake

Food guide pyramid — a visual depiction of U.S. Department of Agriculture recommendations on food choices, which takes into account factors of proportion, moderation, and variety

Foramen, intervertebral — the passage formed by the superior and inferior notches on the pedicles of adjacent vertebrae; its anatomic contents include the spinal nerve, nerve roots, recurrent meningeal (sinuvertebral) nerves, blood vessels, lymphatics, and connective tissue

Fremitus — vibration of the chest wall induced by the vocal cords

Full scope physician — a medical or osteopathic physician licensed to practice medicine and surgery

Functio laesa — loss of normal function; a cardinal sign of inflammation

Functional ailment — an ailment with symptoms that are persistent, painful, and real, but where no underlying organic problem can be found

Gatekeeper — a health care provider designated by a health care plan to act as the patient's entry into their health care services; many managed care plans require that patients have a referral from their gatekeeper physicians in order to access specialty providers and laboratory or treatment services; gatekeepers are used to contain costs and to ensure the appropriateness of services

Genu valgus — an abnormal postural variant in which the knees are unusually close together, with the toes pointing outward

Genu varus — an abnormal postural variant in which the knees are separated, with toes pointing inward

Globalize — to make broad overarching claims on the basis of limited anecdotal evidence

Grahamism — a system of mid-nineteenth century alternative healing that placed strong emphasis on natural foods

Headache, tension — a headache characterized by muscular tension in the posterior neck, extending upward to include the occiput

Headache, cervicogenic — a headache whose site of origin is in the cervical spine

Headache, migraine — a vascular headache, usually unilateral and of vascular etiology, often in conjunction with nausea, vomiting, and irritability, and often preceded by visual or other sensory abnormalities

Healing partnership — a doctor–patient relationship based on mutual respect, which includes active effort by the patient and openness to questions on the part of the doctor

Hemianesthesia — complete loss of sensation on one side of the body

Heroic medicine — extreme measures intended to elicit healing, including bloodletting, use of leaches, purging, and excessive drugging

High tech — tools and procedures that rely primarily on advanced machinery and the infrastructure that supports it

Holistic — viewing humankind in its totality within a wide ecological spectrum, emphasizing the view that ill health or disease is brought about by an imbalance, or disequilibrium, of the individual in the total ecologic system, and not only by the causative agent and pathologic evolution

Homeopathy — a system of healing based on the use of minute dilutions of substances for medicinal purposes

Hydropathy — treatment of disease by the application of water; water cure

Hyperalgesia — an increased response to a stimulus that is normally painful

Hyperlipidemia — a prolonged elevation of blood lipids

Hypochondriasis — deep anxiety about one's health, which may manifest in a variety of symptoms not attributable to organic disease

Hypomobility — restriction of joint movement; the fixation component of subluxation

Hypermobility — excessive joint movement, often involving laxity of ligaments

Iatrogenic disorder — any adverse mental or physical condition induced in a patient by unwanted effects of a therapeutic intervention

Image intensifier — a tube used in videofluoroscopy to amplify the intensity of the image, reducing the amount of radiation necessary to perform the procedure

Indemnity insurance — traditional prepaid health care insurance, in which health care expenses are reimbursed on a fee-for-service basis, usually with some percentage due from the patient as a copayment

Independent medical examination (IME) — an examination in which a claimant for worker's compensation, personal injury protection benefits, or some other form of compensation for a health condition is assessed and an opinion provided for the payor of the claim as an independent evaluation of the merit and value of the claim

Independent practitioner — a health care provider legally permitted to practice without a supervisory or collaborative relationship with a medical physician or other provider

Informed consent — a legal doctrine that requires that health care providers obtain consent for treatment based on an informed and knowledgeable understanding by the patient of the risks, benefits, and alternatives to treatment

Innate intelligence — the inborn healing wisdom of the body

Interphalangeal — between the bones of a finger

Inspection — visual observation

Ischemia — local deficiency of blood supply due to obstruction of the circulation to a part of the body

Ischemic penumbra — a state of decreased blood flow not sufficiently low to cause neuronal death, but low enough to bring about electrical silence

JCAHO — The Joint Commission on Accreditation of Health Care Orgazinations evaluates and accredits more than 15,000 health care organizations in the United States, including hospitals, health care networks and health care organizations that provide home care, long-term care, behavioral health care, laboratory, and ambulatory care services; an independent, not-for-profit organization, the Joint Commission is the nation's oldest and largest standards-setting and accrediting body in health care

Joint dysfunction — joint mechanics showing functional disturbances without structural changes

Joint fixation (restriction) — the temporary immobilization of a joint in a position that it may normally occupy during any phase of normal movement

Joint play — the qualitative evaluation of the joint's resistance to movement when it is in a neutral position

Kickback — the offering, paying, soliciting, or receiving of any form of direct remuneration intended to induce referrals

Kinematics — the study of the mechanics of biologic motion

Kinetic chain — the orderly function of all musculoskeletal structures required to perform an activity

Labial — relating to the lips; *m* is a labial sound

Laminar — layered

Lantz model — a theoretical model of the vertebral subluxation complex developed by Charles Lantz that describes a hierarchy of organization and a pattern of interrelatedness among its components; components of this model are connective tissue pathology, vascular abnormalities, inflammatory response, and pathophysiology, as well as the five components of the Faye model—neuropathophysiology, kinesiopathology, myopathology, histopathology, and the biochemical component

Legg-Calvé-Perthes disease — avascular necrosis of the femoral epiphysis

Level playing field — a political arrangement in which the claims of competing parties are evaluated according to a fair, mutually agreed-upon set of rules

Liability — legal exposure, either civil or criminal, to a patient or a payor of care, for errors in diagnosis or treatment, or for misbilling or other financial violations such as kickbacks

Lingual — relating to the tongue; *t* is a lingual sound

Locked-in syndrome — a condition in which the patient is awake and retains mental content but cannot express himself/herself because of paralysis of efferent motor pathways that interfere with speech or limb movement; it usually involves a lesion of the motor pathways in the base of the pons or midbrain, while the dorsal gray matter is spared from injury

Long-term depression — a longlasting decrease in synaptic efficacy, which can be established by both high- and low-frequency conditioning stimuli

Long-term potentiation (LTP) — increased synaptic efficiency following a high-frequency conditioning discharge by the primary afferent neuron

Low tech — tools and procedures that rely primarily on human effort, rather than on advanced machinery

Magnetic resonance imaging (MRI) — a technique that produces images of the body through analysis of signals produced after the area of interest is placed in a magnetic field and exposed to radiofrequency pulses; images may be produced in axial, sagittal, coronal, or oblique planes; MRI does not employ ionizing radiation

Malingering — intentional falsification or overstatement of illness or injury

Malnutrition — faulty nutrition resulting from malassimilation, poor diet, or overeating

Malpractice — liability for causing injury to a patient which arises due to a failure to meet the standard of care for the practitioner's profession

Managed care — a form of insurance coverage for health care expenses and case management that seeks to oversee and guide appropriate care; in exchange for cost savings, members agree to see plan providers and to abide by cost-containment mechanisms such as precertification for certain procedures

Manipulation — a passive manual maneuver during which a joint is quickly brought beyond its restricted physiologic range of movement and beyond its elastic barrier, without exceeding the boundaries of anatomic integrity.

Manipulation under anesthesia (MUA) — a manipulative procedure, performed in a hospital or ambulatory surgical center, during which the patient is anesthetized

Manipulable subluxation — a subluxation in which altered alignment, movement, or function can be improved by manual thrust procedures

Manual therapy — procedures by which the hands directly contact the body to treat the articulations of soft tissues

Maximum medical improvement — the point at which no further recovery from injury or illness can reasonably be expected

McMullen reverse fencer reflex — a chiropractic technique used to detect subluxation in the neonate, which is a variation of the fencer reflex; the child is hung upside down (held by the ankles) and under normal circumstances will turn the head toward the side of the flexed leg and arm, rather than toward the side of the extended leg and arm

Mechanoreceptor — a receptor that is excited by mechanical pressures or distortions, as those responding to sound, touch, and muscular contractions

Medicaid — the U.S. federal government health care plan for the poor. Medicaid is administered by state governments

Medical staff affiliates — licensed, registered, or otherwise certified professionals trained to perform a select group of activities under the direct supervision of a member of a hospital medical staff; included in this group are clinical psychologists, registered nurses, nurse anesthetists, nurse midwives, nurse practitioners, and professional medical assistants; also known as allied health practitioners

Medicare — the U.S. federal government health plan for the elderly and disabled

Medline — a computerized biomedical research database maintained by the National Library of Medicine in Bethesda, Maryland, and partially supported by the U.S. federal government

Meric technique — a chiropractic system in which a clinical problem is considered in terms of the "zone" (body section innervated by a pair of spinal nerves) where it occurs; all tissue of one type within a zone is considered a "mere"

Mercy guidelines — the Guidelines for Chiropractic Quality Assurance and Practice Parameters, developed at the Mercy Center Consensus Conference

Meta-analysis — a structured, systematic integration of the results of different randomized clinical trials

Metaphysical healing — the "mind–body–spirit" theories that influenced alternative medicine and the early concepts of osteopathy and chiropractic

Mineral — a nonorganic substance from the earth's crust. Major minerals and trace minerals are required for normal physiologic function

Miscoding — using a CPT code incorrectly, which becomes a legal concern when it is done intentionally or negligently and results in overpayment

Mixers — term applied to chiropractors (and early osteopaths) who departed from "hands only" or "straight" utilization of manual adjustments, utilizing methods ranging from physiological therapeutics to obstetrics, minor surgery, and prescriptions

Mnemonic — a memory aid

Mobilization — movement applied singularly or repetitively within or at the physiologic range of joint motion, without imparting a thrust or impulse, with the goal of restoring joint mobility

Moro reflex — in response to a startling stimulus (e.g., loud noise), the infant extends the extremities and then rapidly flexes them, as well as opening the eyes; this is normal up to 4 months; beyond that point, absence indicates possible neurological insult, and asymmetry indicates possible fracture; also known as Startle reflex

Morphology — structure; framework

Motion — movement of a body part; one of five fundamental examination procedures

Motion segment — a functional unit made up of two adjacent articulating surfaces and the connecting tissues binding them to each other

Muscle energy technique — a soft tissue technique involving voluntary contraction of the patient's muscles in a precisely controlled direction, at varying levels of intensity, against a distinctly executed counterforce applied by the practitioner

Myofascial release — a variety of soft tissue techniques for evaluating and treating the fascia

National Institutes of Health (NIH) — one of the world's foremost biomedical research centers, this branch of the U.S. Department of Health and Human Services has 24 separate institutes, centers, and divisions at its campus in Bethesda, Maryland

Natural healing — the ability of the body to heal itself; the process by which health is restored through nonpharmaceutical methods

Neonate — a newborn child

Nerve compression hypothesis — the proposition that a nerve can become compressed through impingement from intersegmental spinal biomechanical derangements

Nerve interference — 1. compression of the spinal nerves in the environs of the intervertebral foramen; 2. initiation of pain in the spinal joints that is capable of creating secondary aberrant reflex effects such as increases in motor neuron or sympathetic neural activity

Nerve sheath — a structure consisting of an inner filamentous endoneurium, a thin but dense collagenous perineurium, and an areolar epineurium that protects the nerve and facilitates movement

Nerve tracing — the act of using digital pressure to follow a line of hyperpathia from a painful body part to the spine or vice versa; the earliest recorded method of chiropractic analysis; lines of hyperpathia may or may not correspond to named nerves

Nervi nervorum — the intrinsic innervation of nerves and their sheaths

Neurocalometer (NCM) — a heat-sensing instrument consisting of two thermocouple probes and a galvanometer, which indicates left-to-right thermal asymmetry as the examiner glides the instrument up or down the spine

Neurodystrophic hypothesis — the proposition that neural dysfunction is stressful to viscera and to other body structures, which may modify immune responses and alter the trophic function of involved nerves

Neurogenic inflammation — sterile inflammation that develops as a result of efferent nociceptor function

Neuroma — a tumor-like mass of regenerating axons that can result from nerve injury

Ninth amendment — a part of the U.S. Bill of Rights, the Ninth Amendment states: "The enumeration in the Constitution of certain rights shall not be construed to deny or disparage others retained by the people"; this language has been interpreted to provide certain privacy rights, such as the right to an abortion but has not been interpreted to provide a constitutional right to the health care of one's choice

NIOSH — the National Institute for Occupational Safety and Health is a U.S. Federal agency established by the Occupational Safety and Health Act of 1970. NIOSH is part of the Centers for Disease Control and Prevention (CDC) and is responsible for conducting research and making recommendations for the prevention of work-related illness and injuries

Nociception — activity in a neural structure considered capable of leading to or contributing to a sensation of pain

Nociceptive — the quality displayed by an active nociceptor. This term is often misused to modify "stimulus"; a stimulus cannot be nociceptive, but it can be noxious

Nociceptor — a receptor preferentially sensitive to a noxious stimulus or to a stimulus that would become noxious if prolonged

Nociceptor, Group III — a neural element innervating noncutaneous somatic tissues whose axons are small in diameter and lightly myelinated (A fiber)

Nociceptor, Group IV — a neural element innervating noncutaneous somatic tissues whose axons are small in diameter and unmyelinated (C fiber)

Nonphysical causation — mental, emotional, social, or spiritual influences on the etiology of illness

Nonphysicians — a JCAHO classification for health care providers with a limited scope of practice (e.g., podiatrists, dentists, and chiropractors), who are granted a limited degree of hospital clinical privileges; nonphysicians are required to co-admit with a medical or osteopathic physician having full active staff membership and admission privileges

Nonsteroidal anti-inflammatory drugs (NSAIDs) — a broad class of drugs that reduce inflammation and decrease pain by reducing tissue concentrations of prostaglandins, hormones that produce inflammation and pain; NSAIDs are used for treatment of joint pain, inflammation, and stiffness; this class includes specific generic drugs, such as ibuprofen, indomethacin, ketoprofen, naproxen, and sulindac

Noxious stimulus — a stimulus that damages normal tissue; while most noxious stimuli are painful, some are not, including radiation injury and cutting the wall of the small intestine

Objective — that which can be detected with the doctor's own senses (see Subjective)

Oculomotion — movement of the eyes, controlled by the extraocular muscles

Office of Alternative Medicine (OAM) — established as part of the National Institutes of Health by a 1992 congressional mandate, the purpose OAM of is to "facilitate the evaluation of alternative medical treatment modalities" for the purpose of determining their effectiveness and to help integrate such treatments into mainstream medical practice; OAM has funded research projects and established 10 "exploratory centers for alternative medicine" at U.S. universities

Ongoing activity — neural discharge in the absence of evident stimulus

Open-ended inquiry — an interview method that encourages the patient to tell the story in his own words

Ophthalmologist — a medical physician specializing in the diseases of the eye

OSHA — established by the U.S. Congress in 1970, the Occupational Safety and Health Administration develops, implements, and enforces rules for workplace safety

Osteoarthritis — a chronic disease involving the joints characterized by joint pain, destruction of articular cartilage, and impaired function

Osteopath or Osteopathic Physician (DO) — a full-scope physician with training in osteopathic manipulation

Osteopathic lesion — a disturbance of musculoskeletal structure and/or function that may include accompanying distrubances of other biologic mechanisms

Osteoporosis — abnormal thinning of bone, seen most frequently in older persons

Otitis media — inflammation of the middle ear. The serous type is generally chronic, while the purulent type is generally acute

Outcome measure — a qualitative or quantitative indicator of the effect of a clinical intervention on one or more aspects of a patient's health

Pain — an unpleasant sensory and emotional experience associated with actual or potential tissue damage, or described in terms of such damage

Palmar grasp reflex — when the examiner's finger is placed in the baby's hand, the fingers curl in response; this is normal for 3 to 6 months; persistence beyond that point may indicate cerebral insult; absence of the palmar grasp reflex in the neonate may indicate central nervous system disease or insult

Palpation — manual examination of a body part; one of five fundamental examination methods

Paradigm — an explanatory model that helps clarify a complex process

Paradigm shift — a fundamental change in an explanatory model

Parenchyma — the tissue or structure of an organ

Passive analysis — the first step in ergonomic evaluation of workplace data, largely involving review and analysis of workplace documents (see Active analysis)

Pathophysiology — abnormal physiology; the stage before pathology or disease

Patient-centered approach — a mutually respectful doctor–patient relationship in which the doctor's emotional, social, or financial needs are not permitted to override the best interest of the patient

Peer review — a system of review used by hospitals, managed care, and insurance companies in which health care records are reviewed to determine if services provided are medically necessary, meet standards of care, and fulfill other cost-containment criteria established by the payor of care

Percussion — inducing vibration into a part of the body

Periarticular — surrounding a joint

Phoria — weakness of the extraocular muscles

Physiatrist — a medical physician specializing in physical medicine and rehabilitation

Physical rehabilitation — treatment intended to achieve restoration of optimal strength, stability, and integrity in the injured worker through a planned functional program; can include aerobic, flexibility, and strength training

Physiologic barrier — the end point of a joint's active range of motion

Plasma extravasation — passive and active transmission of plasma elements through a blood vessel wall

Pleximeter — the finger that is struck in the act of percussion

Plexor — the striking finger in the act of percussion

Pocket mask — a protective barrier with a one-way valve that allows a health practitioner to apply respiratory resuscitation without risk of disease exposure

Popular health movement — a grassroots movement which emerged in the mid-nineteenth century, embracing many unconventional forms of healing, and which emphasized a partnership role between practitioners and patients

Post-facilitation stretch — a proprioceptive neuromuscular technique primarily used to stretch chronically shortened muscles

Post isometric relaxation — a soft tissue technique in which the doctor lengthens the muscle, after which the muscle is isometrically contracted and then relaxed by the patient

Primitive reflexes — reflexes that demonstrate immaturity of the nervous system; normally present for approximately the first 6 months of life; persistence beyond that point is indicative of neurologic dysfunction; examples include the palmar grasp, rooting, steppage, and tonic neck reflexes

Proprioception — sensory nerve information pertaining to movement, position, or tension of muscle, tendon, ligament, bone, or joint tissues

Proprioceptive training — exercise used to build the coordination of proprioceptors and muscles to promote proper biomechanic function

Proteolytic enzymes — enzymes that split proteins by hydrolysis of peptide bonds; clinically, proteolytic enzyme supplements have an anti-inflammatory effect

Psychiatrist — a medical physician specializing in mental illness and dysfunction

Psychogenic — arising from the mind rather than the body

Radiograph — an x-ray photograph

Radiography — the process of producing x-ray photographs

Radiolucent — easily penetrated by x-rays; Radiolucent structures appear dark on radiographs

Randomized controlled trial (RCT) — an experimental study for assessing the effects of a particular variable (e.g., a drug or treatment) where subjects are randomly assigned to either of two groups, experimental or control; the experimental group receives the procedure while the control group does not

Rarefaction — a loss of tissue substance in which the structure becomes less dense

Radiopaque — not easily penetrated by x-rays; radiopaque structures appear white on radiographs

RDA — the recommended daily allowance is the level of a nutrient necessary to meet the needs of practically all healthy persons

Receptive field — the area from which a receptor can be activated by a given stimulus

Red flag — a finding in a patient's history or physical examination that should raise suspicion for the presence of a serious underlying condition

Reflex arc — a pattern of nerve transmission consisting of a stimulus-activated receptor, transmission over an afferent pathway to an integration center, transmission over an efferent pathway to the effector, and induction of a reflex response

Rhoncus — a deep rattling in the proximal airway due to obstruction or constriction

Roentgen, Wilhelm — the discoverer of x-rays and recipient of the first Nobel Prize for physics

Rooting reflex — upon stroking a baby's cheek, its head should turn toward the side of stroking; this is normal during the first 3 to 4 months of life; persistence beyond that point may indicate a severe central nervous system problem; absence of the rooting reflex in the neonate may indicate central nervous system disease or insult

Rubor — a localized redness; a cardinal sign of inflammation

Scope of practice — the range of diagnostic and treatment procedures that a given licensed professional is allowed to use; scope provided by the definition of the healing art in the state statute

Self-care — methods used to restore or maintain one's own health

Self-referral — an arrangement in which the referring doctor has an ownership interest in an ancillary facility to which he makes referrals; self-referral is illegal under the U.S. Medicare law

Sensitization — a phenomenon induced by stimulation of nociceptors and characterized by increased sensitivity to mechanical and chemical stimuli and by the development of ongoing activity

Seven-Day food diary — a contemporaneously compiled list recording all foods and beverages consumed during a week

Sham manipulation — a manual procedure that does not impart significant motion into a vertebral joint, used as a control variable in studies of spinal adjusting and manipulation

Sherrington's Law of Reciprocal Innervation — contraction of muscles is accompanied by the simultaneous inhibition of their antagonists; also known as reciprocal inhibition

Shoulder instability — the pathologic condition in which the humeral head tends to slip out of the glenoid socket; dislocation is the most severe presentation of shoulder instability

Soft tissue — tissues including muscles, tendons, bursae, ligaments, and fascia

Somatic dysfunction — impaired or altered function of the skeletal, arthrodial, myofascial, vascular, lymphatic, or neuronal components of one or more motion segments; this impaired or altered somatic function can result in visceral disturbance as well as musculoskeletal pain; term was introduced in 1970 to replace "ostepathic lesion"

Somatic dyspnea — air hunger or shortness of breath which can be alleviated or abolished by the correction of vertebral subluxation complex or other somatic dysfunction

Somatoautonomic reflex — see Somatovisceral reflex hypothesis

Somatosomatic reflex hypothesis — the proposition that stimulus at one level of musculoskeletal system produces reflex activity in the nervous system, which then manifests elsewhere in the musculoskeletal system

Somatosympathetic reflex — see Somatovisceral reflex hypothesis

Somatovisceral reflex hypothesis — the proposition that a stimulus to nerves or receptors related to spinal structures produces reflexive responses influencing function in the visceral organs such as those in the digestive, cardiovascular, or respiratory systems; synonyms include somatosympathetic and somatoautonomic

Sonography — the method of producing images of internal structures by exposing the area of interest to ultrasonic impulses and reconstructing the resulting echoes into an image

Spinal motion segment — two adjacent vertabrae and the connecting tissues that bind them to each other

Spinography — a technique for evaluating spinal biomechanics which employs geometric analysis of radiographs

Standard of care — the consensus within a professional community regarding the appropriate methods of diagnosis and treatment that can reasonably be applied to management of a patient's presenting difficulties; the standard of care sets the legal obligation providers are held to in malpractice actions

Startle reflex — see Moro reflex

Steppage reflex — with the baby held upright, the dorsum of the foot lightly strikes the underside or top of a table; in response, the baby places the foot down; persistence of this reflex varies; average duration is 2 to 4 months; beyond that point, absence indicates possible neurological insult

Straights — chiropractors who chose not to use any supplements to spinal adjustments

Subjective — discernible by the patient but not directly discernible by the doctor (see Objective)

Subluxation, chiropractic — 1. an alteration of alignment, movement, integrity, and/or physiologic function of a motion segment, while the joint surfaces remain in contact; resulting neurophysiologic disturbance may be local or widespread; 2. an aberrant relationship between two adjacent structures that may have functional or pathologic sequelae

Subluxation, orthopedic — a partial or incomplete dislocation

Subluxation complex — See Vertebral subluxation complex

Subluxation syndrome — an aggregate of signs and symptoms that relate to pathophysiology or dysfunction of spinal and pelvic motion segment or to peripheral joints

Sustainability — the ability of a system to maintain healthy function over an extended period of time

Target diet — a visual depiction of recommended food choices, in which the foods near the center of the circle should be eaten most frequently

Thoracic outlet syndrome — compression of the brachial plexus nerve trunks; signs and symptoms of thoracic outlet syndrome may include neck pain, occipital headaches, intermittent arm pain, numbness, paresthesias, fatigue, and weakness

Thrill — a palpable vibration of turbulence caused by a loss of laminar flow in a vessel

Tibial torsion — with the patellas positioned normally, the toes turn inward (medially), due to primary rotation of the tibia. This is normal up to age 6 to 18 months

Tone — the rate or intensity of function of any tissue or organ, reflecting the integrity of transmission of neurologic information to and from that tissue or organ

Tonic neck reflex — when a baby is placed supine with the head turned to one side, it extends the extremities on that side; this is normal up to 4 to 6 months of age; persistence beyond 6 months indicates possible neurologic insult; also known as Fencer reflex

Transforaminal ligaments — ligamentous bands crossing the intervertebral foramen

Transverse friction massage — a soft tissue technique usually administered to a ligament or muscle; light friction may be used with caution on a recent partial tear or ligamentous sprain, while stronger friction is generally appropriate in the chronic stage

Trophic nerve function — the function of nerves related to nutrition and growth; trophic substances produced by nerves have been found to be essential for the maintenance of proper tissue structure and function

Tumor — localized swelling; a cardinal sign of inflammation

24-Hour recall diary — a written list compiled by a patient recording everything he or she ate or drank the previous day, noting the time, place, type of food, and amount consumed

Ultrasonography — see Sonography

Unbundling — taking CPT codes intended to reference multiple procedures with a single code, and instead billing each procedure using a separate code; this practice results in a higher payment and is illegal

Upcoding — using a more involved CPT code than the appropriate code for the service actually provided; billing for a complex office visit when the patient was only seen for a brief office visit, for example, is upcoding. This results in a higher payment and is illegal

USDA — U.S. Department of Agriculture

Utilization review — a fiscal control mechanism whereby a health insurer reviews claims to determine if the treatment provided is appropriate and supported by a diagnosis documented by appropriate testing; its purpose is to detect overutilization or services which are not medically necessary or appropriate

Vertebral subluxation complex — subluxation of one or more spinal motion segments resulting from mechanical, emotional, or chemical stressors, and resulting in aberrant tone and eventual pathologic changes in the constituent tissues of the involved motion segments; pathologic changes may also take place in other body tissues influenced by the resultant neural disturbance

Vertebrobasilar insufficiency — a lack of normal blood supply to the brain stem caused by narrowing or blockage of one or both vertebral arteries and/or the basilar artery; can result in symptoms such as dizziness, fainting, or double vision

Videofluoroscopy — a technique for producing x-ray motion pictures which are recorded on videotape

Visceral disease simulation — the proposition that somatic dysfunction or vertebral subluxation can often simulate, or mimic, the symptoms of visceral disease; synonyms include pseudovisceral disease, organ disease mimicry, somatic visceral disease mimicry syndromes, and somatic simulation syndromes

Viscerosomatic reflex hypothesis — the proposition that a stimulus to nerves or receptors related to visceral structures produces reflexive responses influencing function in the musculoskeletal system

Vitamin — an organic substance found in food and required for normal physiologic function

Vitamins, fat-soluble — include vitamins A, D, E, and K; these tend to be stored in the body, are readily absorbable with dietary fats and unlikely to be excreted in the urine

Vitamins, water-soluble — include the B vitamins (B_1, B_2, B_6, B_{12}), niacin, pantothenic acid, biotin, folic acid, inositol, and choline, and vitamin C; these are not stored in the body and are readily excreted in the urine

VDT worker — an employee whose job includes work on a video display terminal, such as a computer

Vocational rehabilitation — programs designed to aid injured workers unable to perform their usual and customary pre-injury work. This often involves retraining in a less physically demanding job

Wallenberg syndrome — loss of pain and temperature sensation of the face on the ipsilateral side of the lesion, and of the body on the contralateral side, usually resulting from a lesion to the brain stem within the distribution of the posterior cerebral circulation

Wilk case — *Wilk v. AMA et al* is the landmark antitrust suit in which chiropractor plaintiffs prevailed over the American Medical Association, ending a decades-long officially sanctioned medical boycott of chiropractic

Worker's compensation — a system of benefits designed to protect and assist workers suffering adverse health affects as a result of their employment

World Health Organization (WHO) — the United Nations health agency, with headquarters in Geneva, Switzerland

Whiplash — a cervical acceleration-deceleration injury, often the result of a motor vehicle collision

Windup — the phenomenon of increasing response of a spinal cord cell to repeated stimuli

Zygapophysis — an articular process of a vertebra

Index